Risk of Type 2 Diabetes Mellitus: Cardiorenometabolic Syndrome and Its Components

Risk of Type 2 Diabetes Mellitus: Cardiorenometabolic Syndrome and Its Components

Guest Editors

Andrej Belančić
Bojan Jelaković
Martina Matovinović

MDPI • Basel • Beijing • Wuhan • Barcelona • Belgrade • Novi Sad • Cluj • Manchester

Guest Editors
Andrej Belančić
Department of Clinical Pharmacology
Clinical Hospital Centre Rijeka
Rijeka
Croatia

Bojan Jelaković
Department for Nephrology, Hypertension, Dialysis and Transplantation
University Hospital Center Zagreb
Zagreb
Croatia

Martina Matovinović
Department of Endocrinology
University Hospital Center Zagreb
Zagreb
Croatia

Editorial Office
MDPI AG
Grosspeteranlage 5
4052 Basel, Switzerland

This is a reprint of the Special Issue, published open access by the journal *Diabetology* (ISSN 2673-4540), freely accessible at: https://www.mdpi.com/journal/diabetology/special_issues/39OW6R377A.

For citation purposes, cite each article independently as indicated on the article page online and as indicated below:

Lastname, A.A.; Lastname, B.B. Article Title. *Journal Name* **Year**, *Volume Number*, Page Range.

ISBN 978-3-7258-4713-6 (Hbk)
ISBN 978-3-7258-4714-3 (PDF)
https://doi.org/10.3390/books978-3-7258-4714-3

Contents

diabetology

MDPI

Editorial

The Risk of Type 2 Diabetes Mellitus: Cardiorenometabolic Syndrome and Its Components—A Call to Action

Andrej Belančić [1,*], Martina Matovinović [2] and Bojan Jelaković [3,4]

1 Department of Basic and Clinical Pharmacology and Toxicology, Faculty of Medicine, University of Rijeka, 51000 Rijeka, Croatia
2 Department of Internal Medicine, Division of Endocrinology, University Hospital Center Zagreb, 10000 Zagreb, Croatia; martina_10000@yahoo.com
3 School of Medicine, University of Zagreb, 10000 Zagreb, Croatia; jelakovic.bojan@gmail.com
4 Department of Nephrology, Hypertension, Dialysis and Transplantation, University Hospital Centre Zagreb, 10000 Zagreb, Croatia
* Correspondence: andrej.belancic@uniri.hr

1. Introduction

Cardiorenometabolic syndrome, a constellation of interrelated risk factors including insulin resistance, central obesity, dyslipidemia, and hypertension, is rapidly becoming one of the defining global health challenges of our time. Metabolic syndrome (MetS), as the unifying clinical entity underpinning this syndrome, significantly increases the risk of development of both type 2 diabetes mellitus (T2DM) and cardiovascular diseases (CVDs)—the latter of which remains the leading cause of death and disability worldwide. Although equally important, renal complications such as chronic kidney disease are frequently underrecognized, despite their central role in disease progression and increased mortality. If MetS is left unaddressed, the downstream effects are devastating: escalating healthcare costs, diminished quality of life, and avoidable mortality [1].

Amidst this troubling epidemiological landscape, projections are sobering: global obesity rates are expected to rise from 650 million to over 2 billion individuals by 2035, and T2DM cases are estimated to increase from 500 million to 1.3 billion by 2050 [2]. These figures are not only alarming from a clinical perspective—they are also economic and social red flags, especially in low- and middle-income countries, where healthcare systems are already under strain. It is within this critical context that we present this Special Issue, which is dedicated to the evolving narrative of MetS and its increasingly complex web of determinants. The contributions included in this Issue span population health interventions, molecular mechanisms, pharmacogenetics, and behavioral sciences, reflecting the truly multidisciplinary nature of the challenge at hand [3].

2. A Sneak Peek at the Published Body of Literature

Understanding and managing MetS requires coordinated insight from multiple domains of research and clinical practice. One area of increasing importance is the role of healthcare delivery systems and population health initiatives in mitigating the glycemic burden and improving cardiometabolic outcomes. Models incorporating clinical pharmacists and multidisciplinary care teams have shown promise in improving key metabolic parameters, especially HbA1c, and may offer scalable solutions in both primary and secondary prevention. These approaches align closely with value-based care principles, where clinical efficacy must be matched by cost-effectiveness and system-level sustainability.

At the other end of the spectrum, the cellular and molecular mechanisms underlying MetS are gaining attention as targets for therapeutic innovation. Hyperglycemia, endothelial dysfunction, and post-translational protein modifications—such as O-GlcNAcylation—are increasingly understood to contribute directly to vascular pathology in diabetes and MetS [4]. Additionally, chronic hyperglycemia and systemic inflammation significantly impact glomerular filtration and renal endothelial integrity, further emphasizing the bidirectional relationship between metabolic dysregulation and kidney health. These insights not only improve our understanding of disease progression, but also provide new molecular targets for pharmacological intervention. The role of epigenetics and non-coding RNAs, particularly microRNAs released through exosomes, also presents exciting diagnostic and therapeutic possibilities. These circulating biomarkers have the potential to non-invasively reflect adipose and systemic metabolic dysfunction, thus bridging the gap between obesity, insulin resistance, and overt T2DM [5].

Genetic susceptibility remains a cornerstone of our understanding of MetS and T2DM risk. Advances in polygenic risk scoring and genome-wide association studies are contributing to a more refined stratification of at-risk individuals [6]. However, in order to move from population-level insights to patient-centered care, there is a need to translate genetic findings into actionable, individualized treatment strategies. This includes tailoring drug choices based on pharmacogenetic profiles and anticipating drug–drug or gene–environment interactions, which could significantly alter therapeutic outcomes in patients with multiple metabolic risk factors [7].

Behavioral and lifestyle determinants continue to be essential in determining both the origin and progression of MetS. Psychological eating patterns, emotional dysregulation, and sedentary lifestyles remain pervasive, and addressing these through integrated behavioral health strategies is critical. Exercise interventions, particularly those combining aerobic and resistance modalities, have been shown to improve not only glycemic control, but also broader cardiovascular outcomes. Coupling these interventions with patient education and adherence support can enhance their long-term efficacy and relevance across diverse populations [8].

In Croatia, for example, national organizations like the Croatian Hypertension League, in collaboration with several partner societies, are actively engaged in combating the cardiorenometabolic burden. Through public health campaigns such as "Mission 70/26" and "Do You Know What Is Your Number?", the League and its collaborators focus on improving blood pressure, lipid control, and other modifiable risk factors by enhancing health literacy. These efforts serve as scalable models for community engagement and population-level risk reduction [9].

3. Conclusions: A Roadmap Going Forward

As the field of cardiorenometabolic syndrome continues to evolve, it is clear that no single intervention, biomarker, or therapeutic can offer a panacea. Rather, a cohesive, multidisciplinary, and personalized approach is required to meet the complexity of the disease. In this Special Issue, we have deliberately chosen to highlight studies that either already impact or are poised to reshape current clinical practices.

Given the global rise of obesity and T2DM and their intertwined relationship with cardiovascular and renal outcomes, a holistic approach to individuals with obesity, metabolic syndrome, or prediabetes is essential to curb progression to type 2 diabetes and mitigate downstream cardiorenal complications [10]. Efforts such as those by the Croatian Hypertension League serve as inspiring examples of how local leadership and targeted education can drive meaningful change [9]. Moreover, this Special Issue serves not only as a scholarly update, but also as a strategic call to action for healthcare providers, researchers, policymakers, and patients alike. The field is brimming with innovation—from molecular biomarkers to digital health interventions—and it is imperative that all stakeholders remain vigilant and informed. We hope that the work presented here will engage a broad readership—from students and early-career scientists to seasoned clinicians and decision-makers—and ultimately lead to meaningful improvements in patient care, policy development, and global health outcomes.

Author Contributions: Conceptualization: A.B., B.J. and M.M.; writing—original draft: A.B.; preparation: A.B.; writing—review and editing: A.B., B.J. and M.M. All authors have read and agreed to the published version of the manuscript.

Conflicts of Interest: The authors declare no conflicts of interest.

References

1. Alberti, K.G.M.M.; Zimmet, P.; Shaw, J. Metabolic Syndrome—A New World-Wide Definition. A Consensus Statement from the International Diabetes Federation. *Diabet. Med.* **2006**, *23*, 469–480. [CrossRef] [PubMed]
2. Belančić, A.; Klobučar, S.; Rahelić, D. Current Obstacles (with Solutions) in Type 2 Diabetes Management, Alongside Future Directions. *Diabetology* **2023**, *4*, 376–378. [CrossRef]
3. The Lancet Diabetes Endocrinology. Metabolic health: A priority for the post-pandemic era. *Lancet Diabetes Endocrinol.* **2021**, *9*, 189. [CrossRef] [PubMed]
4. Bolanle, I.O.; Durham, G.A.; Hobkirk, J.P.; Loubani, M.; Sturmey, R.G.; Palmer, T.M. Do T2DM and Hyperglycaemia Affect the Expression Levels of the Regulating Enzymes of Cellular O-GlcNAcylation in Human Saphenous Vein Smooth Muscle Cells? *Diabetology* **2024**, *5*, 162–177. [CrossRef]
5. Vukelić, I.; Šuša, B.; Klobučar, S.; Buljević, S.; Liberati Pršo, A.-M.; Belančić, A.; Rahelić, D.; Detel, D. Exosome-Derived microRNAs: Bridging the Gap Between Obesity and Type 2 Diabetes in Diagnosis and Treatment. *Diabetology* **2024**, *5*, 706–724. [CrossRef]
6. Ercegović, V.; Džimbeg, M.; Gelemanović, A. Genetic Susceptibility of Type 2 Diabetes and Metabolic Syndrome. *Diabetology* **2025**, *6*, 11. [CrossRef]
7. Knežević, S.; Filippi-Arriaga, F.; Belančić, A.; Božina, T.; Mršić-Pelčić, J.; Vitezić, D. Metabolic Syndrome Drug Therapy: The Potential Interplay of Pharmacogenetics and Pharmacokinetic Interactions in Clinical Practice: A Narrative Review. *Diabetology* **2024**, *5*, 406–429. [CrossRef]
8. Mousavi Zadeh, S.A.; Caminiti, G.; Aracri, M.; Pieri, M.; Mitterhofer, A.P.; De Lorenzo, A.; Bernardini, S.; Farsetti, P.; Volterrani, M.; Barone, R.; et al. Comparative Analysis of Cardiovascular Outcomes in Type 2 Diabetes Patients Engaging in Aerobic, Resistance, and Combined Training: A Systematic Review. *Diabetology* **2025**, *6*, 38. [CrossRef]
9. Jelaković, B.; Pećin, I.; Lang, V.B.; Braš, M.; Capak, K.; Jelaković, A.; Kralj, V.; Miličić, D.; Soldo, A.; Bubaš, M. Improving blood pressure and dyslipidemia control by increasing health literacy in Croatia-missions 70/26 & Do you know what is your number. *Blood Press* **2024**, *33*, 2371863. [CrossRef] [PubMed]
10. Handelsman, Y. Diabetes, cardiorenal, and metabolic multispecialty practice recommendations and early intensive management of cardio-renal-metabolic disease. *Am. J. Manag. Care* **2024**, *30*, S189–S196. [CrossRef] [PubMed]

diabetology MDPI

Article

Impact of an Ambulatory Clinical Pharmacy Population Health Initiative on HbA1c Reduction and Value-Based Measures: A Retrospective, Single-Center Cohort Study

Savannah Nelson [1,*], Tasha A. Butler [1], Amanda Martinez [1], Jessica Bianco [1], Delilah Blanco [1] and Nicholas W. Carris [2,*]

1 Tampa General Hospital, Tampa, FL 33606, USA; tashabutler@tgh.org (T.A.B.); dblanco@tgh.org (D.B.)
2 Taneja College of Pharmacy, University of South Florida Taneja, Tampa, FL 33602, USA
* Correspondence: snelson@tgh.org (S.N.); carris@usf.edu (N.W.C.); Tel.: +1-(813)-844-8218 (S.N.); +1-(813)-974-6333 (N.W.C.)

Abstract: Background: Studies of pharmacists' clinical programs have demonstrated improvements in controlling chronic diseases. However, significantly less data are available regarding pharmacist impact in a value-based Patient-Centered Medical Home (PCMH). The present study assessed a population health initiative to incorporate pharmacists for the management of type 2 diabetes (T2D), hypertension, and hyperlipidemia in a PCMH. **Methods**: This was a single-center retrospective cohort study of patients with T2D and baseline glycated hemoglobin (HbA1c) greater than 9%. Patients were excluded if they received care from an endocrinology provider or were lost to follow-up during the observation window of 1 January 2023 through 31 July 2023. Patients were analyzed in two cohorts: (1) patients who received any outpatient care from a clinical pharmacist (pharmacist cohort) and (2) patients who did not receive any outpatient care from a clinical pharmacist (usual care cohort). The primary outcome was the proportion of patients achieving an HbA1c of less than 8%. Secondary outcomes included blood pressure control and receipt of guideline-directed statin therapy. **Results**: Ninety-one patients were identified, twenty-nine in the pharmacist cohort and sixty-two in the usual care cohort. The overall population was older (mean age ~66 years), 59% female, and racially diverse (<50% Caucasian). HbA1c less than 8% was achieved in 34% of patients in the pharmacist cohort and 29% of patients in the usual care cohort ($p = 0.001$). A blood pressure goal of less than 140/90 mmHg was achieved more frequently in the pharmacist cohort (90% vs. 61%, $p = 0.006$), but guideline-directed statin therapy was similar between groups (90% vs. 79%, $p = 0.215$). **Conclusions**: Pharmacists can play an integral role within a PCMH to improve value-based measures for HbA1c and blood pressure control. Further research is needed to assess the impact of pharmacist care on statin use and economic outcomes.

Keywords: diabetes mellitus; type 2; glycated hemoglobin; patient-centered care; pharmacists; population health; quality indicators

1. Introduction

Historically, Medicare reimbursed providers via a fee-for-service structure that provided payment per individual service provided. Since the passage of the Affordable Care Act in 2010, there has been a shift in reimbursement to focus on the quality of care rather than the quantity of care, with the aim to lower cost and improve health outcomes for individual patients and populations [1]. To measure this quality of care, Medicare plans use value-based measures, such as those set by the Healthcare Effectiveness Data and Information Set (HEDIS) and Centers for Medicare & Medicaid Services (CMS). The achievement of these intermediate measures can help increase overall value-based reimbursement rates to the clinic but also presents an opportunity to minimize the long-term complications of various chronic diseases.

The Patient-Centered Medical Home (PCMH) is one care model used to achieve the goals of value-based care. The PCMH model puts the patient at the center of care to deliver cost-effective, high-quality, team-based management of chronic conditions [2]. Pharmacists provide expertise in pharmacotherapy as part of team-based care to help meet the value-based goals of the PCMH. The ability of pharmacists to provide coordinated medication expertise to improve access to high-quality care has been shown in many settings [3]. One review of 39 randomized controlled trials including a total of 5474 patients found that pharmacist involvement in type 2 diabetes (T2D) care resulted in a mean glycated hemoglobin (HbA1c) decrease of 0.05% to 2.1%, with 16 studies finding a statistically significant difference [4]. Additionally, a retrospective matched cohort study of 1960 patients found that patients seen by a pharmacist were more likely to achieve the HEDIS HbA1c goal of less than 8% within 3 months (OR = 2.44, $p < 0.0001$) [5]. Moreover, a retrospective pre-post intervention study of 105 patients with T2D found that pharmacists improved the key quality measures of statin use and completion of diabetic eye exams [6].

One study found that pharmacists in primary care can fill gaps in care to increase the likelihood of quality measure achievement [7]. While this study included seven quality measures, only one addressed chronic disease treatment (HbA1c control). Therefore, while pharmacist impact has been shown to lower HbA1c and improve chronic disease control generally, data are scant in demonstrating pharmacist impact on improving value-based measures in a PCMH when addressing T2D, hypertension, and hyperlipidemia concurrently, as many pharmacist-driven programs may desire to do.

Therefore, this study aimed to assess a population health initiative to incorporate pharmacists for the management of T2D, hypertension, and hyperlipidemia in a PCMH, specifically by assessing the value-based measures of HbA1c less than 8%, blood pressure less than 140/90 mmHg, and statin use.

2. Materials and Methods

2.1. Setting

Tampa General Medical Group (TGMG, Tampa, FL, USA) consists of multiple primary care clinics associated with a large academic medical center. TGMG has an affiliation with the University of South Florida (USF) Health, providing a unified management and coordination of care that aims to deliver cost-effective care and successful value-based care, with recognition by the National Committee for Quality Assurance (NCQA) as a PCMH. A pharmacist-led population health initiative was implemented at these clinics to reduce HbA1c in patients with uncontrolled T2D (HbA1c greater than 9%). Pharmacists worked in a collaborative practice model to evaluate the safety and efficacy of drug therapy, order and interpret laboratory tests, and adjust medication regimens.

2.2. Pharmacist Care Model

Patients evaluated in this study were seen by one of nine ambulatory care pharmacists at one of 17 TGMG primary care clinics. Patients were either referred by their primary care provider for diabetes education and management, regardless of baseline HbA1c, or auto-enrolled in pharmacy services based on HbA1c being greater than 9% within the year 2022. Upon initial consultation for pharmacotherapy services, pharmacists set up an in-person or telehealth appointment to complete a comprehensive medication review, including previous antihyperglycemic regimens trialed. Each subsequent visit consisted of a subjective review of self-reported blood glucose readings or continuous glucose monitor (CGM) data, screening for hypoglycemic events, discussion of lifestyle and exercise habits, and medication regimen adjustments as allowed in the collaborative practice agreement. Pharmacists also assessed for additional therapies, including a statin therapy for atherosclerotic cardiovascular disease (ASCVD) prevention, antihypertensives for blood pressure control, and other health maintenance recommendations, such as immunizations and referrals to ophthalmology, podiatry, and dental providers.

2.3. Study Design

This was a retrospective, single-center cohort study of adult patients seen at TGMG Family Care Centers. Patients were reviewed for inclusion from quality improvement and Medicare Advantage plan reports of patients identified as having uncontrolled T2D during the year 2022. Uncontrolled diabetes was defined by the CMS star rating measure C11: Diabetes Care—Blood Sugar Controlled as HbA1c greater than 9%. Patients whose primary payor was either UnitedHealthcare (UHC, Minneapolis, MN, USA) or Florida Blue Medicare Advantage Plan were included if they were 18 years of age or older with uncontrolled T2D, had a baseline visit and HbA1c measure in 2022, and had at least one follow-up visit and HbA1c measure during the study period. Patients were excluded if they received outpatient care from an endocrinology provider within the study period, as such patients likely represent a more complex subgroup of patients with T2D. This study was determined to be exempt by the institutional review board at the University of South Florida. The STROBE guidelines were used to ensure the reporting of this observational cohort study [8].

Laboratory values and encounter data were extracted via chart review of the electronic medical record using a standardized data collection sheet. Diabetes management encounters assessed as part of the chart review were completed by pharmacists or primary care providers (i.e., physicians, advanced practice registered nurses, physician assistants) and were either in-person or via telehealth. Baseline demographics, HbA1c, medications, comorbidities, and blood pressure were collected from the last encounter in 2022 and each encounter during the study period of 1 January 2023 through 31 July 2023 (Figure 1). Patients were included in the pharmacist cohort if they had at least one visit with an outpatient clinical pharmacist for diabetes management during the study period in which they received care according to the pharmacist care model described above. These patients were also co-managed by their primary care provider. Patients were included in the usual care cohort if they received care from their primary care provider with no care provided by an outpatient clinical pharmacist during the study period.

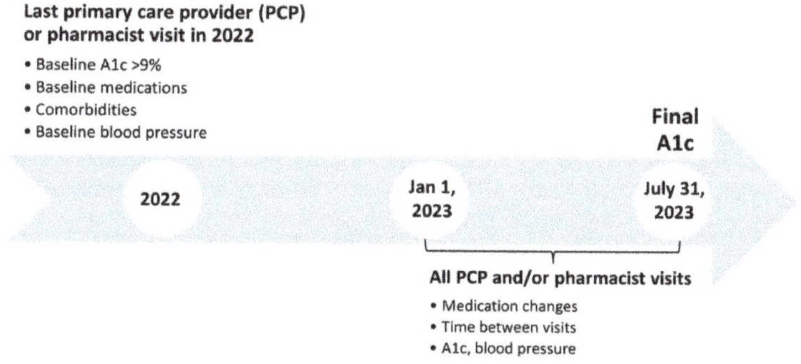

Figure 1. Study design.

2.4. Outcomes

The primary outcome of this study was the proportion of patients achieving HbA1c of less than 8% in the pharmacist cohort versus the usual care cohort. Baseline HbA1c was defined as the last HbA1c measure greater than 9% obtained within the year 2022. Follow-up HbA1c was defined as the last HbA1c measure obtained during the study period. Secondary outcomes included the proportion of patients achieving blood pressure control at the last clinic visit within the study period (defined per HEDIS measure, less than 140/90 mmHg) [9] and the proportion of patients receiving any statin therapy (defined per the HEDIS measure) [10,11]. Additional secondary outcomes included the proportion of patients with at least a 1% reduction in HbA1c from baseline, frequency and interval of visits for diabetes management within the study period, and the number of medication adjustments (defined as any dose modification, initiation, or discontinuation of antihyperglycemics, antihypertensives, or statins).

2.5. Statistical Analysis

Continuous baseline characteristics and outcomes were reported as mean with standard deviation, and categorical baseline characteristics and outcomes were reported as the number (%). The student's *t*-test was used to compare means between cohorts for continuous variables, the Wilcoxon rank sum test was used to compare between cohorts for ordinal variables, and the chi-square test was used to compare between cohorts for categorical variables. Microsoft Excel Version 2310 (Microsoft, Redmond, WA, USA) was used for data collection and analysis, with *p*-values less than 0.05 considered significant.

3. Results

Electronic reports of patients seen at TGMG Family Care Centers in 2022, whose primary payor was UHC, Florida Blue, or Medicare Advantage, identified 630 patients with T2D. Of these, 91 patients met inclusion and exclusion criteria, with the most common reason for exclusion being that they did not have uncontrolled diabetes (Figure 2). Of the 91 included patients, 29 were in the pharmacist cohort and 62 in the usual care cohort.

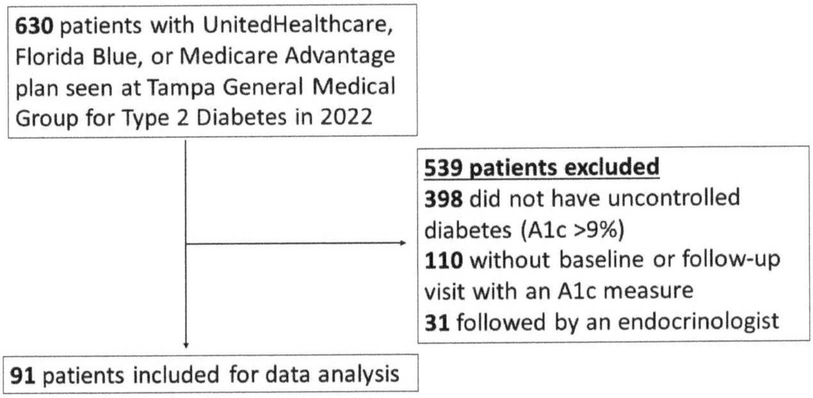

Figure 2. Inclusion and exclusion criteria.

Baseline characteristics were similar between cohorts (Table 1), with a mean age of 66 years and baseline HbA1c of 10.5%. Most patients were Caucasian or African American. Baseline medications were similar among cohorts, except metformin was used more often in the usual care cohort (66% versus 41%, $p = 0.026$), and sodium-glucose cotransporter-2 inhibitors were used more often in the pharmacist cohort (55% versus 32%, $p = 0.037$). More patients in the pharmacy cohort were followed by a pharmacist in the year prior to the study period (76% versus 27%, $p < 0.001$). Both cohorts had similar comorbid conditions, with the most common comorbidities being hypertension and hyperlipidemia. Blood pressure control was similar between groups at baseline (pharmacist cohort, 62%; usual care cohort, 63%; $p = 0.939$), as was statin use (pharmacist cohort, 86%; usual care cohort, 76%; $p = 0.255$).

By the end of the study period, 34% of patients in the pharmacist cohort met the primary outcome of having an HbA1c of less than 8%, compared to 29% of those in the usual care cohort ($p = 0.001$) (Table 2). The mean time between baseline and final HbA1c measurement was shorter in the pharmacist cohort, with a mean of 221 days (SD 86) versus 286 days (SD 128) in the usual care cohort ($p = 0.015$). For the secondary outcome of percent reductions in HbA1c, 52% of patients in the pharmacist cohort had an HbA1c reduction of at least 1% versus 63% in the usual care cohort ($p = 0.512$).

Table 1. Baseline characteristics.

Characteristic [a]	Pharmacist Cohort (n = 29)	Usual Care	p-Value
Age, mean (SD)	65 (12.9)	67 (8.7)	0.333
HbA1c, mean (SD)	10.4 (1.2)	10.5 (1.5)	0.766
Race			
Caucasian	13 (45)	29 (47)	0.862
African American	14 (48)	19 (31)	0.103
Other	2 (7)	7 (11)	0.513
Ethnicity			
Hispanic	5 (17)	7 (11)	0.434
Payer			
UnitedHealthcare	11 (38)	23 (37)	0.939
Florida Blue	3 (10)	10 (16)	0.462
Medicare Advantage	15 (52)	29 (47)	0.660
Followed by pharmacy in year prior to study period	22 (76)	17 (27)	<0.001
Medications			
Metformin	12 (41)	41 (66)	0.026
Sulfonylurea	4 (14)	14 (23)	0.327
Thiazolidinedione	2 (7)	5 (8)	0.846
DPP-4 inhibitor	0 (0)	7 (11)	0.060
SGLT2 inhibitor	16 (55)	20 (32)	0.037
GLP-1 and/or GIP agonist	17 (59)	23 (37)	0.054
Insulin	20 (69)	34 (55)	0.201
ACEi or ARB	23 (79)	47 (76)	0.712
Comorbidities			
Hypertension	23 (79)	52 (84)	0.712
Hyperlipidemia	19 (66)	37 (60)	0.594
Clinical ASCVD	14 (48)	21 (34)	0.594
Heart failure	4 (14)	6 (10)	0.188
Chronic kidney disease	5 (17)	15 (24)	0.559
Obesity	9 (31)	21 (34)	0.789
Statin use	25 (86)	47 (76)	0.255
BP < 140/90	18 (62)	39 (63)	0.939

Abbreviations: ACEi = angiotensin-converting enzyme inhibitor; ARB = angiotensin II receptor blocker; ASCVD = atherosclerotic cardiovascular disease; BP = blood pressure; DPP-4 = dipeptidyl peptidase 4; GLP-1 = glucagon-like peptide 1; GIP = glucose-dependent insulinotropic peptide; SGLT2 = sodium-glucose cotransporter-2. [a] All data are Nos. (%) unless otherwise indicated.

Table 2. Primary and secondary outcomes.

	Pharmacist Cohort (n = 29)	Usual Care	p-Value
Primary Outcome			
HbA1c < 8%, No. (%)	10 (34)	18 (29)	0.001
Secondary Outcomes			
HbA1c reduction of at least 1%, No. (%)	15 (52%)	39 (63%)	0.512
Days between baseline and follow-up HbA1c, mean (SD)	221 (85.6)	286 (128.0)	0.015
Number of visits, mean (SD)	5.8 (3.4)	1.8 (0.8)	<0.001
Days between visits, mean (SD)	34 (18.0)	72 (31.4)	<0.001
Medication changes, mean (SD)	3.5 (3.2)	1.2 (1.2)	<0.001
Statin use, No. (%)	26 (90)	49 (79)	0.214
Final BP < 140/90, No. (%)	26 (90)	38 (61)	0.006

Abbreviations: BP = blood pressure.

Patients in the pharmacist cohort were seen more often for diabetes management, with a mean number of visits of 5.8 (SD 3.4) versus 1.8 (SD 0.83) with usual care ($p < 0.001$). The mean time between visits was 34 days (SD 17.98) for pharmacist care versus 72 days (SD 31.42) for usual care ($p < 0.001$). Patients managed by pharmacists had more changes to their medication regimen during the study period, with a mean number of medication changes of 3.5 (SD 3.15) versus 1.2 (SD 1.19) with usual care ($p < 0.001$). At the end of the study period, 90% of patients had blood pressure control of less than 140/90 mmHg in the pharmacist cohort versus 61% of patients in the usual care cohort ($p = 0.006$). Finally, 90% of patients in the pharmacist cohort versus 79% of patients in the usual care cohort received statin therapy ($p = 0.215$).

4. Discussion

This study found that a pharmacist-led population health initiative improved the attainment of value-based quality measures in a PCMH among patients with uncontrolled T2D at baseline. Patients receiving care from a pharmacist were significantly more likely to have HbA1c less than 8% within 6 months versus patients not receiving pharmacist care. The mean time to the CMS-defined HbA1c control goal was significantly shorter in the pharmacist cohort versus usual care by approximately 2 months. Additionally, this study highlighted the impact of pharmacist care on other value-based measures, such as blood pressure control and guideline-directed statin therapy. While the difference in blood pressure control was statistically significant, the study may have been underpowered to detect a difference in treatment with a statin versus usual care. Based on a post hoc power calculation with the available sample size and an alpha equal to 0.05, the present study had 19.5% power to show a statistically significant difference between groups (pharmacist cohort with ~90% statin use versus usual care, with ~80% statin use).

The most likely factor contributing to the difference in outcomes was the greater frequency of visits and medication changes in the pharmacist cohort versus the usual care cohort. As the patients in the pharmacist cohort were also seen by their primary care provider, achievement of clinical measures cannot be attributed to pharmacist involvement alone but rather the team-based approach fostered by the population health initiative. It is also possible that patients seen by a pharmacist were more motivated to participate in their own care or had fewer access barriers to regular visits. For example, 17 (27%) patients in the usual care cohort saw a pharmacist in the previous year but were unreachable by pharmacists during the study period. The higher percentage of patients followed by a pharmacist in the year prior to the study period in the pharmacist cohort (76% versus 27%) may also explain why a greater proportion of these patients were already on newer, effective antihyperglycemic medications, such as sodium-glucose cotransporter-2 inhibitors and glucagon-like peptide-1 receptor agonists, at baseline. Despite this difference, a greater percentage of patients in the pharmacist cohort achieved HbA1c control.

While several studies report similar findings regarding the beneficial impact pharmacists have on HbA1c control [12,13], the present study provides key insight into the potential mechanism of this benefit, that being more frequent visits and medication changes. Increased frequency of monitoring presents more opportunity for medication counseling, reinforcement of adherence, medication adjustments, and avoidance of therapeutic inertia. Notably, the pharmacy workflow included referral back to usual care once the HbA1c goal was achieved. A study by Bou-Ghazale et al. supports this approach, as it found no difference in mean HbA1c levels after the cessation of pharmacist involvement in care after a mean of 10.5 months [14]. However, this may have also resulted in a greater mean HbA1c in the usual care group, given the potential for longer follow-up.

Limitations of this study include a retrospective study design, limited sample size, and short follow-up time. The period between baseline and the final HbA1c measurement was shorter in the pharmacist cohort, leaving potential further reductions in HbA1c uncaptured. However, the short follow-up time indicates that extended time periods are not needed for pharmacists to impact quality measures. This study also did not assess specific medication adjustments made by pharmacists, apart from the numerical amount made during the study period. Future studies are needed to assess the long-term impact of pharmacist involvement on value-based measures, including the long-term control of chronic disease, patient loss of control following referral back to usual care, and the downstream effect on clinical and economic outcomes. This study did not assess specific interventions made by pharmacists, such as the interpretation of CGM devices, lifestyle counseling, comprehensive medication review, and financial assistance, due to a lack of a specific tracking mechanism. Future investigations should assess the frequency of these interventions and their respective effects on specific outcome measures.

5. Conclusions

Overall, improvements in measures related to diabetes, hypertension, and (numerically) hyperlipidemia through a collaborative practice model within the primary care treatment team demonstrate a successful implementation of the pharmacist population health initiative in the PCMH. The implication of these outcomes extends beyond the achievement of payor-driven value-based measures to why they are important, with the potential to reduce the cardiovascular risk and microvascular complications expected among patients with T2D [15].

The pharmacist-led population health initiative studied was associated with improved HbA1c control among patients with uncontrolled T2D at baseline. Additionally, patients seen by pharmacists were more likely to meet value-based quality measures for blood pressure control. These findings support pharmacists as an integral member in team-based care provided in the PCMH model at primary care clinics with a large academic medical center. Further research is needed to assess the impact of pharmacist care on statin use and economic outcomes.

Author Contributions: Conceptualization, T.A.B., A.M., J.B. and D.B.; methodology, T.A.B.; formal analysis, S.N.; investigation, S.N.; resources, J.B. and A.M.; data curation, S.N. and N.W.C.; writing—original draft preparation, S.N.; writing—review and editing, S.N, A.M, J.B, D.B. and N.W.C.; supervision, A.M., J.B. and D.B.; project administration, S.N. All authors have read and agreed to the published version of the manuscript.

Funding: This research received no external funding.

Institutional Review Board Statement: This study was determined to be exempt by the institutional review board at the University of South Florida due to the retrospective chart review study design.

Informed Consent Statement: Patient consent was waived due to the retrospective chart review study design.

Data Availability Statement: The data presented in this study are available upon request from the corresponding author due to privacy restrictions.

Conflicts of Interest: N.W.C. received research funding [received and managed by university] from Sanofi Winthrope Industrie. The funders had no role in the design of the study; in the collection, analyses, or interpretation of data; in the writing of the manuscript; or in the decision to publish the results. The remaining authors have no relevant conflicts of interest.

References

1. Centers for Medicare & Medicaid Services. What Are the Value-Based Programs? Available online: https://www.cms.gov/medicare/quality/value-based-programs (accessed on 26 December 2023).
2. Centers for Disease Control and Prevention. Patient-Centered Medical Home (PCMH) Model. Available online: https://www.cdc.gov/cardiovascular-resources/php/pcmh-model/index.html (accessed on 26 December 2023).
3. Coe, A.B.; Choe, H.M. Pharmacists supporting population health in patient-centered medical homes. *Am. J. Health Syst. Pharm.* **2017**, *74*, 1461–1466. [CrossRef] [PubMed]
4. Pousinho, S.; Morgado, M.; Plácido, A.I.; Roque, F.; Falcão, A.; Alves, G. Clinical pharmacists' interventions in the management of T2D mellitus: A systematic review. *Pharm. Pract.* **2020**, *18*, 2000. [CrossRef] [PubMed]
5. Benedict, A.W.; Spence, M.M.; Sie, J.L.; Chin, H.A.; Ngo, C.D.; Salmingo, J.F.; Vidaurreta, A.T.; Rashid, N. Evaluation of a Pharmacist-Managed Diabetes Program in a Primary Care Setting Within an Integrated Health Care System. *J. Manag. Care Spec. Pharm.* **2018**, *24*, 114–122. [CrossRef]
6. Joseph, T.; Hale, G.; Moreau, C.; Rosario, E.D.; Logan, N.; Perez, A. Evaluating a Pharmacist-Led Intervention on Cardiovascular- and Diabetes-Related Quality Measures in a Primary Care-Based Accountable Care Organization. *J. Pharm. Pract.* **2022**, *35*, 363–368. [CrossRef] [PubMed]

7. Sinclair, J.; Bentley, O.S.; Abubakar, A.; Rhodes, L.A.; Marciniak, M.W. Impact of a pharmacist in improving quality measures that affect payments to physicians. *J. Am. Pharm. Assoc.* **2019**, *59*, S85–S90. [CrossRef] [PubMed]
8. Vandenbroucke, J.P.; von Elm, E.; Altman, D.G.; Gøtzsche, P.C.; Mulrow, C.D.; Pocock, S.J.; Poole, C.; Schlesselman, J.J.; Egger, M.; Strobe Initiative. Strengthening the Reporting of Observational Studies in Epidemiology (STROBE): Explanation and elaboration. *Epidemiology* **2007**, *18*, 805–835. [CrossRef] [PubMed]
9. National Committee for Quality Assurance. Blood Pressure Control for Patients With Diabetes (BPD). Available online: https://www.ncqa.org/hedis/measures/blood-pressure-control-for-patients-with-diabetes/ (accessed on 26 December 2023).
10. National Committee for Quality Assurance. Statin Therapy for Patients With Cardiovascular Disease and Diabetes (SPC/SPD). Available online: https://www.ncqa.org/hedis/measures/statin-therapy-for-patients-with-cardiovascular-disease-and-diabetes/ (accessed on 26 December 2023).
11. American Diabetes Association Professional Practice Committee. Cardiovascular Disease and Risk Management: Standards of Care in Diabetes-2024. *Diabetes Care* **2024**, *47*, S179–S218. [CrossRef] [PubMed]
12. Coutureau, C.; Slimano, F.; Mongaret, C.; Kanagaratnam, L. Impact of Pharmacists-Led Interventions in Primary Care for Adults with Type 2 Diabetes on HbA1c Levels: A Systematic Review and Meta-Analysis. *Int. J. Environ. Res. Public. Health* **2022**, *19*, 3156. [CrossRef] [PubMed]
13. Cowart, K.; Sando, K. Pharmacist Impact on Treatment Intensification and Hemoglobin A1C in Patients With T2D Mellitus at an Academic Health Center. *J. Pharm. Pract.* **2019**, *32*, 648–654. [CrossRef] [PubMed]
14. Bou-Ghazale, L.; Oldham, E.; Bundeff, A.W.; Hwang, A.Y. Evaluation of the change in HbA1c for patients in an employee health program formerly managed by a pharmacist-run ambulatory care clinic. *Am. J. Health Syst. Pharm.* **2023**, *80*, 1564–1569. [CrossRef] [PubMed]
15. ElSayed, N.A.; Aleppo, G.; Aroda, V.R.; Bannuru, R.R.; Brown, F.M.; Bruemmer, D.; Collins, B.S.; Hilliard, M.E.; Isaacs, D.; Johnson, E.L.; et al. Prevention or Delay of T2D and Associated Comorbidities: Standards of Care in Diabetes-2023. *Diabetes Care* **2023**, *46*, S41–S48, Erratum in *Diabetes Care* **2023**, *46*, 1716–1717. [CrossRef] [PubMed]

diabetology

MDPI

Article

Potential Impact of Metabolic Syndrome Control on Cardiovascular Risk in Elderly Patients with Diabetes: A Cross-Sectional Study

Tânia Nascimento [1,2], Margarida Espírito-Santo [1,2], Adriana Gonçalves [1], Ezequiel Pinto [1,2], Ana Luísa De Sousa-Coelho [1,2] and Maria Dulce Estêvão [1,2,*]

[1] Escola Superior de Saúde, Universidade do Algarve (ESSUAlg), Campus de Gambelas, 8005-139 Faro, Portugal; tinascimento@ualg.pt (T.N.); mfesanto@ualg.pt (M.E.-S.); a65362@ualg.pt (A.G.); epinto@ualg.pt (E.P.); alcoelho@ualg.pt (A.L.D.S.-C.)

[2] Algarve Biomedical Centre Research Institute (ABC-RI), Campus de Gambelas, 8005-139 Faro, Portugal

* Correspondence: mestevao@ualg.pt

Abstract: Metabolic syndrome (MS), a complex pathology with features like abnormal body fat distribution, insulin resistance, and dyslipidaemia, contributes to higher cardiovascular (CV) risk. A cross-sectional study including 87 individuals assessed CV risk score in elderly patients with type 2 diabetes and MS in Algarve, Portugal. The 10-year CV risk score was estimated using the ADVANCE risk score calculator. The reductions in CV risk score were estimated by adjusting the data inputted on the online tool to achieve systolic blood pressure (SBP) <130 or <120 mmHg, and LDL cholesterol <70 mg/dL Beyond waist circumference, the mean number of clinical features of MS was 3.14 ± 0.84, without significant sex differences. The mean CV risk score was 22.5% (CI: 20.3–24.7). Sex-specific analysis showed higher risk score in males (24.2%, CI: 21.3–27.0) vs. females (19.7%, CI: 16.2–23.3; $p = 0.028$). Hypothetical risk score reductions show that lowering SBP to <130 mmHg could significantly lower the risk score by an average of 9.2% (CI: 7.7–10.7), whereas 34.5% of the participants would be out of the diagnostic criteria for MS. When comparing each potential intervention with current risk score, all interventions significantly reduce the 10-year CV risk score. The study highlights the potential of blood pressure control in reducing CV risk score and the importance of multifaceted risk score reduction strategies.

Keywords: cardiovascular risk; ADVANCE risk score calculator; metabolic syndrome; type 2 diabetes mellitus; elderly

1. Introduction

Metabolic syndrome (MS) is defined by the International Diabetes Federation (IDF) as a complex pathology characterized by several general features, such as abnormal body fat distribution, insulin resistance, atherogenic dyslipidaemia, proinflammatory state, and prothrombotic state [1]. Persistent insulin resistance often leads to the development of type 2 diabetes mellitus (T2DM), a metabolic disease characterized by chronic hyperglycaemia, due to an impaired capacity of glucose utilization as an energy source, along with impaired gluconeogenesis and glycogenolysis [2,3]. This can lead to both micro- and macrovascular complications in the long term. Microvascular complications include retinopathy (leading to total vision loss), neuropathy (leading to impaired wound healing and amputations in the lower limbs), nephropathy (possible renal failure), and sexual dysfunction (namely erectile dysfunction in males) [4]. Macrovascular complications include peripheral and coronary artery disease, arrhythmias, diabetic cardiomyopathy, and cerebrovascular disease. As previously reported [5,6], the predisposition to T2DM and the prevalence, progression, and pathophysiology of micro- and macrovascular diseases are different between males and females. Also, several putative sex-specific risk factors should be considered regarding these pathologies. Cardiovascular (CV) diseases are the leading cause of death in patients with T2DM and there is evidence that there are also sex-specific differences regarding CV risk factors [7–9]. In this scenario, it is important to consider these differences and compare the CV risk score across sexes and how males and females react to similar therapeutic strategies.

Ageing of the population is a global phenomenon and Portugal is one of the European countries experiencing a considerable increase in the proportion of elderly people (i.e., individuals aged 65 and over). The ageing index, which measures the ratio of the elderly to the young population, has seen an exponential rise over the years, reaching 185.3% in 2022 [10]. This demographic shift has led to an increase in age-related diseases, including metabolic disorders such as T2DM [11], which is a relevant pathology when considering the occurrence of MS. In this context and considering the life-threatening risk associated with T2DM or, in a broader sense, with MS, it becomes relevant to invest in the prevention of possible complications arising from these health conditions.

Currently, several tools are available to assess CV risk score like the Framingham risk score, the Systematic Coronary Risk Evaluation (SCORE), or QRISK®. The Framingham Risk Score [12] was the first CV risk assessment tool developed with primary prevention in mind, while the SCORE is an algorithm based on 12 European cohort studies and a tool recommended by the European Society of Cardiology [13]. QRISK®, recommended by the National Institute for Health and Care Excellence in the United Kingdom (UK) in its third version [14], now includes, in addition to socio-demographic variables (age, sex) and typical clinical variables (smoking, systolic blood pressure (SBP), or cholesterol), the administration of medications such as glucocorticoids and antipsychotics. These tools consider various factors that can contribute to increased CV risk, including the presence of diabetes, blood pressure (BP) levels, low density lipoprotein cholesterol (LDL cholesterol) levels, age, sex, smoking status, prescribed medications, and the presence of complications. These tools show several advantages, such as a personalized risk assessment and guidance to clinical decision related to the need of lifestyle modifications or the prescription of medication. However, they also have limitations, namely variable accuracy because they are based on average population data. Also, these tools may lead to over-reliance and do not consider all risk factors, such as family history or genetic markers [15–17].

The ADVANCE calculator evaluates the CV risk score in T2DM patients diagnosed with MS [18]. This tool is a specific calculator to assess the 10-year risk of suffering a CV event, for patients with T2DM. Using this calculator, we aimed to estimate how reducing systolic blood pressure (SBP) and/or LDL cholesterol to the recommended levels could decrease the CV risk score and potentially revert the MS diagnosis in elderly patients.

2. Materials and Methods

2.1. Characteristics of the Study

A descriptive cross-sectional study was conducted to assess CV risk score in elderly patients with T2DM and MS. The study analysed a non-random convenience sample of 87 patients, consecutively enrolled, who agreed to participate, residing in the Algarve region (Southern Portugal), aged between 65 and 86 years old, diagnosed with MS according to the IDF criteria [1]. Patients were recruited at the diabetes clinic of the Association for the Study of Diabetes Mellitus and Support for Diabetics in the Algarve (AEDMADA, according to the Portuguese designation), by direct invitation at the time of their consultations for diabetes monitoring. All patients signed an informed consent for their data to be used in this study.

2.2. Data Collection

Clinical data were extracted from the patients' clinical files. These data included sociodemographic characteristics (age, sex, education level), lifestyle factors (exercise frequency, and tobacco and alcohol consumption), clinical profiles (hypertension, dyslipidaemia, duration of diabetes), complications from diabetes (retinopathy, nephropathy, neuropathy), cardiometabolic parameters (weight, body mass index (BMI), waist circumference (WC), SBP, and diastolic blood pressure (DBP)), biochemical parameters (fasting glucose, HbA1c, albumin, creatinine, and cholesterol levels), and the total number of medications used by each patient. BMI was categorized as underweight (<18.5 kg/m^2), normal weight (18.5–24.9 kg/m^2), overweight (25–29.9 kg/m^2), moderate obesity (30–34.9 kg/m^2), severe obesity (35–39.9 kg/m^2), and very severe obesity (≥40 kg/m^2) [19].

2.3. Cardiovascular Risk Score Calculations and Estimations

The 10-year CV risk score was estimated using the ADVANCE risk score calculator [18], an online tool specifically designed for patients with T2DM. This tool also provides estimates on risk score reduction achievable through specific adjustments in SBP and LDL cholesterol levels. Missing data points for the time of T2DM diagnosis and albumin/creatinine ratio were filled with mean population values, obtained from the ADVANCE calculator used, whenever data were not available.

The reductions in CV risk score were estimated by adjusting the data inputted into the online tool to achieve SBP either below 130 mmHg or 120 mmHg, and lowering LDL cholesterol below 70 mg/dL. These reductions were based on the recommendations from the American Diabetes Association (ADA) [3]. The impact of combined adjustments of SBP (<120 mmHg) and LDL cholesterol (<70 mg/dL) was also analysed. Although ADA proposes that BP target values should be individualized, target values of SBP < 130 mmHg should be considered whenever possible [20]. Nevertheless, reducing SBP below 120 mmHg was also considered as it may benefit CV risk score [21,22].

The possibility of starting antiplatelet therapy was not considered in the potential interventions, as the information for this in-depth analysis of the clinical history was not available.

2.4. Statistical Analysis

Data were presented using absolute and relative frequencies, mean (M), median (Md), standard deviation (SD), and interquartile range (IQR). We used the Kolmogorov–Smirnov test to assess to check for compliance of the data with the normal distribution. Group comparisons were made using Pearson chi-square, Mann–Whitney, and Student's *t*-test, according to the results of the normality test. When the results of the chi-square test were considered non-valid due to low expected frequency count, Fisher's or Fisher–Freeman–Halton's exact tests were computed. Correlations were computed using Spearman's correlation coefficient and paired sample comparisons were made using the Wilcoxon's rank test.

Statistical significance for all procedures was set at 0.05. All analyses were carried out using IBM SPSS Statistics 29.0.

3. Results

3.1. Sociodemographic Characteristics of the Population and Metabolic Syndrome Diagnosis

To assess the CV risk score in elderly patients with T2DM, 87 patients (62% males; n = 54) aged 65 years or more were included in this study. The mean age was 75 ± 5 years, without significant differences between the sexes ($p = 0.133$) (Table 1). Regarding academic level, most participants had completed elementary school (67.8%), followed by middle school (14.9%), and high school (6.9%). Only 4.6% of the participants completed a higher degree course. The mean time since the T2DM diagnosis was 13 ± 8 years. On average, patients were taking 6 ± 3 medicines. Table 1 presents the sociodemographic, clinical and lifestyle characteristics of the participants.

The anthropometric variables were significantly different between the sexes (Table 1). Males had a higher body weight (83.8 ± 10 kg) compared to females (75.4 ± 12.9 kg; $p < 0.001$), and a larger WC (100 ± 5 cm for males vs. 92 ± 10 cm for females; $p < 0.001$). Overall mean BMI was 29.8 ± 3.9 kg/m^2. Even if the differences in average BMI were not statistically significant between sexes ($p = 0.07$), the BMI classification indicates a higher prevalence of males with a BMI above the normal range ($p = 0.008$).

Table 1. Sociodemographic, clinical, and lifestyle characteristics for all participants and by sex.

Characteristics		Total Sample (n = 87)	Males (n = 54)	Females (n = 33)	*p*-Value
Age (years) M ± SD		71.6 ± 5.2	70.8 ± 4.8	72.8 ± 5.6	0.113 [a]
Academic level:	Cannot read or write; n (%)	5 (5.7)	3 (5.6)	2 (6.1)	0.697 [b]
	Primary school (4 years); n (%)	59 (67.8)	33 (61.1)	26 (78.8)	
	Middle school (5–9 years); n (%)	13 (14.9)	10 (18.5)	3 (9.1)	
	High school (10–12 years); n (%)	6 (6.9)	5 (9.3)	1 (3.0)	
	College level degree; n (%)	4 (4.6)	3 (5.6)	1 (3.0)	
Years after T2DM diagnosis	M ± SD	12.9 ± 8.0	12.5 ± 8.2	13.5 ± 7.7	0.371 [a]
Number of medications	M ± SD	6.0 ± 2.9	5.7 ± 2.8	6.5 ± 3.0	0.240 [a]
Weight (kg)	M ± SD	80.6 ± 11.8	83.8 ± 10.0	75.4 ± 12.9	**0.001** [c]
Waist circumference (cm)	M ± SD	96.8 ± 8.3	99.7 ± 5.1	92.0 ± 10.2	**<0.001** [a]
BMI (kg/m^2)	M ± SD	29.8 ± 3.9	29.1 ± 2.7	31.0 ± 5.2	0.07 [c]
BMI (category):	Normal weight; n (%)	5 (5.7)	1 (1.9)	4 (12.1)	**0.008** [b]
	Overweight; n (%)	45 (51.7)	33 (61.1)	12 (36.4)	
	Moderate obesity; n (%)	28 (32.2)	18 (33.3)	10 (30.3)	
	Severe obesity; n (%)	7 (8.0)	2 (3.7)	5 (15.2)	
	Very severe obesity; n (%)	2 (2.3)	0	2 (6.1)	
Systolic BP (mmHg)	M ± SD	153.6 ± 22.4	153 ± 22.6	154.5 ± 22.7	0.776 [c]
Diastolic BP (mmHg)	M ± SD	80.4 ± 11.0	79.5 ± 10.3	81.8 ± 12.0	0.349 [c]
Total cholesterol (mg/dL)	M ± SD	184.3 ± 37.8	180.2 ± 36.8	191 ± 39.1	0.195 [a]
HDL cholesterol (mg/dL)	M ± SD	46.5 ± 12.0	45.4 ± 12.5	48.4 ± 11.2	0.261 [a]
LDL cholesterol (mg/dL)	M ± SD	106.9 ± 27.6	105.1 ± 26.6	109.9 ± 29.5	0.441 [a]
Triglycerides (mg/dL)	M ± SD	143.5 ± 57.2	146.1 ± 56.7	139.4 ± 58.6	0.47 [a]
HbA1c (%)	M ± SD	8.3 ± 1.1	8.1 ± 1.0	8.6 ± 1.2	0.072 [a]
Fasting glycaemia (mg/dL)	M ± SD	164.7 ± 45.4	165.6 ± 51.4	163.2 ± 33.9	0.726 [a]
Smokes tobacco	n (%)	2 (2.3)	2 (3.7)	0	**<0.001** [d]
Drinks alcohol	n (%)	59 (67.8)	47 (87.0)	12 (36.4)	**<0.001** [d]
Exercises regularly	n (%)	53 (60.9)	34 (63.0)	19 (57.6)	0.656 [b]
Hypertension	n (%)	79 (90.8)	50 (92.6)	29 (87.9)	0.471 [f]
Dyslipidaemia	n (%)	49 (56.3)	31 (57.4)	18 (54.5)	0.827 [b]
Retinopathy	n (%)	27 (31.0)	16 (29.6)	11 (33.3)	0.812 [b]
Neuropathy	n (%)	2 (2.3)	2 (3.7)	0	0.524 [f]
Nephropathy	n (%)	3 (3.4)	2 (3.7)	1 (3.0)	0.680 [d]

M—mean; SD—standard deviation; BMI—body mass index; BP—blood pressure. Sex differences computed with: [a]—Mann–Whitney's test; [b]—chi-square test; [c]—Student's *t*-test; [d]—Fisher–Freeman–Halton exact test; [f]—Fisher's exact test. Statistical significance ($p < 0.05$) is boldfaced.

Significant differences between sexes were also observed in tobacco and alcohol consumption (Table 1). Only males reported smoking (3.7%), and a higher percentage of males reported alcohol consumption (87.0%) compared to females (36.4%) ($p < 0.001$). Regular exercise was reported by 60.9% of the total sample, without significant sex differences ($p = 0.656$).

Clinical parameters such as SBP and DBP, cholesterol levels, triglycerides, HbA1c, and fasting glycaemia showed no significant differences between the sexes. The prevalence of clinical conditions such as hypertension, dyslipidaemia, retinopathy, neuropathy, and nephropathy also did not differ significantly according to sex.

To determine whether the patients gathered the required components of MS, specific clinical and biochemical characteristics were considered (Table 2). According to the IDF criteria, MS diagnosis includes central obesity (waist circumference ≥94 cm for males, and ≥80 cm for females) plus any two of the following four factors: elevated triglycerides, reduced high density lipoprotein cholesterol (HDL cholesterol), elevated BP, and elevated fasting glycemia [1]. In addition to the increased waist circumference (Table 1), the mean number of clinical features identified in the participants was 3.14 ± 0.84 (Table 2). There were no significant differences between sexes in the number of characteristics or in the prevalence of any of the MS characteristics.

Table 2. Prevalence of MS characteristics for all participants and by sex.

Metabolic Syndrome Characteristics	Total Sample (n = 87)	Males (n = 54)	Females (n = 33)	*p*-Value
BMI showing obesity; n (%)	37 (42.5)	20 (37.0)	17 (51.5)	0.264 [a]
Triglycerides $\geq$ 150 mg/dL; n (%)	35 (40.2)	23 (42.6)	12 (36.4)	0.655 [a]
HDL cholesterol < 40 mg/dL in males or <50 mg/dL in females; n (%)	38 (43.7)	19 (35.2)	19 (57.6)	**0.040** [a]
Blood pressure $\geq$ 130/85 mmHg	78 (89.7)	48 (88.9)	30 (90.9)	1 [a]
Fasting glucose $\geq$ 100 mg/dL	85 (97.7)	52 (96.3)	33 (100)	0.524 [b]
No. of clinical features for MS diagnosis in addition to increased waist circumference:				
M $\pm$ SD	3.1 $\pm$ 0.8	3.0 $\pm$ 0.7	3.4 $\pm$ 1.0	
Md (IQR)	3.0 (1.0)	3.0 (0.0)	3.0 (1.0)	0.109 [c]

M—mean; SD—standard deviation; Md—Median; IQR—interquartile range. Sex differences computed with: [a]—chi-square test; [b]—Fisher's exact test; [c]—Mann-Whitney's test. Statistical significance ($p < 0.05$) is boldfaced.

3.2. Calculation of the ADVANCE Risk Score

The ADVANCE risk score, a CV disease risk prediction tool specifically developed for patients with T2DM, takes into consideration diabetes-specific variables [23]. The estimated risk percentages for myocardial infarction, stroke, or vascular death over a 10-year period were calculated using the ADVANCE risk score online tool (Table 3). The mean risk score for all participants was 22.5% (CI: 20.3–24.7). Sex-specific analysis reveals a significantly higher current risk score in males (24.2%, CI: 21.3–27.0) than in females (19.7%, CI: 16.2–23.3) ($p = 0.028$).

Table 3. Risk score for myocardial infarction, stroke, or vascular death in the next 10 years, and potential interventions.

Risk for Myocardial Infarction, Stroke, or Vascular Death in the Next 10 Years (%)	ADVANCE Risk Score Mean (95% Confidence Interval) Total Sample (n = 87)	Males (n = 54)	Females (n = 33)	Sex Differences *p*-Value
Current risk score	22.5 (20.3–24.7)	24.2 (21.3–27)	19.7 (16.2–23.3)	**0.028**
Risk score if SBP < 130 mm Hg *	13.4 (11.8–15.1)	14.6 (12.4–16.8)	11.7 (9.1–14.4)	0.061
Risk score if SBP < 120 mm Hg *,**	11.8 (10.3–13.3)	13.0 (11.1–14.9)	9.8 (7.6–11.9)	**0.024**
Risk score if LDL cholesterol < 70 mg/dL *	18.8 (16.6–20.9)	20.3 (17.6–23.1)	16.3 (12.9–19.8)	**0.026**
Risk score if SBP < 120 mmHg and LDLC < 7 0 mg/dL *	9.7 (8.4–11.0)	10.8 (9.1–12.6)	7.9 (6.1–9.7)	**0.013**

SBP—systolic blood pressure; LDLC—LDL cholesterol. Sex differences computed with Mann-Whitney's test. *—Paired comparison with current risk score is statistically significant ($p < 0.001$) for all participants, males, and females; **—Paired comparison with BP < 130 mm Hg is statistically significant ($p < 0.001$) for all participants, males, and females. Risk score comparisons between interventions computed with Wilcoxon's rank test. Statistical significance ($p < 0.05$) is boldfaced.

Potential risk score reductions indicate that reducing SBP levels below 130 mmHg could decrease the risk score by an average of 9.2% (CI: 7.7–10.7), resulting in a risk score of 13.4% (CI: 11.8–15.1) for the total sample. This potential risk score after the intervention is statistically significant ($p < 0.001$) when compared to current risk score (22.5%), albeit it does not show significant differences between the sexes ($p = 0.061$). In contrast, sex differences are observed in potential interventions that successfully lower SBP below 120 mmHg ($p = 0.024$), lower LDL cholesterol below 70 mg/dL ($p = 0.026$), or lower both SBP below 120 mmHg and LDL cholesterol below 70 mg/dL ($p = 0.013$) (Table 3). Thus, males seem to maintain a higher risk score than females, except when the intervention is more conservative (SBP < 130 mm Hg).

When comparing each potential intervention with the current risk score, all interventions significantly reduce the risk score for myocardial infarction, stroke, or vascular death over the next 10 years ($p < 0.001$). Nevertheless, mean risk score reduction is not significantly different between sexes when considering all potential interventions.

As expected, the most substantial risk score reduction is observed when combining both BP and LDL cholesterol interventions, which places overall risk score at 9.7% (CI: 8.4–11.0) for the total sample, at 10.8% (CI: 9.1–12.6) for males, and at 7.9% (CI: 6.1–9.7) for females. This intervention yields statistically significant decreases from the current baseline ($p < 0.001$, with an overall decrease of 12.7%, CI: 9.4–14.3), placing males at a higher risk than females ($p = 0.013$). Nevertheless, the decrease in the risk score is not statistically different between males and females ($p = 0.512$): 13.3% (CI: 9.2–15.2) for males and 11.8% (CI: 6.7–15.1) for females.

The calculated current risk score for myocardial infarction, stroke, or vascular death over the next 10 years shows a positive correlation with both age (r = 0.728, $p < 0.001$) and time since T2DM diagnosis (r = 0.681, $p < 0.001$), when sex is controlled for. This association was to be expected, as time elapsed since T2DM diagnosis and sex are variables used in the calculation of the ADVANCE score. The associations are maintained when controlling for sex, suggesting that older patients and those who have the disease longer have a higher risk for CV events. Also, when sex is controlled for, risk score reduction still shows important significant correlations: risk score reduction observed when SBP is less than 130 mmHg is positively correlated with age (r = 0.411, $p = 0.003$) and time since T2DM diagnosis (r = 0.425, $p = 0.002$); risk score reduction observed when SBP is less than 120 mmHg is also positively correlated with age (r = 0.510, $p < 0.001$) and time since the diagnosis (r = 0.503, $p < 0.001$); risk score reduction observed when LDL cholesterol is less than 70 mg/dL is positively correlated with time since the T2DM diagnosis (r = 0.319, $p = 0.024$), but not with age (r = 0.197, $p = 0.171$). Our results suggest that older patients can benefit more from SBP control, but not necessarily from reducing LDL cholesterol levels. Patients who have had T2DM for a longer duration benefit from interventions that favour lower SBP and LDL cholesterol. According to our data, an effective intervention that lowers SBP to less than 130 mmHg in our sample would result in 34.5% of participants (n = 30) no longer meeting the diagnostic criteria for MS.

4. Discussion

Given the increased susceptibility of elderly adults to CV diseases and their associated complications, it becomes crucial to identify and address modifiable risk factors to mitigate these health concerns. This study examines a cohort of Portuguese elderly individuals diagnosed with both T2DM and MS. The aim is to estimate their CV risk score and identify suitable clinical targets, i.e., key modifiable factors such hypertension and dyslipidaemia, to reduce this calculated risk score.

As individuals age, which is a non-modifiable factor, the prevalence of T2DM tends to increase. In Portugal, diabetes affects more than a quarter of the population aged between 60 and 79 years, with a higher prevalence observed in males [11]. According to data from the Portuguese population survey, approximately one-fifth of the general population and more than half of the elderly (those aged 65 and over) have only four years of schooling [24]. This low level of education is consistent with the studied sample, suggesting that this sample may be considered as representative of the elderly Portuguese population.

Our study demonstrates that aggressive BP control, particularly lowering SBP below 120 mmHg, can significantly reduce the estimated 10-year CV risk score for all participants. Lowering BP to less than 130 mmHg also appears to have a significant impact on reducing 10-year CV risk score. Considering the risks associated with more aggressive control (to less than 120 mmHg) in patients with T2DM, this study shows that the values recommended by the ADA [20] and the European Society of Cardiology [25] for BP control (less than 130 mmHg) may have beneficial effects in reducing CV risk. More importantly, the combined effect of SBP and LDL cholesterol interventions results in the most significant risk score reduction. Our findings emphasize the potential benefits of multifaceted intervention strategies that target both BP and lipid levels to mitigate CV risk in patients with T2DM and MS, as already reported in other studies [25].

The ADA recommends using the American College of Cardiology/American Heart Association ASCVD risk calculator for calculating the 10-year CV risk. However, it states that although this calculator includes T2DM as a risk factor, it does not consider the duration of the disease or the presence of long-term complications [20]. The tool used in this study (ADVANCE) includes both factors in the calculation of CV risk score [18], making it a potentially effective guide for therapeutic strategies and goal setting in individuals with T2DM. In the present study, a positive correlation was observed between the time since the T2DM diagnosis ($r = 0.681$, $p < 0.001$) and these events, after controlling for sex. This suggests that patients with a longer duration of the disease have a higher risk. The positive correlations between age, time since T2DM diagnosis, and estimated CV risk score underscore the progressive nature of CV risk accumulation over time in individuals with T2DM. Older individuals and those with a longer duration of T2DM exhibit a higher baseline risk for CV events, highlighting the importance of early and sustained intervention strategies to prevent or delay adverse outcomes in this vulnerable population [26]. De Jong et al. [27], in a prospective cohort study of UK Biobank participants, described that a 5-year increase in the duration of T2DM was associated with a CV risk increase of around 20%. Yao et al. [28] also reported that the duration of diabetes increases the 10-year CV risk. Thus, it seems crucial to consider the time of diagnosis when calculating the 10-year CV risk in these patients.

The current study revealed significant differences in body weight, BMI, and abdominal circumference between males and females. The results obtained in relation to overweight or obesity are in line with the data reported in the WHO European Regional Obesity Report 2022 [29], since the prevalence is higher in males than in females, but when we analyse the data relating to obesity, there is a reversal, since females have higher levels of obesity. These results are also consistent with studies carried out in Portugal [30,31]. These findings underscore the importance of considering sex-specific factors in the assessment and management of MS among elderly individuals with T2DM. CV risk management must consider several factors, including the patient's sex, since this will be a factor to consider in risk stratification, the therapy implemented, and the expected outcomes in terms of metabolic health [25]. Although the differences in BMI between the sexes were not statistically significant, the higher prevalence of males above the normal BMI range highlights the need for targeted interventions to address overweight and obesity and its associated CV risks in the elderly population with diabetes [32,33]. This finding could prompt a discussion on the role of BMI as a predictor of CV risk score and the importance of comprehensive risk assessment beyond traditional measures. In a study that included 23,961 Chinese patients with diabetes, Hu et al. found that every 5 years of early diagnosis increased the risk of heart disease by 14%. This association was even higher in patients with obesity [34], showing that BMI should be a factor to consider when calculating CV risk score.

The observed disparities in smoking and alcohol consumption between sexes underscore the influence of lifestyle behaviours on CV health outcomes. According to 2019 data from the National Statistics Institute, tobacco was considered the primary risk factor for premature death and lost years of healthy life in Portuguese males [35]. In this national report, although the number of smokers decreased, an increase in the consumption of alcoholic beverages, compared to previous years, was observed. Smoking and alcohol consumption significantly impact the components of MS and CV risk, leading to the definition of intervention strategies targeting modifiable risk factors in elderly patients with T2DM [25]. The fact that habits of tobacco and alcohol consumption were higher in males than females may be an important contributor to the increased risk score observed in males.

Despite the absence of significant differences between the sexes in clinical parameters such as BP, cholesterol levels, and glycaemic control, it is essential to consider the cumulative impact of these factors on CV risk in elderly individuals with diabetes [25]. The finding of no significant sex differences in the prevalence of MS characteristics highlights the uniform burden of metabolic features among the individuals regardless of their sex.

Relimpio et al. [36] carried out a study of diabetic patients attending a T2DM clinic in Spain with the aim of assessing the influence of age and other factors on the presence of MS. The average HbA1c in elderly patients (>70 years) was slightly lower (7.0 ± 2.1% for males and 7.2 ± 1.5% for females) than that found in the present study. Abdominal perimeter, on the other hand, showed higher average values (100.0 ± 7.8 cm for males and 106.5 ± 11.6 cm for females), although the average BMI was like the one found. Most of the cardiometabolic parameters did not show differences between the sexes either. Another study carried out in Spain with 501 diabetic patients followed in an endocrinology clinic showed similar results. Around 75% of the patients had a diagnosis of hypertension, the average SBP was 143 ± 17 mmHg, and the average DBP was 80 ± 10 mmHg [37], very similar to what we found. A study in Jordan also showed results of uncontrolled cardiometabolic parameters in patients with T2DM. Around 62% of the patients were obese and 87% had a high abdominal circumference. The prevalence of hypertension was 74.6% and the rate of uncontrolled hypertension was higher in the elderly (>60 years) [38]. Naseri et al. involved 321 patients with T2DM and analysed various cardiometabolic parameters of these patients. Although their mean age was much lower than that our study (53.86 ± 11.54), their HbA1c values were higher than those found in the present study (HbA1c = 9.27 ± 2.4%). On the other hand, the BP values were like those obtained, where 70.5% of the patients had high BP values, with an average SBP of 146.94 ± 23.19 mmHg [39].

There were also no significant differences between sexes in the prevalence of microvascular complications of T2DM. In fact, the diagnosis of neuropathy and nephropathy was relatively lower than that described in the literature [4,40]. However, as mentioned in the literature, the prevalence of these complications was higher in males than in females [41]. A study conducted in Portugal with the aim of assessing the prevalence of CV disease and CV risk factors in patients with T2DM followed up in hospital included 715 patients with an average age of 66.6 years and an average duration of the disease of 17.4 years and described neuropathy as the second most common complication in these patients (26.4%) [42]. The results obtained, especially in the case of neuropathy, may be because these patients are followed up in a specialised clinic and therefore have tighter control of the pathology and its complications, or on the other hand, because neuropathy often has few symptoms that patients may not notice (asymptomatic or mildly symptomatic) [40] or consider normal for their age, since all the patients in this study were elderly. The presence of retinopathy, on the other hand, showed results more in line with the literature (31%) [4]. This could be because in the region there are public screening programmes available, which could result in early diagnosis of this microvascular complication.

Dyslipidaemia is a crucial factor in the diagnosis of MS, as defined by the IDF [1], and is a major factor for the development of CV disease [43]. This study suggests that while elderly patients may derive greater benefit from SBP control, the effects of the intervention on LDL cholesterol may not be as pronounced in this population. However, the impact of lowering lipid parameters in the elderly appears to mirror the results observed in the prevention of CV events in younger individuals. No additional safety concerns were identified, supporting the use of lipid-lowering agents in older individuals [44]. In fact, 56.3% of the patients evaluated in this study were treated for dyslipidaemia. It is worth noting that the most recent tools developed to estimate CV risk score in the general and older European population, namely SCORE-2 and SCORE-2-OP, use total cholesterol levels as an indicator of dyslipidaemia. This allows the estimation of absolute 10-year risk reduction for CVD events from risk factor treatment [43,45]. However, while T2DM was considered a predictive factor in the development of these tools, it is not an indicator used in their operationalization. Hence, the ADVANCE tool was chosen to calculate the 10-year risk of fatal CV events in the elderly population with T2DM analysed in this study, based on previous studies [18,46,47]. Also, the European Association of Preventive Cardiology (EAPC) recommends the use of a U-Prevent tool, namely the use of the ADVANCE risk score in patients with T2DM, pointing out that all U-Prevent risk algorithms have been extensively validated in the European population and that geographical updates are applied where appropriate [45,48]. As mentioned, this calculator considers the time since diagnosis and the presence of long-term complications, which are important factors in calculating the 10-year CV risk score. Interestingly, while waist circumference is a mandatory factor for diagnosing MS according to the IDF [1], it is not considered in any CV risk calculation tool. This could be significant, especially in patients with MS. Conversely, scoring systems for non-alcoholic fatty liver disease (NAFLD) such as the Fatty Liver Index (FLI), which are strongly associated with high CV risk score [49], do include waist circumference in their calculation [50]. BMI is a required parameter when calculating 10-year CV risk using the DIAbetes Lifetime perspective (DIAL) model. However, the online calculator model indicates that this tool may underestimate the 10-year and lifetime risk score without a history of CV disease, and that the algorithm is currently being calibrated [51]. Although the recalibration has been published, the new algorithm is not yet available for online calculations [52].

HbA1c levels, indicative of the glycaemic control, have been linked to a decrease in non-fatal CV events, such as stroke, and microvascular and macrovascular complications [53–55]. Consequently, attaining optimal glycaemic control is a current recommendation in the individualized treatment to all persons with T2DM [56]. Nonetheless, the IDF criteria for diagnosing MS consider fasting blood glucose rather than this parameter [1]. Given that HbA1c represents the average blood glucose values over the past three months, it could be a relevant parameter to assessing uncontrolled diabetes [57], and thus a criterion for MS.

The results of this study suggest that effective SBP control alone (<130 mmHg) could result in a significant proportion of participants (34.5%) no longer fulfilling the diagnostic criteria for MS. Furthermore, this possible intervention alone could significantly reduce the CV risk score in the studied population, compared to the current risk score. This highlights the potential role of aggressive risk factor modification in ameliorating metabolic abnormalities and reducing the overall burden of CV risk in diabetic groups. The fact that the calculator used (ADVANCE) does not allow the control of all the parameters considered in the CV risk score calculation and/or MS, such as HbA1c, HDL cholesterol, or total cholesterol, hinders the feasibility of quantitatively calculating the impact of changes in CV risk score for each individual. This would be probably a complex task, since the therapeutic objectives for some of these parameters need to be defined, considering the individual characteristics of the patient. It might be beneficial to include additional parameters not covered here, such as health literacy, as previously suggested [58], to further reduce CV risk.

The clustering of MS may play a significant role in the identifying priority interventions associated with CV risk. This contributes to the emphasis on early detection and intervention to mitigate adverse outcomes in this population. The burden of CV diseases attributable to metabolic risk factors has been growing over the last few decades. This trend is expected to continue, considering global aging and the increase in life expectancy [59].

It is important to acknowledge the limitations of the study, such as the cross-sectional design and the use of population mean for albumin creatinine ratio parameter in the risk score calculation on ADVANCE calculator due to the lack of information regarding this parameter. Another limitation of the present study is related to the size of our sample, which limited the conclusions drawn from the statistical treatment of the data, especially when considering the comparison between males and females.

Future research is essential. This includes longitudinal studies to assess the prospective trajectory of MS and its relationship with CV outcomes in elderly individuals with T2DM. It would also be beneficial to develop or upgrade tools that allow the adjustment of other important modifiable parameters in the CV risk score of patients with T2DM and MS, such as HDL cholesterol, triglycerides, fasting glucose, and/or HbA1c levels.

5. Conclusions

The current study examines the intricate relationship between MS, T2DM, and CV risk in the elderly population. Our findings highlight the heightened CV risk score faced by individuals with T2DM and MS, particularly as they age and the duration of their disease increases. Sex disparities found in the CV risk score highlight the need for tailored interventions that address specific risk factors in both male and female populations.

This study shows the considerable potential of aggressive BP control in reducing the CV risk score, with notable reductions observed across the entire study cohort. The synergistic effect of simultaneously addressing SBP and LDL cholesterol levels further emphasizes the importance of multifaceted risk reduction strategies in optimizing patient outcomes.

Further research is needed to explore additional therapeutic approaches and modifiable factors that aim to enhance CV health in elderly patients with T2DM and MS.

Author Contributions: Conceptualization, T.N. and M.E.-S.; methodology, T.N., M.E.-S. and M.D.E.; formal analysis, T.N., M.E.-S., A.G. and E.P.; investigation, T.N., M.E.-S. and A.G.; writing—original draft preparation, T.N., M.E.-S., A.L.D.S.-C. and M.D.E.; writing—review and editing, all authors. All authors have read and agreed to the published version of the manuscript.

Funding: Agency for Clinical Research and Biomedical Innovation (AICIB) with the support of the solidarity account "Todos Por Quem Cuida (TPQC)", within the scope of the awarded project IMPPACTO, to A.L.D.S.-C.

Institutional Review Board Statement: The study was conducted in accordance with the Declaration of Helsinki and approved by the Cranfield University Ethical Committee (CURES/840/2016).

Informed Consent Statement: Informed consent was obtained from all subjects involved in the study.

Data Availability Statement: The data presented in this study are available on request from the corresponding author due to privacy restrictions.

Conflicts of Interest: The authors declare no conflicts of interest.

References

1. Alberti, K.G.M.M.; Zimmet, P.; Shaw, J.; George, K.; Alberti, M.M.; Aschner, P.; Balkau, B.; Bennett, P.; Boyko, E.; Brunzell, J.; et al. Metabolic Syndrome-a New World-Wide Definition. A Consensus Statement from the International Diabetes Federation. *Diabet. Med.* **2006**, *23*, 469–480. [CrossRef] [PubMed]
2. Kharroubi, A.T.; Darwish, H.M. Diabetes Mellitus: The Epidemic of the Century. *World J. Diabetes* **2015**, *6*, 850–867. [CrossRef] [PubMed]
3. American Diabetes Association Professional Practice Committee. 2. Diagnosis and Classification of Diabetes: Standards of Care in Diabetes—2024. *Diabetes Care* **2024**, *47*, S20–S42. [CrossRef] [PubMed]
4. Faselis, C.; Katsimardou, A.; Imprialos, K.; Deligkaris, P.; Kallistratos, M.; Dimitriadis, K. Microvascular Complications of Type 2 Diabetes Mellitus. *Curr. Vasc. Pharmacol.* **2020**, *18*, 117–124. [CrossRef] [PubMed]
5. Maric-Bilkan, C. Sex Differences in Micro- and Macro-Vascular Complications of Diabetes Mellitus. *Clin. Sci.* **2017**, *131*, 833–846. [CrossRef] [PubMed]
6. Tramunt, B.; Smati, S.; Grandgeorge, N.; Lenfant, F.; Arnal, J.-F.; Montagner, A.; Gourdy, P. Sex Differences in Metabolic Regulation and Diabetes Susceptibility. *Diabetologia* **2020**, *63*, 453–461. [CrossRef] [PubMed]
7. Damaskos, C.; Garmpis, N.; Kollia, P.; Mitsiopoulos, G.; Barlampa, D.; Drosos, A.; Patsouras, A.; Gravvanis, N.; Antoniou, V.; Litos, A.; et al. Assessing Cardiovascular Risk in Patients with Diabetes: An Update. *Curr. Cardiol. Rev.* **2020**, *16*, 266–274. [CrossRef] [PubMed]
8. Neppala, S.; Rajan, J.; Yang, E.; DeFronzo, R.A. Unexplained Residual Risk In Type 2 Diabetes: How Big Is The Problem? *Curr. Cardiol. Rep.* **2024**, *26*, 623–633. [CrossRef] [PubMed]
9. Rajendran, A.; Minhas, A.S.; Kazzi, B.; Varma, B.; Choi, E.; Thakkar, A.; Michos, E.D. Sex-Specific Differences in Cardiovascular Risk Factors and Implications for Cardiovascular Disease Prevention in Women. *Atherosclerosis* **2023**, *384*, 117269. [CrossRef]
10. PORDATA Índice de Envelhecimento. Available online: https://www.pordata.pt/Europa/%C3%8Dndice+de+envelhecimento-1609 (accessed on 5 May 2024).
11. Sociedade Portuguesa de Diabetologia. *Diabetes: Factos e Números—O Ano de 2019, 2020 e 2021—Relatório Anual Do Observatório Nacional Da Diabetes 03/2023*; Sociedade Portuguesa de Diabetologia: Lisboa, Portugal, 2023.
12. Bitton, A.; Physician, A. The Framingham Heart Study's Impact on Global Risk Assessment. *Prog. Cardiovasc. Dis.* **2010**, *53*, 68–78. [CrossRef]
13. Piepoli, M.F. 2016 European Guidelines on Cardiovascular Disease Prevention in Clinical Practice. *Int. J. Behav. Med.* **2016**, *24*, 321–419. [CrossRef] [PubMed]
14. Hippisley-Cox, J.; Coupland, C.; Brindle, P. Development and Validation of QRISK3 Risk Prediction Algorithms to Estimate Future Risk of Cardiovascular Disease: Prospective Cohort Study. *BMJ* **2017**, *357*, j2099. [CrossRef] [PubMed]

15. Badawy, M.A.E.M.D.; Naing, L.; Johar, S.; Ong, S.; Rahman, H.A.; Tengah, D.S.N.A.P.; Chong, C.L.; Tuah, N.A.A. Evaluation of Cardiovascular Diseases Risk Calculators for CVDs Prevention and Management: Scoping Review. *BMC Public Health* **2022**, *22*, 1742. [CrossRef] [PubMed]
16. Quaglini, S.; Stefanelli, M.; Boiocchi, L.; Campari, F.; Cavallini, A.; Micieli, G. Cardiovascular Risk Calculators: Understanding Differences and Realising Economic Implications. *Int. J. Med. Inform.* **2005**, *74*, 191–199. [CrossRef] [PubMed]
17. Rocha, E. Cardiovascular Risk Scores: Usefulness and Limitations. *Rev. Port. Cardiol. (Engl. Ed.)* **2016**, *35*, 15–18. [CrossRef] [PubMed]
18. U Prevent ADVANCE Risk Score. Available online: https://u-prevent.com/calculators/advanceScore (accessed on 5 May 2024).
19. WHO Consultation on Obesity 1999: World Health Organization Obesity: Preventing and Managing the Global Epidemic: Report of a WHO Consultation. Available online: https://iris.who.int/handle/10665/42330 (accessed on 7 May 2024).
20. American Diabetes Association Professional Practice Committee. 10. Cardiovascular Disease and Risk Management: Standards of Medical Care in Diabetes—2022. *Diabetes Care* **2022**, *45*, S144–S174. [CrossRef] [PubMed]
21. The SPRINT Research Group. A Randomized Trial of Intensive versus Standard Blood-Pressure Control. *N. Engl. J. Med.* **2015**, *373*, 2103. [CrossRef]
22. The ACCORD Study Group. Effects of Intensive Blood-Pressure Control in Type 2 Diabetes Mellitus. *N. Engl. J. Med.* **2010**, *362*, 1575. [CrossRef] [PubMed]
23. Gourdy, P.; Schiele, F.; Halimi, J.M.; Kownator, S.; Hadjadj, S.; Valensi, P. Atherosclerotic Cardiovascular Disease Risk Stratification and Management in Type 2 Diabetes: Review of Recent Evidence-Based Guidelines. *Front. Cardiovasc. Med.* **2023**, *10*, 1227769. [CrossRef]
24. PORDATA Instituto Nacional de Estatística I.P. Resident Population Aged 15 and over by Level of Education Completed. Available online: https://www.pordata.pt/ (accessed on 6 May 2024).
25. Marx, N.; Federici, M.; Schütt, K.; Müller-Wieland, D.; Ajjan, R.A.; Antunes, M.J.; Christodorescu, R.M.; Crawford, C.; Di Angelantonio, E.; Eliasson, B.; et al. 2023 ESC Guidelines for the Management of Cardiovascular Disease in Patients with Diabetes. *Eur. Heart J.* **2023**, *44*, 4043–4140. [CrossRef]
26. Kim, M.K.; Lee, K.N.; Han, K.; Lee, S.-H. Diabetes Duration, Cholesterol Levels, and Risk of Cardiovascular Diseases in Individuals With Type 2 Diabetes. *J. Clin. Endocrinol. Metab.* **2024**, dgae092. [CrossRef] [PubMed]
27. de Jong, M.; Woodward, M.; Peters, S.A.E. Duration of Diabetes and the Risk of Major Cardiovascular Events in Women and Men: A Prospective Cohort Study of UK Biobank Participants. *Diabetes Res. Clin. Pract.* **2022**, *188*, 109899. [CrossRef]
28. Yao, X.; Zhang, J.; Zhang, X.; Jiang, T.; Zhang, Y.; Dai, F.; Hu, H.; Zhang, Q. Age at Diagnosis, Diabetes Duration and the Risk of Cardiovascular Disease in Patients with Diabetes Mellitus: A Cross-Sectional Study. *Front. Endocrinol.* **2023**, *14*, 1131395. [CrossRef]
29. WHO. *WHO European Regional Obesity Report 2022*; WHO Regional Office for Europe: Copenhagen, Denmark, 2022; Licence: CC BY-NC-SA 3.0 IGO.
30. Gaio, V.; Antunes, L.; Namorado, S.; Barreto, M.; Gil, A.; Kyslaya, I.; Rodrigues, A.P.; Santos, A.; Bøhler, L.; Castilho, E.; et al. Prevalence of Overweight and Obesity in Portugal: Results from the First Portuguese Health Examination Survey (INSEF 2015). *Obes. Res. Clin. Pract.* **2018**, *12*, 40–50. [CrossRef]
31. Oliveira, A.; Araújo, J.; Severo, M.; Correia, D.; Ramos, E.; Torres, D.; Lopes, C.; Rodrigues, S.; Vilela, S.; Guiomar, S.; et al. Prevalence of General and Abdominal Obesity in Portugal: Comprehensive Results from the National Food, Nutrition and Physical Activity Survey 2015–2016. *BMC Public Health* **2018**, *18*, 614. [CrossRef]
32. Martínez-González, M.A.; García-Arellano, A.; Toledo, E.; Bes-Rastrollo, M.; Bulló, M.; Corella, D.; Fito, M.; Ros, E.; Lamuela-Raventós, R.M.; Rekondo, J.; et al. Obesity Indexes and Total Mortality among Elderly Subjects at High Cardiovascular Risk: The PREDIMED Study. *PLoS ONE* **2014**, *9*, e103246. [CrossRef] [PubMed]
33. Chiazor, E.I.; Evans, M.; van Woerden, H.; Oparah, A.C. A Systematic Review of Community Pharmacists' Interventions in Reducing Major Risk Factors for Cardiovascular Disease. *Value Health Reg. Issues* **2015**, *7*, 9–21. [CrossRef]
34. Hu, C.; Lin, L.; Zhu, Y.; Zhang, Y.; Wang, S.; Zhang, J.; Qi, H.; Li, M.; Zhu, Y.; Huo, Y.; et al. Association Between Age at Diagnosis of Type 2 Diabetes and Cardiovascular Diseases: A Nationwide, Population-Based, Cohort Study. *Front. Endocrinol.* **2021**, *12*, 717069. [CrossRef]
35. Instituto Nacional Estatística. *Inquérito Nacional de Saúde 2019*; Instituto Nacional de Estatística: Lisboa, Portugal, 2020.
36. Relimpio, F.; Martinez-Brocca, M.A.; Leal-Cerro, A.; Losada, F.; Mangas, M.A.; Pumar, A.; Astorga, R. Variability in the Presence of the Metabolic Syndrome in Type 2 Diabetic Patients Attending a Diabetes Clinic: Influences of Age and Gender. *Diabetes Res. Clin. Pract.* **2004**, *65*, 135–142. [CrossRef]
37. Del Cañizo-Gómez, F.J.; Moreira-Andrés, M.N. Cardiovascular Risk Factors in Patients with Type 2 Diabetes: Do We Follow the Guidelines? *Diabetes Res. Clin. Pract.* **2004**, *65*, 125–133. [CrossRef]
38. Salameh, A.B.; Hyassat, D.; Suhail, A.; Makahleh, Z.; Khader, Y.; EL-Khateeb, M.; Ajlouni, K. The Prevalence of Hypertension and Its Progression among Patients with Type 2 Diabetes in Jordan. *Ann. Med. Surg.* **2022**, *73*, 103162. [CrossRef] [PubMed]
39. Naseri, M.W.; Esmat, H.A.; Bahee, M.D. Prevalence of Hypertension in Type-2 Diabetes Mellitus. *Ann. Med. Surg.* **2022**, *78*, 103758. [CrossRef]
40. Hicks, C.W.; Selvin, E. Epidemiology of Peripheral Neuropathy and Lower Extremity Disease in Diabetes. *Curr. Diab Rep.* **2019**, *19*, 86. [CrossRef] [PubMed]

41. Kautzky-Willer, A.; Harreiter, J.; Pacini, G. Sex and Gender Differences in Risk, Pathophysiology and Complications of Type 2 Diabetes Mellitus. *Endocr. Rev.* **2016**, *37*, 278–316. [CrossRef] [PubMed]
42. Cardoso, H.; Tavares Bello, C.; Andrade, L.; Sobral do Rosário, F.; Louro, J.; Nogueira, C.; Rodrigues, E.; Vieira, N.B.; Carqueja, T. High Prevalence of Cardiovascular Disease and Risk Factors among Type 2 Diabetes Patients Followed in a Hospital Setting in Portugal: The PICT2RE Observational Study. *Rev. Port. Cardiol.* **2023**, *42*, 319–330. [CrossRef] [PubMed]
43. SCORE2 working group; ESC Cardiovascular risk collaboration. SCORE2 Risk Prediction Algorithms: New Models to Estimate 10-Year Risk of Cardiovascular Disease in Europe. *Eur. Heart J.* **2021**, *42*, 2439–2454. [CrossRef] [PubMed]
44. Gencer, B.; Marston, N.A.; Im, K.A.; Cannon, C.P.; Sever, P.; Keech, A.; Braunwald, E.; Giugliano, R.P.; Sabatine, M.S. Efficacy and Safety of Lowering LDL Cholesterol in Older Patients: A Systematic Review and Meta-Analysis of Randomised Controlled Trials. *Lancet* **2020**, *396*, 1637. [CrossRef] [PubMed]
45. SCORE2-OP Working Group. ESC Cardiovascular Risk SCORE2-OP Risk Prediction Algorithms: Estimating Incident Cardiovascular Event Risk in Older Persons in Four Geographical Risk Regions. *Eur. Heart J.* **2021**, *42*, 2455–2467. [CrossRef] [PubMed]
46. Kengne, A.P. The ADVA NCE Cardiovascular Risk Model and Current Strategies for Cardiovascular Disease Risk Evaluation in People with Diabetes. *Cardiovasc. J. Afr.* **2013**, *24*, 376. [CrossRef]
47. Kengne, A.P.; Patel, A.; Marre, M.; Travert, F.; Lievre, M.; Zoungas, S.; Chalmers, J.; Colagiuri, S.; Grobbee, D.E.; Hamet, P.; et al. Contemporary Model for Cardiovascular Risk Prediction in People with Type 2 Diabetes. *Eur. J. Cardiovasc. Prev. Rehabil.* **2011**, *18*, 393–398. [CrossRef]
48. Rossello, X.; Dorresteijn, J.A.; Janssen, A.; Lambrinou, E.; Scherrenberg, M.; Bonnefoy-Cudraz, E.; Cobain, M.; Piepoli, M.F.; Visseren, F.L.; Dendale, P. Risk Prediction Tools in Cardiovascular Disease Prevention: A Report from the ESC Prevention of CVD Programme Led by the European Association of Preventive Cardiology (EAPC) in Collaboration with the Acute Cardiovascular Care Association (ACCA) and the Association of Cardiovascular Nursing and Allied Professions (ACNAP). *Eur. J. Prev. Cardiol.* **2019**, *26*, 1534–1544. [CrossRef] [PubMed]
49. Kweon, Y.N.; Ko, H.J.; Kim, A.S.; Choi, H.I.; Song, J.E.; Park, J.Y.; Kim, S.M.; Hong, H.E.; Min, K.J. Prediction of Cardiovascular Risk Using Nonalcoholic Fatty Liver Disease Scoring Systems. *Healthcare* **2021**, *9*, 899. [CrossRef]
50. Bedogni, G.; Bellentani, S.; Miglioli, L.; Masutti, F.; Passalacqua, M.; Castiglione, A.; Tiribelli, C. The Fatty Liver Index: A Simple and Accurate Predictor of Hepatic Steatosis in the General Population. *BMC Gastroenterol.* **2006**, *6*, 33. [CrossRef]
51. U-Prevent. Available online: https://u-prevent.com/calculators/dialModel (accessed on 6 May 2024).
52. Østergaard, H.B.; Hageman, S.H.J.; Read, S.H.; Taylor, O.; Pennells, L.; Kaptoge, S.; Petitjean, C.; Xu, Z.; Shi, F.; Mcevoy, J.W.; et al. Estimating Individual Lifetime Risk of Incident Cardiovascular Events in Adults with Type 2 Diabetes: An Update and Geographical Calibration of the DIAbetes Lifetime Perspective Model (DIAL2). *Eur. J. Prev. Cardiol.* **2023**, *30*, 61–69. [CrossRef] [PubMed]
53. Tan, J.K.; Thumboo, J.; Lim, G.H.; Salim, N.N.M.; Chia, S.Y.; Bee, Y.M. Associations Between Mean HbA1c, HbA1c Variability, and Both Mortality and Macrovascular Complications in Patients with Diabetes Mellitus: A Registry-Based Cohort Study. *Clin. Epidemiol.* **2023**, *15*, 137–149. [CrossRef] [PubMed]
54. Boye, K.S.; Thieu, V.T.; Lage, M.J.; Miller, H.; Paczkowski, R. The Association Between Sustained HbA1c Control and Long-Term Complications Among Individuals with Type 2 Diabetes: A Retrospective Study. *Adv. Ther.* **2022**, *39*, 2208. [CrossRef]
55. Wu, T.E.; Su, Y.W.; Chen, H.S. Mean HbA1c and HbA1c Variability Are Associated with Differing Diabetes-Related Complications in Patients with Type 2 Diabetes Mellitus. *Diabetes Res. Clin. Pract.* **2022**, *192*, 110069. [CrossRef]
56. Maiorino, M.I.; Longo, M.; Scappaticcio, L.; Bellastella, G.; Chiodini, P.; Esposito, K.; Giugliano, D. Improvement of Glycemic Control and Reduction of Major Cardiovascular Events in 18 Cardiovascular Outcome Trials: An Updated Meta-Regression. *Cardiovasc. Diabetol.* **2021**, *20*, 210. [CrossRef]
57. American Diabetes Association Professional Practice Committee. 6. Glycemic Goals and Hypoglycemia: Standards of Care in Diabetes—2024. *Diabetes Care* **2024**, *47*, S111–S125. [CrossRef]
58. Albus, C. Health Literacy: Is It Important for Cardiovascular Disease Prevention? *Eur. J. Prev. Cardiol.* **2018**, *25*, 934–935. [CrossRef]
59. Wang, H.; Liu, J.; Feng, Y.; Ma, A.; Wang, T. The Burden of Cardiovascular Diseases Attributable to Metabolic Risk Factors and Its Change from 1990 to 2019: A Systematic Analysis and Prediction. *Front. Epidemiol.* **2023**, *3*, 1048515. [CrossRef] [PubMed]

diabetology

MDPI

Article

Do T2DM and Hyperglycaemia Affect the Expression Levels of the Regulating Enzymes of Cellular *O*-GlcNAcylation in Human Saphenous Vein Smooth Muscle Cells?

Israel O. Bolanle [1], Gillian A. Durham [1], James P. Hobkirk [2], Mahmoud Loubani [3], Roger G. Sturmey [1] and Timothy M. Palmer [1,*]

[1] Biomedical Institute for Multimorbidity, Centre for Biomedicine, Hull York Medical School, University of Hull, Hull HU6 7RX, UK; olapeju.bolanle@hyms.ac.uk (I.O.B.); gill.durham@hyms.ac.uk (G.A.D.); roger.sturmey@hyms.ac.uk (R.G.S.)

[2] School of Sport Exercise and Rehabilitation Sciences, University of Hull, Hull HU6 7RX, UK; j.hobkirk@hull.ac.uk

[3] Department of Cardiothoracic Surgery, Castle Hill Hospital, Cottingham HU16 5JQ, UK; mahmoud.loubani@nhs.net

* Correspondence: tim.palmer@hyms.ac.uk

Abstract: Protein *O*-GlcNAcylation, a dynamic and reversible glucose-dependent post-translational modification of serine and threonine residues on target proteins, has been proposed to promote vascular smooth muscle cell proliferation and migration events implicated in vein graft failure (VGF). Therefore, targeting the enzymes (glutamine fructose-6P amidotransferase (GFAT), *O*-GlcNAc transferase (OGT), and *O*-GlcNAcase (OGA)) that regulate cellular *O*-GlcNAcylation could offer therapeutic options to reduce neointimal hyperplasia and venous stenosis responsible for VGF. However, it is unclear how type 2 diabetes mellitus (T2DM) and hyperglycaemia affect the expression of these enzymes in human saphenous vein smooth muscle cells (HSVSMCs), a key cell type involved in the vascular dysfunction responsible for saphenous VGF. Therefore, our aim was to assess whether T2DM and hyperglycaemia affect GFAT, OGT, and OGA expression levels in HSVSMCs in vitro. Expression levels of GFAT, OGT, and OGA were determined in low-passage HSVSMCs from T2DM and non-T2DM patients, and in HSVSMCs treated for 48 h with hyperglycaemic (10 mM and 25 mM) glucose concentrations, by quantitative immunoblotting. Expression levels of OGT, OGA, and GFAT were not significantly different in HSVSMC lysates from T2DM patients versus non-T2DM controls. In addition, treatment with high glucose concentrations (10 mM and 25 mM) had no significant effect on the protein levels of these enzymes in HSVSMC lysates. From our findings, T2DM and hyperglycaemia do not significantly impact the expression levels of the *O*-GlcNAcylation-regulating enzymes OGT, OGA, and GFAT in HSVSMCs. This study provides a foundation for future studies to assess the role of *O*-GlcNAcylation on VGF in T2DM.

Keywords: type 2 diabetes mellitus; protein *O*-GlcNAcylation; glutamine fructose-6P amidotransferase; *O*-GlcNAc transferase; *O*-GlcNAcase

1. Introduction

Protein *O*-GlcNAcylation is a post-translational modification (PTM) that occurs on target proteins in response to nutrient and stress (hypoxia, heat shock, and nutrient shortage) changes by attaching a single sugar, β-*N*-acetylglucosamine (*O*-GlcNAc), to target serine or threonine residues [1–3]. Protein *O*-GlcNAcylation alters the cellular functions of these target proteins, promoting inflammation, metabolism, trafficking, and cytoskeletal organisation [1,4,5]. Furthermore, *O*-GlcNAcylation has been linked to a number of other cellular processes, such as the temporal control of insulin signalling, gene transcription, epigenetic changes, and cell signalling dynamics [1,6,7]. The enzymes that regulate *O*-GlcNAcylation have been well characterised and include the rate-limiting enzyme L-glutamine-D-fructose 6-phosphate amidotransferase (GFAT), together with *O*-GlcNAc transferase (OGT) and *O*-GlcNAcase (OGA) that catalyse the attachment and removal of *O*-GlcNAc moieties to target proteins, respectively [1].

Although the mechanisms governing the temporal regulation of *O*-GlcNAc signalling are dynamic and frequently transient, they remain poorly understood [6,8,9]. The abundance of the donor substrate UDP-GlcNAc, as well as the activities of OGT, OGA, and their corresponding adaptor proteins and substrates, are regulated by nutrient availability, which also controls the amounts of cellular *O*-GlcNAcylation [6,10,11]. While the mutual control of OGT and OGA maintains cellular *O*-GlcNAcylation levels, persistent hyperglycaemia can shift the balance in favour of OGT-mediated *O*-GlcNAcylation, which has now been implicated in vein graft failure (VGF) [6,12,13].

It is now becoming clear that protein *O*-GlcNAcylation is a significant cellular modification through which type 2 diabetes mellitus (T2DM) initiates vascular dysfunction that has been implicated in multiple cardiovascular diseases (CVDs) [1,4]. However, it remains unexplored for possible drug development in managing vascular pathologies [14]. Although the enzymes that regulate *O*-GlcNAcylation have been extensively characterised in many cell types and systems [1,4], our understanding of the factors that influence their expression and functions is still expanding. One such factor of critical interest in this study is hyperglycaemia, a hallmark feature of unresolved or poorly controlled T2DM. Several studies have demonstrated a causal relationship between *O*-GlcNAcylation and prolonged hyperglycaemia [15–17].

In patients with coronary artery disease (CAD) with or without T2DM, coronary artery bypass graft (CABG) using an autologous saphenous vein remains the gold standard procedure for restoring blood supply to the heart [18,19]. Patients with T2DM who have CAD, however, are more susceptible to neointimal hyperplasia, vascular remodelling, and stenosis that result in VGF [20]. While the underlying mechanisms responsible for this are unclear, upregulated *O*-GlcNAcylation, which is common in T2DM, has been implicated [21]. However, it is currently unknown if hyperglycaemia or T2DM regulates the expression of these regulating enzymes of *O*-GlcNAcylation in human saphenous vein smooth muscle cells (HSVSMCs), a key cell type involved in the vascular dysfunction responsible for saphenous VGF. Thus, in this study, HSVSMCs from T2DM and non-T2DM patients, as well as HSVSMCs from non-T2DM patients, were treated with high glucose concentrations (10 mM and 25 mM), as described by [15,22]. Following this, the expression of key enzymes that regulate cellular *O*-GlcNAcylation status in vitro was determined.

2. Materials and Methods

2.1. Materials

Anti-MGEA5/OGA (Abcam, Cambridge, UK, Cat No: ab105217); Anti-O-GlcNAc Transferase (DM-17) (OGT, Sigma-Aldrich (Merck), Dorset, UK, Cat No: O6264); GFAT (Santa Cruz Biotechnology, Dallas, TX, USA, Cat No: Sc-377479); Anti-STAT3 antibody (EPR787Y) (STAT3, Abcam, Cambridge, UK, Cat No: ab68153); Anti- glyceraldehyde-3-phosphate dehydrogenase (GAPDH) antibody [6C5] (GAPDH, Abcam, Cambridge, UK, Cat No: ab8245). SmGM2 (supplemented with 5% (v/v) foetal bovine serum, 0.5 ng/mL epidermal growth factor, 2 ng/mL basic fibroblast growth factor, and 5 g/mL insulin; Promocell, Heidelberg, Germany, Cat. No: C-22162); Rabbit monoclonal [SP171] to alpha smooth muscle Actin (α-SMA, Abcam, Cambridge, UK, Cat No: ab ab150301); Rabbit monoclonal [EPR8965] to non-muscle Myosin IIA (SMMHC, Abcam, Cambridge, UK, Cat No: ab 138498); anti-PECAM-1 (CD31) (BD Bioscience, Berkshire, UK, Cat No: BD 555444). IRDye-conjugated secondary antibodies were from LI-COR Biotechnology, Cambridge, UK. A mammalian expression construct for Myc epitope-tagged human OGT (HG17892-NM) was from Sino-Biological Incorporated, Beijing, China. A mammalian expression construct for Myc and FLAG epitope-tagged mouse OGT (MR211167) was from Origene Technologies, Rockville, MD, USA.

2.2. Methods

2.2.1. Isolation of HSVSMCs

As shown in Table 1, surplus HSV tissues were obtained from T2DM and non-T2DM patients undergoing coronary artery bypass graft (CABG) surgery at the Cardiothroacic Surgery Department, Castle Hill Hospital, Cottingham, UK, under NHRA ethical approval (NHS REC:15/NE/0138). Detailed information for each of the patient samples used in this study is provided in Table S1. HSV tissues (length = 0.5 cm to 4 cm) were stored at 4 °C for a maximum of 48 h in DMEM supplemented with 100 IU/mL penicillin, 100 g/mL streptomycin, and 0.25 µg/mL fungizone. VSMCs were explanted from HSV as described by [22]. Briefly, HSV tissue was placed in a 10 cm dish with enough medium to cover it, and a sterile blade was used to remove the perivascular fat, vein branches, connective tissue, and adventitia. The vein was then dissected longitudinally, and the endothelial and tunica intima layers were gently removed with sterile surgical scissors and forceps. Then, HSV tissue was dissected into small fragments (~1 mm^3). These were transferred into a 25 cm^2 tissue culture flask with 2 mL of SmGM2 and cultured at 37 °C in 5% (*v*/*v*) CO_2 in a humidified atmosphere. Once HSVSMCs had migrated from the explant tissue, after approximately two weeks, the growth medium was topped up with 0.5 mL of fresh SmGM2 twice weekly. The addition of 0.5 mL of fresh SmGM2 continued until a total of 5 mL of growth medium had been added; then, 2.5 mL of growth medium was removed and replenished with fresh 2.5 mL of SmGM2 until 90% confluence. Thereafter, HSVSMCs were transferred to a 75 cm^2 tissue culture flask and fed with 10 mL of SmGM2, which was replaced twice weekly until cells reached 90% confluency and expanded for either cryopreservation in liquid nitrogen or downstream experimental applications.

Table 1. Patient information for HSV samples.

	Description	T2DM	Non-T2DM
1	Number of samples	17	38
2	Age range	56–80	48–84
3	Sex	Male—15 Female—2	Male—37 Female—1
4	Ethnicity	White British—17	White British—37 Asian—1
5	Reason for surgery	CAD	CAD

CAD: coronary artery disease; T2DM: type 2 diabetes mellitus. HSV samples were collected between January 2020 and May 2022 from patients undergoing elective coronary artery bypass graft procedure.

2.2.2. Cell Culture

HSVSMCs, human umbilical vein endothelial cells (HUVECs), and human embryonic kidney (HEK) 293T cells were maintained with SmGM2, ECGM-MV2, and DMEM (supplemented with 10% (*v*/*v*) FBS, 100 IU/mL penicillin, 100 g/mL streptomycin, and 2 mM L-glutamine), respectively, in a T75 flask and kept in a cell culture incubator maintained at 37 °C and 5% (*v*/*v*) CO_2 in a humidified atmosphere. For all experiments, cells were allowed to be 80–90% confluent before subculturing.

2.2.3. Characterisation of HSVSMCs by Immunofluorescence Microscopy

To validate the integrity of isolated HSVSMCs, they were examined for the SMC markers α-smooth muscle actin (α-SMA) and smooth muscle-myosin heavy chain (SMMHC) using confocal immunofluorescence microscopy [23,24]. Also, isolated HSVSMCs were examined for an EC marker (anti-PECAM (CD31)) to rule out EC contamination. HUVECs served as the control in this set of experiments. Lab-Tek 4 chambered coverglasses were precoated with poly-D-lysine. Following this, passages 1 and 4 HSVSMCs were seeded in the Lab-Tek 4 chamber coverglass at 10,000 cells/well and allowed to grow until cells reached 40% confluency. Cells were washed three times (for 5–10 s) with 500 µL of ice-cold PBS and fixed with 500 μL of 4% (*w*/*v*) paraformaldehyde in PBS for 10 min at room temperature. Then, fixative was removed, and fixed cells were washed three times with 500 μL of PBS on each occasion. Cell membranes of cells were permeabilised with 500 μL of 0.1% (*v*/*v*) Triton X-100 in PBS for 30 min at room temperature. Cells were then washed three times and blocked with 500 μL of 5% (*w*/*v*) BSA, 0.1% (*v*/*v*) Tween 20 in PBS. After this, cells were labelled and incubated with either anti-SMMHC (1:400) or anti-α-SMA (1:200) primary antibody in 1% (*w*/*v*) BSA in PBST at 4 °C overnight in a humidified chamber. Cells were then washed three times with 500 μL of 5% (*w*/*v*) BSA, 0.1% (*v*/*v*) Tween 20 in PBS to remove unbound primary antibody, and bound antibody was detected by incubation with 200 μL/well goat anti-rabbit IgG (Alexa 568; 1:500) in 1% BSA for 1–4 h at room temperature in the dark. Cells were then washed three times with 500 μL of 0.1% (*v*/*v*) Tween 20 in PBS, followed by three washes with 500 μL of PBS (5 min/wash) in the dark. Permeabilised cells were also stained with 500 μL of 5 μg/mL Hoechst to identify nuclei. To exclude endothelial cell contamination, fixed and permeabilised HSVSMCs and HUVECs from passages 1 and 4 seeded in the Lab-Tek 4 chamber slides were also stained with mouse anti-PECAM (CD31) antibody, followed by incubation with goat anti-mouse IgG. (Alexa 488 1:500). All images were captured at x200 magnification using a LSM710 Zeiss laser scanning confocal microscope and processed using image J software (version 1.54e).

2.2.4. Generation of Cell Lysates

Cells within 70–90% confluency in 6-well plates or 6 cm dishes were transferred to an ice bath, and the growth medium was withdrawn and discarded. The cell monolayer was rinsed twice with 2 to 5 mL of ice-cold PBS, and any leftover PBS was removed using a pipette. Cells were then scraped into 500 μL and 1 mL of ice-cold PBS for 6-well dishes and 6 cm dishes, respectively. Following this, the cell suspension was centrifuged at 500× *g* for 5 min at 4 °C. After this, the supernatant was gently removed without distorting the pellets, and cells were lysed with 70 μL–200 μL of RIPA+ (50 mM HEPES pH 7.4, 150 mM sodium chloride, 1% (*v*/*v*) Triton x100, 0.5% (*v*/*v*) sodium deoxycholate, 0.1% (*w*/*v*) SDS, 10 mM sodium fluoride, 5 mM EDTA, 10 mM sodium phosphate, 0.1 mM PMSF, 10 μg/mL benzamidine, 10 μg/mL soybean trypsin inhibitor, 2% (*w*/*v*) EDTA-free complete protease inhibitor cocktail (1 tablet per 10 mL buffer). Samples were incubated on a rotating wheel at 4 °C for 45 min before centrifugation at 13,500× *g* for 15 min at 4 °C. The resulting supernatant was removed into fresh, labelled 1.5 mL microcentrifuge tubes and stored at −80 °C.

2.2.5. Transfection of HEK 293T Cells

A day before transfection, a poly-D lysine pre-coated 6-well plate was seeded with HEK 293T cells at a density of 5–6.25 × 10^5 cells/well and allowed to be 50–80% confluent. On the day of transfection, growth media was withdrawn and replaced with fresh medium. Then, 2 μg of DNA was dissolved in 500 μL of Opti-MEM I without serum, and 5 μL of Lipofectamine LTX reagent was added to the Opti-MEM-DNA solution. This was mixed gently and allowed to incubate for 30 min at room temperature to form DNA–Lipofectamine LTX Reagent complexes. Following this, 100 μL of the DNA–Lipofectamine LTX Reagent complex was added to each well directly and incubated at 37 °C in a CO_2 incubator for 18–48 h before visualising with the florescence microscope or assaying for transgene expression.

2.2.6. SDS-PAGE and Immunoblotting

Cell lysates were equalised for protein content and resolved in 13% (*w*/*v*) acrylamide. Separated bands were then transferred from the gel to an Amersham™ Protran® 2 μm pore nitrocellulose membrane using the semi-dry Thermofisher transfer device for 1 hr. Membranes were incubated for 1 h at room temperature with a 5% (*w*/*v*) BSA blocking solution diluted in Tris buffered saline-Tween 20 (TBST). Each membrane was then incubated overnight with a specific primary antibody at 4 °C on a rotating wheel. Then, three

TBST washes (5 min per wash) at room temperature were used to remove the unbound primary antibody. Following this, appropriate IRDye-conjugated secondary antibodies diluted in 5% (w/v) dried skimmed milk in TBST were used to incubate the membrane at room temperature for 1 hr. The unbound secondary antibody was then removed by washing three times with TBST. Immunoreactive bands were detected by imaging with a Licor Odyssey DLx.

2.2.7. Statistical Analysis

Statistical analysis was carried out using Graphpad Prism® 6, San Diego, CA, USA. Data are presented as mean ± standard error of mean (S.E.M) and were analysed using an independent t-test and one-way analysis of variance followed by Dunnett's post hoc test to determine significant differences between means, where $p < 0.05$ was considered statistically significant.

3. Results

3.1. Characterisation of Isolated HSVSMCs

Cells isolated and expanded from HSV explants were assessed using immunofluorescence and confocal imaging. Results revealed that these explanted cells (passages 1 and 4) isolated from HSVs are exclusively SMCs, as evidenced by positive staining with both anti-α-SMA (Figure 1) and anti-SMMHC (Figure 2) antibodies characteristic of SMCs. In contrast, HUVECs were negative for both anti-α-SMA and anti-SMMHC under the same conditions (Figures 1 and 2). In addition, the isolated cells did not react with antibodies against the EC marker PECAM-1 under conditions where anti-PECAM-1 staining was detectable in HUVECs (Figure 3), thereby excluding contamination with ECs (bottom panels). Therefore, to summarise, Figures 1–3 showed that cells isolated from explanted HSVs were exclusively SMCs devoid of contamination from ECs.

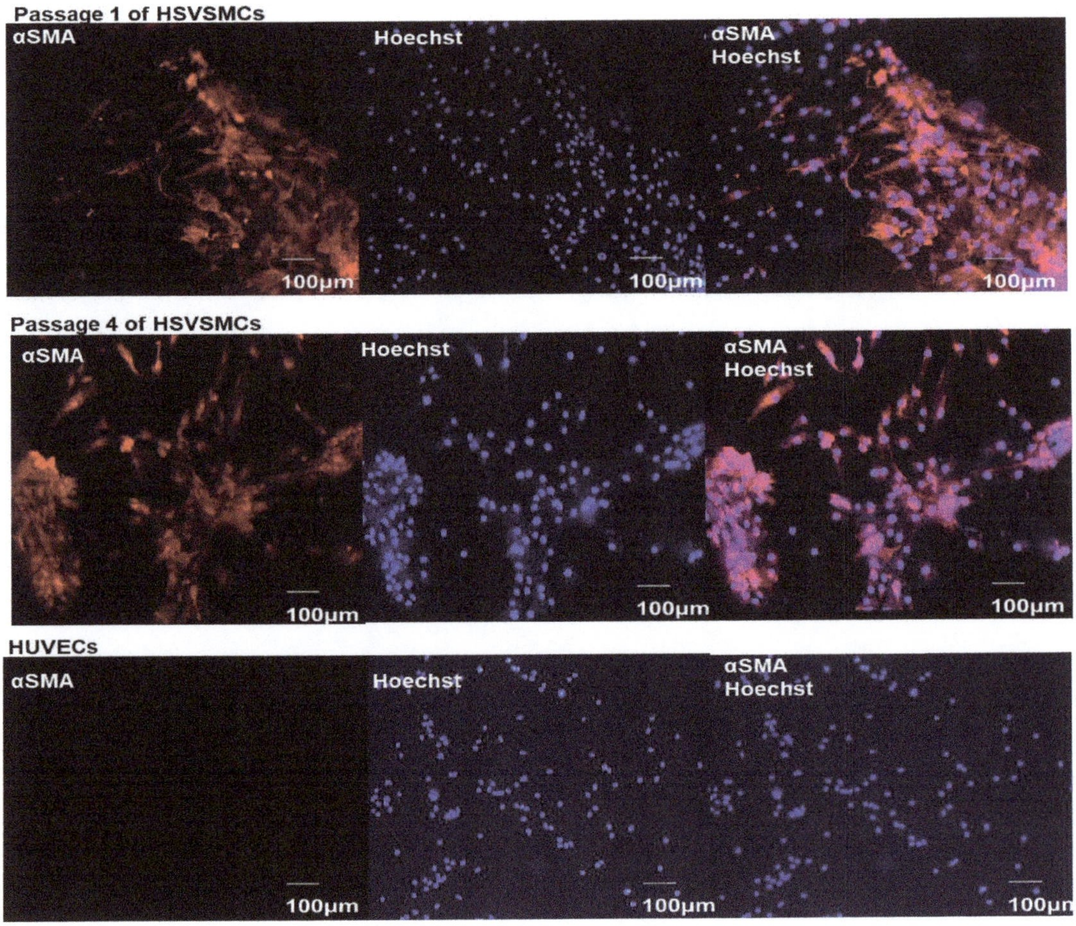

Figure 1. Verification of the identity of HSVSMCs from non-T2DM patients by immunofluorescence microscopy using anti-αSMA. Images reveal expression of SMC-specific marker α-SMA (red) and nuclei Hoechst stain (blue). Scale bar 100 μm, magnification × 200, n = 3. (**Top panel**): Passage 1 of HSVSMCs. (**Middle panel**): Passage 4 of HSVSMCs. (**Bottom panel**): HUVECs. SMA: smooth muscle actin; HSVSMC: human saphenous vein smooth muscle cell; HUVEC: human umbilical vascular endothelial cell.

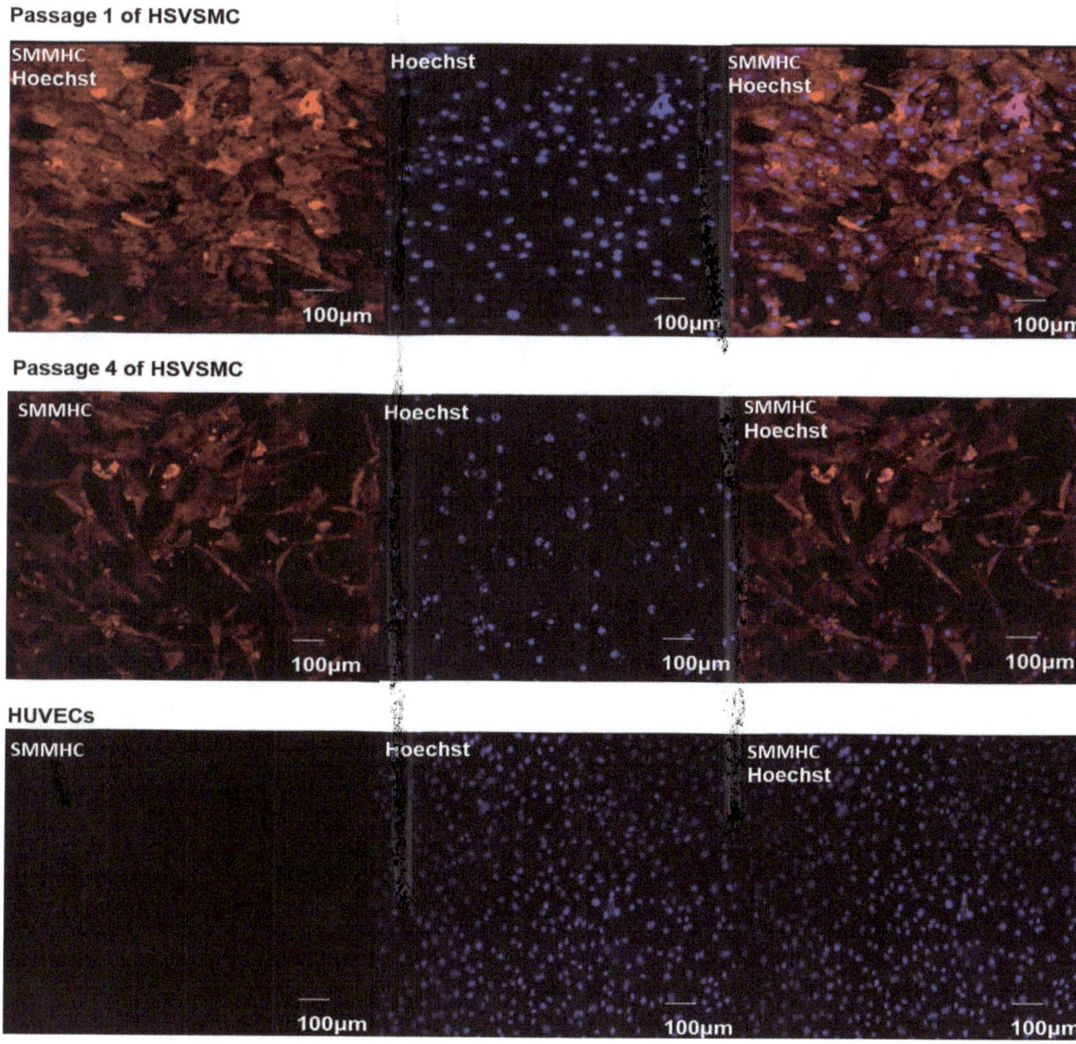

Figure 2. Verification of the identity of HSVSMCs from non-T2DM patients by immunofluorescence microscopy using anti-SMMHC. Images reveal expression of SMC-specific marker SMMHC (red) and nuclei Hoechst stain (blue). Scale bar 100 μm, magnification × 200, n = 3. (**Top panel**): Passage 1 HSVSMCs. (**Middle panel**): Passage 4 HSVSMCs. (**Bottom panel**): HUVECs. SMMHC: non-muscle myosin ll; HSVSMC: human saphenous vein smooth muscle cell; HUVEC: human umbilical vascular endothelial cell.

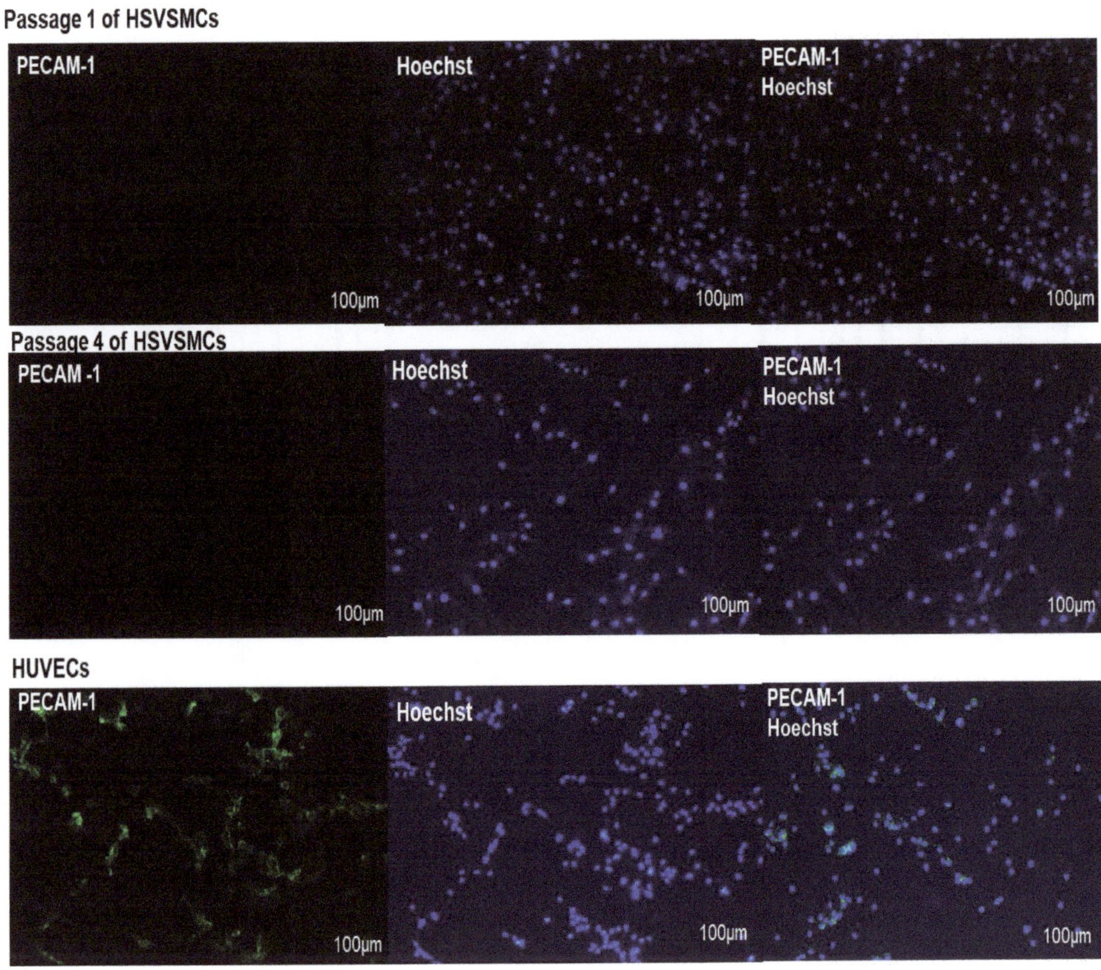

Figure 3. Excluding the presence of endothelial cell contamination in HSVSMCs from non-T2DM patients. Images reveal expression of EC-specific marker anti-PECAM (CD31) (green) and nuclei Hoechst stain (blue). Scale bar 100 μm, magnification × 200, n = 3. (**Top panel**): Passage 1 HSVSMCs. (**Middle Panel**): Passage 4 HSVSMCs. (**Bottom panel**): HUVECs. PECAM: platelet endothelial cell adhesion molecule; HSVSMC: human saphenous vein smooth muscle cell; HUVEC: human umbilical vascular endothelial cell.

3.2. Effect of Passage on the Expression of the Regulating Enzymes of O-GlcNAcylation in HSVSMC

To assess if the expression of *O*-GlcNAcylation enzymes OGA, OGT, and GFAT was altered with passage in HSVSMCs, SDS-PAGE and quantitative immunoblotting were used to compare their relative expression levels across passages 1–4 of HSVSMCs isolated from the same HSV tissue sample. As shown in Figure 4, the expressions of OGA, OGT, and GFAT were not significantly altered (n = 5 biological replicates using P1 as a reference for P2-4 for comparison) across passages 1–4.

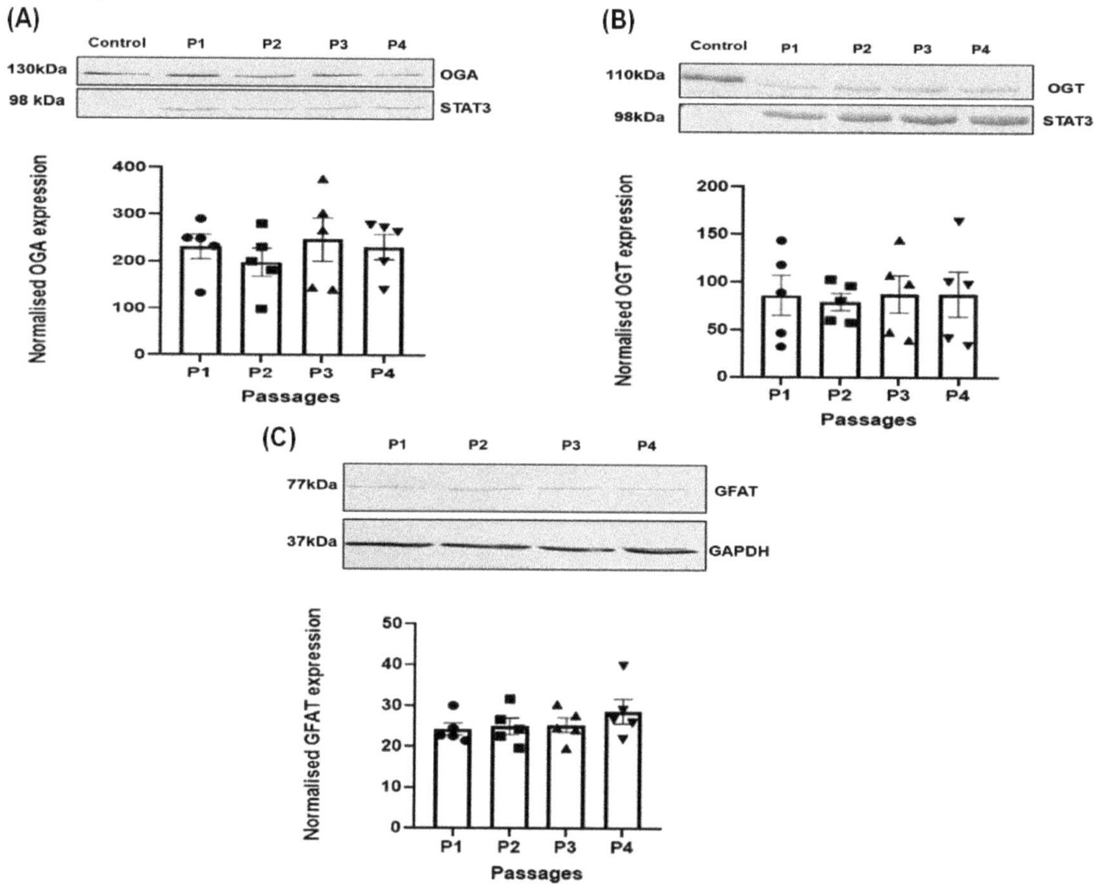

Figure 4. Expression of OGA, OGT, and GFAT across passages 1–4 of HSVSMCs from non-T2DM patients. (**A**) **Upper panel:** representative immunoblots for OGA (130 kDa) and STAT3 (98 kDa) expressions. OGA expression is in HEK293 cells (control) and in serially passaged HSVSMC (p1–p4) from non-T2DM patients. **Lower panel**: Densitometric analysis of OGA expression normalised to STAT3 (loading control). (**B**) **Upper panel**: Representative immunoblots for OGT (110 kDa) and STAT3 (98 kDa). OGT expression is in HEK293 cells (control) and in serially passaged p1-p4HSVSMC from non-T2DM patients. **Lower panel:** Densitometric analysis of OGT expression normalised to STAT3 (loading control). (**C**) **Upper panel**: Representative immunoblots for GFAT (77 kDa) and GAPDH (37 kDa). GFAT expression is in serially passaged p1–p4 HSVSMC from non-T2DM patients. **Lower panel**: Densitometric analysis of GFAT expression normalised to GAPDH (loading control). Normalised data are expressed as the mean ± SEM from n = 5 biological replicates using samples from different patients. Data from p2-4 were compared to p1 for statistical difference at $p < 0.05$. OGA: *O*-GlcNAcase; OGT: *O*-GlcNAc transferase; GFAT: glutamine fructose-6-phosphate amidotransferase; STAT3: signal transducer and activator of transcription 3; GAPDH: glyceraldehyde 3-phosphate dehydrogenase; P1-4: passages 1–4.

3.3. Comparison of OGA, OGT, and GFAT Expression Levels in HSVSMCs from T2DM versus Control Patients

Our understanding of the *O*-GlcNAcylation-regulating enzymes has considerably improved in recent years, in part because of advances in research tools that have aided in better characterisation [1,4]. The necessity to create pharmacological tools to control the regulating enzymes of *O*-GlcNAcylation has become increasingly significant as the involvement of *O*-GlcNAcylation in disease pathologies, most notably diabetes mellitus and CVDs, has continued to emerge [4]. It is, therefore, important to determine if T2DM alters the expression of these regulating enzymes to assess their viability as targets for drug development. Therefore, the expression levels of OGA, OGT, and GFAT were compared in HSVSMCs from T2DM and non-T2DM patients. Results from these experiments, as shown in Figure 5, showed that T2DM did not significantly alter (n = 6 biological replicates comparing values from T2DM and non-T2DM) the expression levels of OGA, OGT, and GFAT, respectively, in HSVSMCs in vitro.

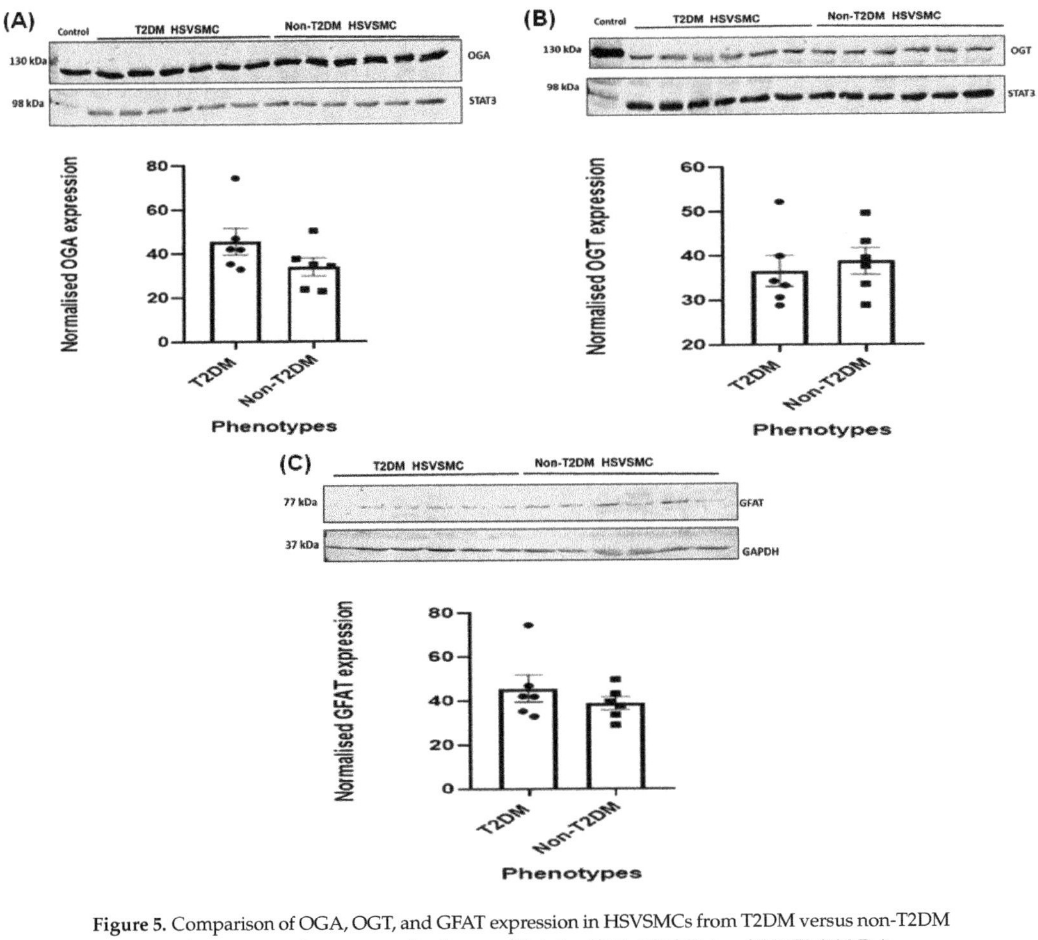

Figure 5. Comparison of OGA, OGT, and GFAT expression in HSVSMCs from T2DM versus non-T2DM patients. (**A**) **Upper panel**: representative immunoblots for OGA (130 kDa) and STAT3 (98 kDa) expressions. OGA expression is in HEK293 cells (control) and lysates of HSVSMC from T2DM patients versus non-T2DM patients. **Lower panel**: Densitometric analysis of OGA expression normalised to STAT 3

(loading control). (**B**) **Upper panel**: Representative immunoblots for OGT (110 kDa) and STAT3 (98 kDa) expressions. OGA expression is in HEK293 cells (control) and lysates of HSVSMC from T2DM patients versus non-T2DM patients. **Lower panel**: Densitometric analysis of OGT expression normalised to STAT3 (loading control). (**C**) **Upper panel**: Representative immunoblots for GFAT (77 kDa) and GAPDH (37 kDa). GFAT expression is in lysates of HSVSMC from T2DM patients versus non-T2DM patients. **Lower panel**: Densitometric analysis of GFAT expression normalised to GAPDH (loading control). Normalised data are expressed as mean ± SEM from n = 6 samples from different patients. Mean values were compared for statistical difference at $p < 0.05$; OGA: *O*-GlcNAcase; OGT: *O*-GlcNAc transferase; GFAT: glutamine fructose-6-phosphate amidotransferase; STAT3: signal transducer and activator of transcription 3; GAPDH: glyceraldehyde 3-phosphate dehydrogenase.

3.4. Effect of Increasing Glucose Concentrations on OGT, OGA, and GFAT Expression Levels in HSVSMCs

Although our understanding of the relationship between hyperglycaemia and *O*-GlcNAcylation is still developing, it is not entirely obvious if a high glucose level alters the expression of the enzymes (OGA, OGT, and GFAT) that regulate cellular *O*-GlcNAcylation. To assess this, expressions of these enzymes were determined after treating HSVSMCs with glucose concentrations mimicking normoglycaemia (5 mM) and hyperglycaemia (10 mM and 25 mM) for 48 h. From our findings, as shown in Figure 6, expression levels of OGA, OGT, and GFAT in HSVSMCs were unaltered by high (10 mM and 25 mM) glucose concentrations versus 5 mM glucose-treated cells.

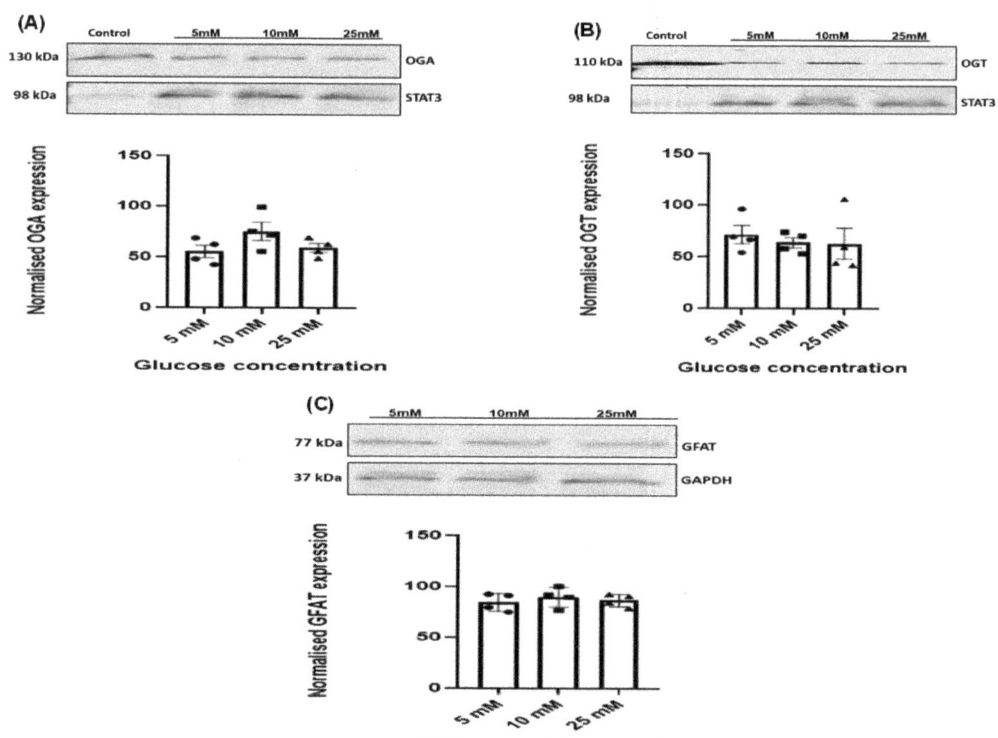

Figure 6. Expression of OGA, OGT, and GFAT by HSVSMCs treated with healthy (5 mM) and high (10 mM and 25 mM) glucose concentrations. (**A**) **Upper panel**: representative immunoblots for OGA

(130 kDa) and STAT3 (98 kDa) expressions. OGA expression is in HEK293 cells (control) and lysates of HSVSMC treated with healthy (5 mM) and high (10 mM and 25 mM) glucose concentrations. **Lower panel**: Densitometric analysis of OGA expression normalised to STAT3 (loading control). (**B**) **Upper panel**: Representative immunoblots for OGT (110 kDa) and STAT3 (98 kDa) expressions. OGA expression is in HEK293 cells (control) and lysates of HSVSMC treated with healthy (5 mM) and high (10 mM and 25 mM) glucose concentrations. **Lower panel**: Densitometric analysis of OGT expression normalised to STAT3 (loading control). (**C**) **Upper panel**: Representative immunoblots for GFAT (77 kDa) and GAPDH (37 kDa). GFAT expression is in lysates of HSVSMC treated with healthy (5 mM) and high (10 mM and 25 mM) glucose concentrations. **Lower panel**: Densitometric analysis of GFAT expression normalised to GAPDH (loading control). Normalised data are expressed as mean ± SEM from n = 4 biological replicates using samples from different patients. Data from cells treated with high (10 mM and 25 mM) glucose concentrations were compared to cells treated with healthy (5 mM) glucose concentration for statistical difference at $p < 0.05$. OGA: *O*-GlcNAcase; OGT: *O*-GlcNAc transferase; GFAT: Glutamine fructose-6-phosphate amidotransferase; STAT3: Signal transducer and activator of transcription 3; GAPDH: Glyceraldehyde 3-phosphate dehydrogenase.

4. Discussion

Vein graft failure after 10 years is about 50%, and this statistic is suggested to be worse (80%) in T2DM patients [25,26]. Therefore, understanding any link between DM and compromised vascular function, specifically in autologous saphenous veins used as conduits in bypass surgery procedures in DM patients, is critical to improving vein graft patency and improving patient outcomes. The findings of this study describe the effect of T2DM and high glucose concentrations on the expression levels of the enzymes that regulate cellular O-GlcNAcylation in HSVSMCs.

Isolation of uncontaminated VSMCs from HSV tissue is critical for data reliability in this project. Other cell types, such as fibroblasts and endothelial cells (EC), are present in the vascular wall, and their contamination of the SMC population must be excluded. As shown in Figures 1 and 2, we have demonstrated that the isolated cells are SMCs because they co-expressed two distinct SMC markers, namely α-SMA and SMMHC. While α-SMA lacks specificity as a SMC marker, SMMHC was also employed as a second marker since SMCs express it from early in development through to maturation [27–29]. To rule out EC contamination in the isolated HSVSMCs, the adhesion protein PECAM-1, which is present in ECs from various origins, including venous Ecs, was used as a marker (Figure 3). PECAM-1 is a known indicator of Ecs, and its expression is primarily concentrated at junctions between adjacent cells [30]. These data confirm the consistent isolation of a pure population of SMCs using an explant technique [22,24]. Furthermore, successive passage of primary cells, including VSMCs, has been shown to significantly alter gene expression profiles [31–34]. As early passage cells have a greater preservation of molecular characteristics found in freshly isolated primary human SMCs [35,36], only early passage (1–4) of HSVSMCs were used in all experiments. This is to eliminate inconsistencies caused by sustained SMC dedifferentiation in vitro, and the results showed that there were no significant differences in the expression of the regulatory enzymes (OGA, OGT, and GFAT) responsible for cellular *O*-GlcNAcylation (Figure 4).

VSMCs have garnered attention as a possible target to treat vascular pathologies due to their role in neointima hyperplasia (NIH) and venous graft stenosis [37–40]. HSV wall thickening is caused by the HSVSMCs shifting from a differentiated to a dedifferentiated phenotype, resulting in uncontrolled cell migration and proliferation responsible for long-term VGF [21]. Moreover, multiple studies have described links between *O*-GlcNAcylation and T2DM [1,15,41–43]. However, the direct impact of T2DM on the regulatory enzymes of *O*-GlcNAcylation in many cell systems is unknown. A clear understanding of how T2DM alters the vascular homeostasis of these enzymes could, therefore, be invaluable to inform the development of therapeutic tools that can help modulate this dynamic post-translational modification in vascular diseases. This is vital because limiting OGT results in downregulation of *O*-GlcNAcylation, the consequences of which are wide-ranging [1]. While it might be predominantly beneficial in cardiac pathologies [1,4,44,45], other studies suggest that downregulating O-GlcNAcylation could be detrimental in cardiac pathologies [45,46].

On the other hand, modulating OGA, the enzyme that reverses the O-GlcNAcylation process, is also critical, and progress has been made in the creation of potential therapeutic drugs aimed at raising cellular O-GlcNAcylation levels [4]. While the rationale for using GFAT inhibitors as prospective medicines for the treatment of CVDs is still being clarified, UDP-GlcNAc acts as a universal precursor for all amino sugars needed to create glycoproteins, glycolipids, and proteoglycans. Consequently, many important cellular processes would be hampered by GFAT suppression, thereby increasing the risk of adverse drug reactions arising from GFAT inhibitors. OGT inhibitor development may, therefore, be a more feasible option [4].

Our study has shown that neither T2DM nor 48 h treatment with high glucose concentrations had any significant effect on the expression levels of OGA, OGT, and GFAT in HSVSMCs (Figure 6). Given that T2DM has been shown to upregulate O-GlcNAcylation in human VECs [15], and the link between T2DM and O-GlcNAcylation has been described [1,4,41–43,47], it is currently unclear as to why T2DM has not affected the expression of these enzymes. However, there could be cell-type-specific differences in how OGT, OGA, and GFAT are regulated. More so, the finding of [48] showed that OGT protein levels are increased in the pancreatic islets of diabetic rats.

McClain et al. [49] have shown that overexpression of OGT in the muscle and fat of transgenic male mice contributed to the development of insulin resistance and T2DM; however, it is unknown if this connection works in reverse. Also, overexpression of OGT in the liver, muscle, and fat tissues of T2DM mice causes insulin resistance [50]. On the other hand, OGA is overexpressed in pancreatic β cells of transgenic mice, which results in reduced glucose tolerance and decreased insulin secretion [51]. Conversely, overexpression of OGA in the liver of diabetic mice has been shown to increase glucose tolerance [52]. Furthermore, it has been demonstrated that insulin resistance and T2DM are caused by the overexpression of GFAT in transgenic mice [53]. In addition, McClain et al. [49] demonstrated that muscles and adipocyte cells develop insulin resistance when bathed with high glucose chronically; however, treatment with DON, a potent inhibitor of GFAT, ameliorated this. Also, a prior study [54] demonstrated that there was no significant difference in the expression of GFAT between T2DM patients and non-diabetic controls in the liver and muscle of rats, which is consistent with the findings of this study. Interestingly, this same study [54] found that GFAT activity was about 40% lower in the muscle and liver of diabetic rats compared to the controls, indicating that expression and activity are not necessarily causally connected. Therefore, the observations highlighted in this paragraph suggest a cell-specific and complex relationship between T2DM and the expression of the enzymes that regulate cellular O-GlcNAcylation.

We acknowledge some limitations of this study. Firstly, we have demonstrated that neither T2DM nor hyperglycaemia caused any significant alteration in the protein expression levels of the regulatory enzymes of cellular O-GlcNAcylation in HSVSMCs from T2DM patients versus non-T2DM controls. However, this finding does not suggest that the activities of these enzymes are not altered by T2DM and hyperglycaemia; hence, this will be investigated in our future studies. Additionally, we will investigate the impact of T2DM and hyperglycaemia on these enzymes (OGA, OGT, and GFAT) and their consequent effect on other PTMs such as phosphorylation. Given that their relationship is inverse in nature, O-GlcNAcylation and phosphorylation control of subcellular colocalisation has been described as a potential mediator of vascular dysfunction [14,55,56]. This is because the production of nitric oxide by eNOS is compromised because eNOS phosphorylation is downregulated due to increased O-GlcNAcylation [14,15,55,56]. Furthermore, it is our aim in future studies to identify and functionally characterise target proteins in HSVSMCs that are more or differentially O-GlcNAcylated in T2DM patients compared to non-diabetic control. Additionally, studies to describe and assess this link in HSVECs will be useful to further understand this dynamic cellular interaction in vascular dysfunction and, consequently, will help identify possible novel target(s) for drug development.

5. Conclusions

Through this study, we have demonstrated that neither T2DM nor hyperglycaemia caused any significant alteration in the expression levels of regulatory enzymes that control *O*-GlcNAcylation in HSVSMCs isolated from excess saphenous vein tissue obtained under consent from T2DM patients versus non-T2DM controls undergoing coronary artery bypass graft procedures. Our findings have now provided preliminary information that will help lay the foundation for further investigations about this dynamic dysregulation in particular cell types and disease states.

Supplementary Materials: The following supporting information can be downloaded at: https://www.mdpi.com/article/10.3390/diabetology5020013/s1, Table S1: Patients' characteristics with medication history and sample ID number.

Author Contributions: I.O.B.: conceptualisation, methodology, investigation, formal analysis, visualisation, funding acquisition, writing—original draft. G.A.D.: investigation, visualisation, writing—review and editing. J.P.H.: writing—ethics and project administration. M.L.: investigation, validation, writing—review and editing. R.G.S.: supervision, validation, writing—review and editing. T.M.P.: conceptualisation, supervision, methodology, project administration, funding acquisition, writing—review and editing. All authors have read and agreed to the published version of the manuscript.

Funding: Research in TMP's laboratory is supported by the Hull and East Riding Cardiac Trust Fund. IOB received scholarships from the Tertiary Education Trust Fund (TETFund), the University of Benin, Nigeria, and the Hull York Medical School, University of Hull, UK.

Informed Consent Statement: Informed consent was obtained from all subjects involved in the study.

Data Availability Statement: Data are available on request from the corresponding author.

Conflicts of Interest: The authors declare no conflict of interest.

References

1. Yang, X.; Qian, K. Protein *O*-GlcNAcylation: Emerging mechanisms and functions. *Nat. Rev. Mol. Cell Biol.* **2017**, *18*, 452–465. [CrossRef] [PubMed]
2. Hart, G.W.; Housley, M.P.; Slawson, C. Cycling of O-linked β-N-acetylglucosamine on nucleocytoplasmic proteins. *Nature* **2007**, *446*, 1017–1022. [CrossRef]
3. Hart, G.W.; Haltiwanger, R.S.; Holt, G.D.; Kelly, W.G. Glycosylation in the nucleus and cytoplasm. *Annu. Rev. Biochem.* **1989**, *58*, 841–874. [CrossRef]
4. Bolanle, I.O.; Riches-Suman, K.; Williamson, R.; Palmer, T.M. Emerging roles of protein *O*-GlcNAcylation in cardiovascular diseases: Insights and novel therapeutic targets. *Pharmacol. Res.* **2021**, *165*, 105467. [CrossRef] [PubMed]
5. Bolanle, I.O.; Palmer, T.M. Targeting protein *O*-GlcNAcylation, a link between type 2 diabetes mellitus and inflammatory disease. *Cells* **2022**, *11*, 705. [CrossRef] [PubMed]
6. Wells, L.; Vosseller, K.; Hart, G.W. Glycosylation of nucleocytoplasmic proteins: Signal transduction and O-GlcNAc. *Science* **2001**, *291*, 2376–2378. [CrossRef] [PubMed]
7. Yi, W.; Clark, P.M.; Mason, D.E.; Keenan, M.C.; Hill, C.; Goddard, W.A., III; Peters, E.C.; Driggers, E.M.; Hsieh-Wilson, L.C. Phosphofructokinase 1 glycosylation regulates cell growth and metabolism. *Science* **2012**, *337*, 975–980. [CrossRef] [PubMed]
8. Slawson, C.; Hart, G.W. O-GlcNAc signalling: Implications for cancer cell biology. *Nat. Rev. Cancer* **2011**, *11*, 678–684. [CrossRef]
9. Ruan, H.B.; Singh, J.P.; Li, M.D.; Wu, J.; Yang, X. Cracking the O-GlcNAc code in metabolism. *Trends Endocrinol. Metab.* **2013**, *24*, 301–309. [CrossRef]
10. Zhu, Y.; Shan, X.; Yuzwa, S.A.; Vocadlo, D.J. The emerging link between O-GlcNAc and Alzheimer disease. *J. Biol. Chem.* **2014**, *289*, 34472–34481. [CrossRef]
11. Bond, M.R.; Hanover, J.A. O-GlcNAc cycling: A link between metabolism and chronic disease. *Annu. Rev. Nutr.* **2013**, *33*, 205–229. [CrossRef] [PubMed]
12. Da Costa, R.M.; Silva, J.F.; Alves, J.V.; Dias, T.B.; Rassi, D.M.; Garcia, L.V.; Lobato, N.D.; Tostes, R.C. Increased *O*-GlcNAcylation of endothelial nitric oxide synthase compromises the anti-contractile properties of perivascular adipose tissue in metabolic syndrome. *Front. Physiol.* **2018**, *9*, 341. [CrossRef] [PubMed]

13. Lazarus, M.B.; Nam, Y.; Jiang, J.; Sliz, P.; Walker, S. Structure of human O-GlcNAc transferase and its complex with a peptide substrate. *Nature* **2011**, *469*, 564–567. [CrossRef] [PubMed]
14. Bolanle, I.O.; Riches-Suman, K.; Loubani, M.; Williamson, R.; Palmer, T.M. Revascularisation of type 2 diabetics with coronary artery disease: Insights and therapeutic targeting of *O*-GlcNAcylation. *Nutr. Metab. Cardiovasc. Dis.* **2021**, *31*, 1349–1356. [CrossRef] [PubMed]
15. Masaki, N.; Feng, B.; Bretón-Romero, R.; Inagaki, E.; Weisbrod, R.M.; Fetterman, J.L.; Hamburg, N.M. *O*-GlcNAcylation Mediates Glucose-Induced Alterations in Endothelial Cell Phenotype in Human Diabetes Mellitus. *J. Am. Heart Assoc.* **2020**, *9*, e014046. [CrossRef] [PubMed]
16. Vasconcelos-dos-Santos, A.; de Queiroz, R.M.; da Costa Rodrigues, B.; Todeschini, A.R.; Dias, W.B. Hyperglycemia and aberrant *O*-GlcNAcylation: Contributions to tumor progression. *J. Bioenerg. Biomembr.* **2018**, *50*, 175–187. [CrossRef] [PubMed]
17. Bond, M.R.; Hanover, J.A. A little sugar goes a long way: The cell biology of O-GlcNAc. *J. Cell Biol.* **2015**, *208*, 869–880. [CrossRef] [PubMed]
18. Yusuf, S.; Zucker, D.; Passamani, E.; Peduzzi, P.; Takaro, T.; Fisher, L.D.; Kennedy, J.W.; Davis, K.; Killip, T.; Norris, R.; et al. Effect of coronary artery bypass graft surgery on survival: Overview of 10-year results from randomised trials by the Coronary Artery Bypass Graft Surgery Trialists Collaboration. *Lancet* **1994**, *344*, 563–570. [CrossRef]
19. National Health Service (NHS) Inform. Coronary Heart Bypass Graft. 2020. Available online: https://www.nhsinform.scot/tests-and-treatments/surgical-procedures/coronary-artery-bypass-graft (accessed on 25 June 2023).
20. Motwani, J.G.; Topol, E.J. Aortocoronary saphenous vein graft disease: Pathogenesis, predisposition, and prevention. *Circulation* **1998**, *97*, 916–931. [CrossRef]
21. De Vries, M.R.; Simons, K.H.; Jukema, J.W.; Braun, J.; Quax, P.H. Vein graft failure: From pathophysiology to clinical outcomes. *Nat. Rev. Cardiol.* **2016**, *13*, 451–470. [CrossRef]
22. Riches, K.; Alshanwani, A.R.; Warburton, P.; O'Regan, D.J.; Ball, S.G.; Wood, I.C.; Turner, N.A.; Porter, K.E. Elevated expression levels of miR-143/5 in saphenous vein smooth muscle cells from patients with Type 2 diabetes drive persistent changes in phenotype and function. *J. Mol. Cell. Cardiol.* **2014**, *74*, 240–250. [CrossRef] [PubMed]
23. Peters, S.C.; Reis, A.; Noll, T. Preparation of endothelial cells from microand macrovascular origin. In *Practical Methods in Cardiovascular Research*; Springer: Berlin/Heidelberg, Germany, 2005; pp. 610–629.
24. Madi, H.A.; Riches, K.; Warburton, P.; O'Regan, D.J.; Turner, N.A.; Porter, K.E. Inherent differences in morphology, proliferation, and migration in saphenous vein smooth muscle cells cultured from nondiabetic and Type 2 diabetic patients. *Am. J. Physiol.-Cell Physiol.* **2009**, *297*, C1307–C1317. [CrossRef] [PubMed]
25. McKavanagh, P.; Yanagawa, B.; Zawadowski, G.; Cheema, A. Management and prevention of saphenous vein graft failure: A review. *Cardiol. Ther.* **2017**, *6*, 203–223. [CrossRef] [PubMed]
26. Campeau, L.J.; Lesperance, J.; Hermann, J.; Corbara, F.; Grondin, C.M.; Bourassa, M.G. Loss of the improvement of angina between 1 and 7 years after aortocoronary bypass surgery: Correlations with changes in vein grafts and in coronary arteries. *Circulation* **1979**, *60*, 1–5. [CrossRef] [PubMed]
27. Riches-Suman, K.; Hussain, A. Identifying and targeting the molecular signature of smooth muscle cells undergoing early vascular ageing. *Biochim. Biophys. Acta (BBA)-Mol. Basis Dis.* **2022**, *1868*, 166403. [CrossRef] [PubMed]
28. Owens, G.K.; Kumar, M.S.; Wamhoff, B.R. Molecular regulation of vascular smooth muscle cell differentiation in development and disease. *Physiol. Rev.* **2004**, *84*, 767–801. [CrossRef]
29. Miano, J.M.; Cserjesi, P.; Ligon, K.L.; Periasamy, M.; Olson, E.N. Smooth muscle myosin heavy chain exclusively marks the smooth muscle lineage during mouse embryogenesis. *Circ. Res.* **1994**, *75*, 803–812. [CrossRef]
30. Woodfin, A.; Voisin, M.B.; Nourshargh, S. PECAM-1: A multi-functional molecule in inflammation and vascular biology. *Arterioscler. Thromb. Vasc. Biol.* **2007**, *27*, 2514–2523. [CrossRef]
31. Weissberg, P.L.; Cary, N.R.; Shanahan, C.M. Gene expression and vascular smooth muscle cell phenotype. *Blood Press. Suppl.* **1995**, *2*, 68–73.
32. Clempus, R.E.; Sorescu, D.; Dikalova, A.E.; Pounkova, L.; Jo, P.; Sorescu, G.P.; Lasseègue, B.; Griendling, K.K. Nox4 is required for maintenance of the differentiated vascular smooth muscle cell phenotype. *Arterioscler. Thromb. Vasc. Biol.* **2007**, *27*, 42–48. [CrossRef]
33. Mouriaux, F.; Zaniolo, K.; Bergeron, M.A.; Weidmann, C.; De La Fouchardiere, A.; Fournier, F.; Droit, A.; Morcos, M.W.; Landreville, S.; Guérin, S.L. Effects of long-term serial passaging on the characteristics and properties of cell lines derived from uveal melanoma primary tumors. *Investig. Ophthalmol. Vis. Sci.* **2016**, *57*, 5288–5301. [CrossRef]
34. Neumann, E.; Riepl, B.; Knedla, A.; Lefèvre, S.; Tarner, I.H.; Grifka, J.; Steinmeyer, J.; Schölmerich, J.; Gay, S.; Müller-Ladner, U. Cell culture and passaging alters gene expression pattern and proliferation rate in rheumatoid arthritis synovial fibroblasts. *Arthritis Res. Ther.* **2010**, *12*, R83. [CrossRef]
35. Frid, M.G.; Shekhonin, B.V.; Koteliansky, V.E.; Glukhova, M.A. Phenotypic changes of human smooth muscle cells during development: Late expression of heavy caldesmon and calponin. *Dev. Biol.* **1992**, *153*, 185–193. [CrossRef]
36. Gimona, M.; Herzog, M.; Vandekerckhove, J.; Small, J.V. Smooth muscle specific expression of calponin. *FEBS Lett.* **1990**, *274*, 159–162.

37. Ortiz-Munoz, G.; Martin-Ventura, J.L.; Hernandez-Vargas, P.; Mallavia, B.; Lopez-Parra, V.; Lopez-Franco, O.; Munoz-Garcia, B.; Fernandez-Vizarra, P.; Ortega, L.; Egido, J.; et al. Suppressors of cytokine signaling modulate JAK/STAT-mediated cell responses during atherosclerosis. *Arterioscler. Thromb. Vasc. Biol.* **2009**, *29*, 525–531. [CrossRef]
38. Xiang, S.; Dong, N.G.; Liu, J.P.; Wang, Y.; Shi, J.W.; Wei, Z.J.; Hu, X.J.; Gong, L. Inhibitory effects of suppressor of cytokine signaling 3 on inflammatory cytokine expression and migration and proliferation of IL-6/IFN-γ-induced vascular smooth muscle cells. *J. Huazhong Univ. Sci. Technol. Med. Sci.* **2013**, *33*, 615–622. [CrossRef] [PubMed]
39. Xiang, S.; Liu, J.; Dong, N.; Shi, J.; Xiao, Y.; Wang, Y.; Hu, X.; Gong, L.; Wang, W. Suppressor of cytokine signaling 3 is a negative regulator for neointimal hyperplasia of vein graft stenosis. *J. Vasc. Res.* **2014**, *51*, 132–143. [CrossRef] [PubMed]
40. Wang, D.; Uhrin, P.; Mocan, A.; Waltenberger, B.; Breuss, J.M.; Tewari, D.; Mihaly-Bison, J.; Huminiecki, Ł.; Starzyński, R.R.; Tzvetkov, N.T.; et al. Vascular smooth muscle cell proliferation as a therapeutic target. Part 1: Molecular targets and pathways. *Biotechnol. Adv.* **2018**, *36*, 1586–1607. [CrossRef] [PubMed]
41. Lazarus, B.D.; Love, D.C.; Hanover, J.A. Recombinant O-GlcNAc transferase isoforms: Identification of O-GlcNAcase, yes tyrosine kinase, and tau as isoform-specific substrates. *Glycobiology* **2006**, *16*, 415–421. [CrossRef]
42. Liu, C.; Dong, W.; Li, J.; Kong, Y.; Ren, X. O-GlcNAc Modification and Its Role in Diabetic Retinopathy. *Metabolites* **2022**, *12*, 725. [CrossRef]
43. Ma, J.; Hart, G.W. Protein *O*-GlcNAcylation in diabetes and diabetic complications. *Expert Rev. Proteom.* **2013**, *10*, 365–380. [CrossRef]
44. Umapathi, P.; Mesubi, O.O.; Banerjee, P.S.; Abrol, N.; Wang, Q.; Luczak, E.D.; Wu, Y.; Granger, J.M.; Wei, A.C.; Reyes Gaido, O.E.; et al. Excessive *O*-GlcNAcylation causes heart failure and sudden death. *Circulation* **2021**, *143*, 1687–1703. [CrossRef]
45. Chatham, J.C.; Zhang, J.; Wende, A.R. Role of O-linked N-acetylglucosamine protein modification in cellular (patho) physiology. *Physiol. Rev.* **2021**, *101*, 427–493. [CrossRef] [PubMed]
46. Jensen, R.V.; Andreadou, I.; Hausenloy, D.J.; Bøtker, H.E. The role of *O*-GlcNAcylation for protection against ischemia-reperfusion injury. *Int. J. Mol. Sci.* **2019**, *20*, 404. [CrossRef]
47. Park, K.; Saudek, C.D.; Hart, G.W. Increased expression of β-N-acetylglucosaminidase in erythrocytes from individuals with pre-diabetes and diabetes. *Diabetes* **2010**, *59*, 1845–1850. [CrossRef]
48. Akimoto, Y.; Hart, G.W.; Wells, L.; Vosseller, K.; Yamamoto, K.; Munetomo, E.; Ohara-Imaizumi, M.; Nishiwaki, C.; Nagamatsu, S.; Hirano, H.; et al. Elevation of the post-translational modification of proteins by O-linked N-acetylglucosamine leads to deterioration of the glucose-stimulated insulin secretion in the pancreas of diabetic Goto–Kakizaki rats. *Glycobiology* **2007**, *17*, 127–140. [CrossRef] [PubMed]
49. McClain, D.A.; Lubas, W.A.; Cooksey, R.C.; Hazel, M.; Parker, G.J.; Love, D.C.; Hanover, J.A. Altered glycan-dependent signaling induces insulin resistance and hyperleptinemia. *Proc. Natl. Acad. Sci. USA* **2002**, *99*, 10695–10699. [CrossRef]
50. Yang, X.; Ongusaha, P.P.; Miles, P.D.; Havstad, J.C.; Zhang, F.; So, W.V.; Kudlow, J.E.; Michell, R.H.; Olefsky, J.M.; Field, S.J.; et al. Phosphoinositide signalling links O-GlcNAc transferase to insulin resistance. *Nature* **2008**, *451*, 964–969. [CrossRef] [PubMed]
51. Soesanto, Y.; Luo, B.; Parker, G.; Jones, D.; Cooksey, R.C.; McClain, D.A. Pleiotropic and age-dependent effects of decreased protein modification by O-linked N-acetylglucosamine on pancreatic β-cell function and vascularization. *J. Biol. Chem.* **2011**, *286*, 26118–26126. [CrossRef]
52. Dentin, R.; Hedrick, S.; Xie, J.; Yates, J., III; Montminy, M. Hepatic glucose sensing via the CREB coactivator CRTC2. *Science* **2008**, *319*, 1402–1405. [CrossRef]
53. Yki-Järvinen, H.; Virkamäki, A.; Daniels, M.C.; McClain, D.; Gottschalk, W.K. Insulin and glucosamine infusions increase O-linked N-acetyl-glucosamine in skeletal muscle proteins in vivo. *Metabolism* **1998**, *47*, 449–455. [CrossRef] [PubMed]
54. Robinson, K.A.; Weinstein, M.L.; Lindenmayer, G.E.; Buse, M.G. Effects of diabetes and hyperglycemia on the hexosamine synthesis pathway in rat muscle and liver. *Diabetes* **1995**, *44*, 1438–1446. [CrossRef] [PubMed]
55. Fulton, D.; Gratton, J.P.; McCabe, T.J.; Fontana, J.; Fujio, Y.; Walsh, K.; Franke, T.F.; Papapetropoulos, A.; Sessa, W.C. Regulation of endothelium-derived nitric oxide production by the protein kinase Akt. *Nature* **1999**, *399*, 597–601. [CrossRef] [PubMed]
56. Montagnani, M.; Chen, H.; Barr, V.A.; Quon, M.J. Insulin-stimulated activation of eNOS is independent of Ca^{2+} but requires phosphorylation by Akt at Ser1179. *J. Biol. Chem.* **2001**, *276*, 30392–30398. [CrossRef]

diabetology

Review

Genetic Susceptibility of Type 2 Diabetes and Metabolic Syndrome

Vladimir Ercegović [1,2,†], Monika Džimbeg [2,3,†] and Andrea Gelemanović [4,*]

1 School of Medicine, University of Split, 21000 Split, Croatia
2 Youth Association for P4 Medicine PROMISE, 10000 Zagreb, Croatia
3 Faculty of Pharmacy and Biochemistry, University of Zagreb, 10000 Zagreb, Croatia
4 Mediterranean Institute for Life Sciences (MedILS), University of Split, 21000 Split, Croatia
* Correspondence: agelemanovic@medils.unist.hr
† These authors contributed equally to this work.

Abstract: Type 2 diabetes (T2D) and metabolic syndrome (MetS) represent complex, multifactorial conditions that pose significant challenges to public health and healthcare costs worldwide. These two conditions share common risk factors such as obesity, dyslipidemia, and hypertension and, as a consequence, are frequently jointly diagnosed in an individual. More specifically, it is estimated that around 85% of T2D patients also have MetS, while patients diagnosed with MetS are five times as likely to develop T2D. While lifestyle and environmental factors, such as poor diet and physical inactivity, play a crucial role, genetic susceptibility also has a substantial influence on the overall risk. Recent advancements in genome-wide association studies (GWAS) have had a major impact on identifying numerous genetic loci associated with these conditions. This narrative review summarizes key findings from T2D and MetS genome-wide association studies, highlighting key genetic loci and pathways and their clinical implications. The objective of this review is to provide a comprehensive understanding of the known genetic underpinnings of T2D and MetS to inform future research and open potential therapeutic and preventive strategies.

Keywords: type 2 diabetes; metabolic syndrome; genetic susceptibility; genome-wide association study

1. Introduction

Today, non-communicable diseases (NCDs) are considered a major global public health issue, and the majority of premature deaths are associated with NCDs. In particular, there is a tremendous rise in so-called metabolic diseases, which include type 2 diabetes (T2D), hypertension, hyperlipidemia, and obesity [1]. Overall, T2D is considered a common diagnosis that has significantly increased in prevalence across the globe [2,3]. With a prevalence of over 537 million, T2D is regarded as one of the biggest public health crises of the twenty-first century [3,4]. Global data from 2021 reported 37.8 million diabetes-related years of life lost (YLLs) and 41.4 million diabetes-related years lived with disability (YLDs), identifying a 90.5% increase in age-standardized prevalence of diabetes in the past three decades and an additional increase of 59.7% until 2050 [5].

This varied condition results from a plethora of pathophysiological mechanisms and molecular pathways that are, in most cases, cell-type specific [6,7]. It is known that T2D causes a persistent state of hyperglycemia (high glucose in the bloodstream), with glucose intolerance, due to the inability of the body to adequately respond to insulin, consequently leading to an increase in insulin production by the pancreatic islets and a subsequent insulin shortage [7,8]. Moreover, evidence is being accumulated that the β-cell is adversely influenced by the fatty acid influx and the increase in cholesterol and its toxic effects [8,9]. Furthermore, T2D is commonly associated with being obese and adopting Western lifestyles [10]. The complications of T2D include macrovascular complications such as cardiovascular disease, almost a third of patients experience retinopathy, while half of patients develop chronic kidney disease, and up to 50% of those affected develop neuropathy [11–13]. Studies have shown that being obese is a critical risk factor for T2D, influencing an earlier onset and further progression of the disease [11].

T2D and cardiovascular diseases are more likely to occur in patients who have been diagnosed with metabolic syndrome (MetS), a group of metabolic disorders, and in fact, around 85% of T2D patients also have MetS [14]. MetS consists of a cluster of abdominal obesity, elevated arterial blood pressure, atherogenic dyslipidemia, elevated plasma glucose, proinflammatory states, and prothrombotic states [15,16].

Patients diagnosed with MetS are five times as likely to develop T2D and two times as likely to develop cardiovascular disease and have an increased risk of fatty liver disease, certain cancers, and sleep apnea [17–20]. Lifestyle and environmental factors play a substantial role in developing MetS, with it being connected to overeating, a higher caloric intake, and performing less physical activity [21–23]. Essential mechanisms that kickstart the progression of MetS are insulin resistance, neurohormonal activity, and chronic inflammation [24,25].

Since T2D and MetS share multiple underlying pathophysiological characteristics, it is of great interest to evaluate the genetic susceptibility of these overlapping diseases, with genetic variations reducing disease risk. Furthermore, raising awareness in the population about genetic susceptibility to diseases could open new opportunities for preventive medicine among those with genetic risk factors. Identifying genetic risk factors for T2D and MetS also opens the possibility of making stratified risk models, targeted drug development, and a deeper understanding of disease mechanisms to improve patient outcomes and public health strategies. Thus, the aim of this review is to summarize the plethora of existing genetic studies and to improve the current understanding of genetic risk factors and pathological pathways associated with the development of T2D and MetS worldwide across different genomic ancestries and ethnicities.

2. Methodology

We conducted a search using the largest biomedical database, PubMed, with the following keywords: "type 2 diabetes" OR "metabolic syndrome" together with "genome-wide association studies", including their synonyms and abbreviations. By screening the identified literature, we opted to include several large (based on sample size) published genome-wide association studies, focusing on recently published studies. By extracting information on genes and single nucleotide polymorphisms (SNPs), we evaluated the number of genes and SNPs that were uniquely identified and replicated in several studies. To visualize the obtained results, data are presented as stacked bar plots created in R v4.3.2 (https://www.r-project.org/, accessed on 1 October 2023) using package *ggpubr*. To retrieve the interaction among identified genes and to evaluate the functional over-representation of selected genes, we used the online tool StringDB (https://string-db.org/, accessed on 21 October 2024) for protein–protein interactions and enrichment analysis. Finally, to visualize the obtained network, we used Cytoscape v3.7.1 (https://cytoscape.org/, accessed on 21 October 2024). In addition, we searched the online repository of human genome-wide association studies (GWAS) called GWAS Catalog (https://www.ebi.ac.uk/gwas/, accessed on 13 January 2025) using the following keywords as the main traits of interest:

"type 2 diabetes mellitus" OR "metabolic syndrome". Upon selection of only T2D and MetS traits, summary statistics of 86 and 13 studies were available for retrieval, respectively.

3. Importance of Studying the Genetic Background of Multifactorial Diseases

By definition, multifactorial diseases originate from the combined effects of multiple genetic and environmental factors. Unlike single-gene (Mendelian) diseases, conditions like T2D and MetS are polygenic and involve complex interactions between numerous genes and lifestyle factors. To understand the hereditary factors that contribute to the risk, development, and treatment response of multifactorial diseases, genetic background should be investigated. In brief, three main types of genetic variations: (1) single nucleotide polymorphisms (SNPs) as the most common type of genetic variation, which involves a change in a single nucleotide; (2) insertions and deletions (indels), which involve small insertions or deletions in the genome; and (3) copy number variations (CNVs), which involve duplication or deletion of a larger part of the genome. To understand the genetic risk factors of complex diseases, these variations can be evaluated through case–control genetic studies, linkage studies, or genome-wide association studies (GWAS). These experimental designs range from studying the genetic background of unrelated individuals (case–control studies) to examining how these genetic factors are inherited within families (linkage studies and twin studies). GWAS represent the most powerful tool for studying complex diseases as it investigates the entire genome for genetic variants (most commonly SNPs) associated with the disease in large populations, results of which then necessarily need to be replicated in another independent validation cohort. Replication should ideally also be performed in diverse populations so that both common and population-specific genetic variants can be identified. GWAS have so far identified numerous genetic loci associated with many multifactorial diseases and complex traits; however, the contribution of each genetic variant is often small, highlighting the polygenic nature of these conditions [26,27]. Summary statistics of relevant genetic variants can be used in the development of polygenic risk scores (PRSs) that represent an aggregated effect of multiple genetic variants, which can stratify individuals based on their genetic risk and guide future preventive strategies and therapies.

The heritability of T2D is estimated to be between 20% and 80% [28], which varies even more for MetS depending on the trait used [29]. This indicates that genetic factors play a significant role in the development of these conditions, but since these estimates vary, further research is needed to refine these estimates, especially across diverse populations.

To better understand the biological mechanisms underlying T2D and MetS, identified genetic variants from GWAS studies should be considered through follow-up functional studies. These can provide a mechanistic insight into how specific genetic variants influence insulin secretion, glucose metabolism, lipid regulation, and inflammation as key pathways relevant for T2D and MetS. Understanding the molecular mechanisms of these complex diseases can direct and prioritize resources into the investigation of the most promising targets and the development of preventative measures and/or therapeutic interventions.

4. Genetic Risk Factors for Type 2 Diabetes (T2D)

In recent decades, significant progress has been made in identifying genes associated with the potential risk for T2D. These recent discoveries in GWAS for T2D may facilitate the creation of innovative approaches for predicting and preventing diabetes as well as other negative clinical outcomes [30].

The majority of identified genes have been found in European populations, of which *TCF7L2* was most commonly replicated across different populations. This transcription factor is part of the Wnt signaling pathway and acts as a regulator of lipid and glucose metabolism [31]. Among other most commonly replicated genes in European populations are *CAMK1D* and *CDC123* (protein kinase/β-cell function), *CDKAL1* (β-cell function), *CDKN2A*, *CDKN2B* (cyclin-dependent kinase inhibitor/β-cell function), *CHCHD9* (unknown), *FTO* (metabolic regulator/insulin action), *HHEX* (transcriptional repressor), *HMGA2* (transcriptional regulator), *HNF1A* (pancreatic and liver transcriptional activator), *HNF1B* (transcription factor/β-cell function), *IGF2BP2* (binding protein/β-cell function), *IRS1* (insulin signaling element/insulin action), *JAZF1* (zinc finger/β-cell function), *KCNJ11* (potassium channel/β-cell function), *KLF14* (transcription factor/insulin action), *MTNR1B* (melatonin receptor/β-cell function), *NOTCH2* (membrane receptor), *PPARG* (nuclear receptor/insulin action), *SLC30A8* (zinc efflux transporter/β-cell function), *THADA* (thyroid adenoma-associated protein/β-cell function), *TP53INP1* (proapoptotic protein/unknown), and *WFS1* (transmembrane protein/β-cell function) [32]. Additionally, numerous studies have identified and replicated genes in Asian populations, such as *KCNK16* (potassium channel/β-cell function), *ZFAND3* (functional evidence for regulation of β-cell mass), *GCC1* (functional evidence for regulation of β-cell mass), *PAX4* and *GLIS3* (transcription factor involved in development of pancreatic islet β-cell), *KCNQ1* (potassium channel/β-cell function), and *HNF4A* (nuclear transcription factor) [32,33]. Notably, some genes, such as *KCNQ1*, are shared between these populations. Overall, these replicated genes across different studies and populations (Figure 1) are functionally enriched in processes such as regulation of insulin secretion, glucose homeostasis, and pancreas development (Gene Ontology); maturity-onset diabetes (KEGG Pathways); and regulation of beta-cell development (Reactome Pathways).

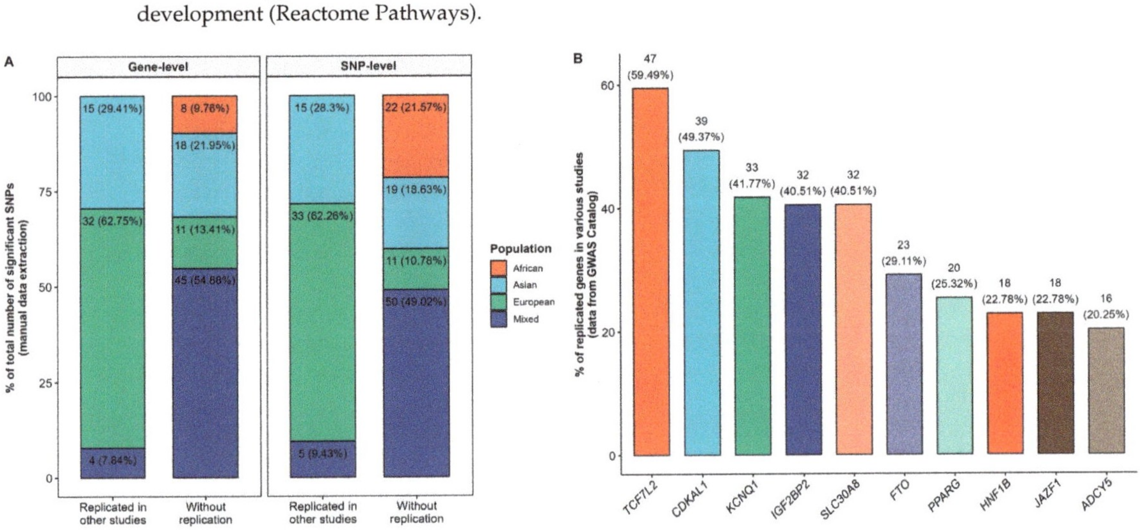

Figure 1. Summary of identified genetic risk factors associated with type 2 diabetes (T2D). (**A**) Manually extracted genes and SNPs from the largest recently published genome-wide association studies. Data are presented as numbers and percentages of genes and SNPs uniquely identified and replicated across different studies. (**B**) Available summary statistics were downloaded from the GWAS Catalog (https://www.ebi.ac.uk/gwas/, accessed on 13 January 2025). The top 10 most replicated genes are visualized with the numbers and percentages of studies in which they were found to have a significant association with T2D. Complete data used for generating these plots can be found in Supplementary Table S1.

Some of the largest GWAS conducted are on T2D, as it represents a major healthcare burden. Only a few of the largest (in terms of sample size) published GWAS in recent years will be mentioned here. In 2018, Xue et al. identified 139 common and four rare variants, of which 33 are functional genes, highlighting *CAMK1D*, *TP53INP1*, and *ATP5G1* through epigenetic regulation mechanisms [2]. Ding et al. showed a nominally significant association with the *GPSM1* gene in the Asian population, for which functional studies pointed towards a regulatory role in skeletal muscle, which is important for maintaining glucose homeostasis [34]. One of the largest consortia, which included studies such as Million Veteran Program, DIAMANTE, Biobank Japan, and many others, leading to over 220,000 cases and over 1.1 million controls, identified over 500 significant associations, half of which were previously unreported. This study also performed an extensive transcriptome-wide study, included polygenic risk score assessment, and opened pathways for exploring the linkage between T2D and vascular outcomes [35]. One study on UK Biobank data performed age-stratified analysis, highlighting the importance of gene–environment interaction studies, where several SNPs mapped to *CDKN2B-AS1* and *TCF7L2* genes were most strongly associated with very late onset of T2D (cases diagnosed after 70 years of age), which suggests personalized approaches to diagnostic, prevention and treatment strategies [36,37].

Two large-scale GWAS papers were published in 2024. The study by Suzuki et al. included almost 430,000 T2D cases (out of over 2.5 million individuals, of which 40% were non-European) and identified 611 genetic loci, of which 145 were novel [38]. Elashi et al. investigated a Middle Eastern population, including almost 2800 cases and 8700 controls from the Qatar Biobank, and managed to identify almost 200 known T2D loci. Interestingly, effect sizes and allele frequencies matched with those of European populations; in addition, they identified a cohort-specific locus between *APOBEC3H* and *CBX7* genes, for which previous reports suggest that SNPs in this region are linked with coronary artery calcified atherosclerotic plaque in diabetes subjects of African American ancestry [39].

4.1. *TCF7L2*

TCF7L2 is the dominant locus associated with T2D risk. The transcription factor 7-like 2, formerly known as TCF4 or transcription factor 4, belongs to the T-cell factor/lymphoid enhancer binding factor (TCF/LEF) family. This family comprises transcription factors that interact with DNA via a high-mobility group (HMG) domain. The *TCF7L2* gene in humans is located on chromosome 10q25.3 and consists of 18 exons, exhibiting a complex splicing pattern across various tissues. This intricate splicing mechanism indicates that the alternative utilization of isoforms in the 3′ region leads to the production of distinct protein isoforms, which possess both agonistic and antagonistic transactivation capabilities [31]

A comprehensive meta-analysis examining genetic associations across various populations revealed that the *TCF7L2* variants linked to type 2 diabetes (T2D) operate under a multiplicative genetic model. This analysis indicates that *TCF7L2* is implicated in nearly 20% of T2D cases [31].

The mechanisms through which *TCF7L2* exerts its effect on T2D are still not well understood. *TCF7L2* plays a critical role in the development and metabolism of adipose tissue. Its regulation of adipogenesis, in conjunction with Wnt signaling pathways, is more intricate than previously understood. In vivo studies have shown that the loss of *TCF7L2* in adipocytes leads to increased adipocyte hypertrophy, along with peripheral and hepatic insulin resistance. *TCF7L2* acts as a key transcriptional regulator of the adipocyte metabolic program by directly influencing the expression of genes associated with lipid and glucose metabolism [31].

4.2. *KCNQ1*

The *KCNQ1* gene was identified and replicated through various GWA studies, and most importantly, it showed significance in diverse populations. This gene is located within the imprinted domain at 11p15.5, a region confirmed for its role in congenital growth phenotypes. Variants within the introns of *KCNQ1* have been linked to increased susceptibility to diabetes when maternally inherited. This locus encompasses at least two distinct regions, intron 10 and intron 15, associated with type 2 diabetes risk, primarily through their impact on islet function [40,41].

KCNQ1 encodes the Kv7.1 voltage-gated potassium channel subunit, which is expressed in human β-cells, although its role in insulin secretion remains uncertain. *KCNQ1* is expressed in the brain, heart muscle, adipose tissue, and pancreas, as well as in the insulin-secreting INS-1 cell line. Notably, the risk allele of *KCNQ1* for type 2 diabetes is linked to impaired insulin secretion, suggesting that this dysfunction underpins the allele's contribution to diabetes susceptibility [40,41].

Studies have shown that inhibition of the KCNQ1 channel with the selective inhibitor chromanol 293B enhances tolbutamide-induced insulin secretion in INS-1 cells. Furthermore, overexpression of *KCNQ1* in the MIN6 mouse β-cell line has been associated with impaired insulin secretion triggered by glucose, pyruvate, or tolbutamide. These findings suggest that heightened *KCNQ1* activity may impair insulin secretion by inducing premature repolarization of the action membrane potential in pancreatic β-cells. Consequently, the *KCNQ1* risk allele may promote the development of type 2 diabetes by increasing *KCNQ1* expression in β-cells, leading to disrupted insulin secretion [41].

5. Genetic Risk Factors for Metabolic Syndrome (MetS)

The most commonly replicated genes associated with MetS are *APOC1* (apolipoprotein C1, which plays a central role in HDL/VLDL metabolism), *CETP* (involved in the transfer of cholesteryl ester from HDL to other lipoproteins), *GCKR* (regulatory protein that inhibits glucokinase in liver and pancreatic islet cells), *TRIB1* (negative regulator of the lipopolysaccharide-mediated signaling pathway), and *ZPR1* (communicates proliferative growth signals from the cytoplasm to the nucleus) (Figure 2), which are functionally enriched for high-density lipoprotein particles (Gene Ontology) and cholesterol metabolism (KEGG Pathways).

Prior to GWAS, the literature on shared genetic variants associated with metabolic syndrome was limited [42]. Kissebah et al. conducted a genome-wide linkage analysis involving 500 families, identifying quantitative trait loci on chromosomes number 3 and 17. These loci are located near the solute carrier family 2 gene, which encodes the facilitated glucose transporter (*GLUT2*), and the adiponectin gene [42]. Additionally, Lehman et al. (2005) conducted a bivariate linkage analysis that examined multiple pairs of metabolic syndrome components and found associations with a broad region on chromosome 7 linked to various metabolic traits and specifically discovered an association at 7q11.23 across several combinations [43]. This region was later confirmed to be linked to lipoprotein sizes by Chasman et al. in a GWAS study in 2009 [44].

With the metabolism of lipids being an important energy source for homeostasis, the dysregulation of the lipid metabolism can result in multiple metabolic disorders. *CETP* and *LPL*, genes responsible for the control of homeostasis of lipids, have been associated with MetS [45], opening a potential new treatment target of drugs for MetS [46]. Kraja et al. (2011) utilized data from the STAMPEED consortium, which encompassed seven studies and included 22,161 participants of European ancestry, with the study involving bivariate genome-wide association analyses of metabolic traits and examining every possible pairwise combination of MetS phenotypes, classifying individuals that exceeded set thresholds as affected. The study identified 28 SNPs linked to either MetS or specific trait pairs located in or near 15 genes associated with these traits at genome-wide significance levels. Remarkably, all but two of the bivariate associations featured a lipid abnormality, indicating that genetic effects on lipid levels are more pronounced than those on other traits. The variants most influential in the correlations among traits were found in or near genes such as *ZNF259*, *BUD13*, *CETP*, *APOA5*, *LPL*, *TRIB1*, *LOC100128154*, and *LOC100129500*, with variants impacting MetS directly including *CETP*, *LPL*, and the *APOA* cluster (*APOA5*, *ZNF259*, and *BUD13*), which are recognized for their significant roles in lipid metabolism [47]. For the Korean population, the *APOA5* SNPs showed a substantial impact [48]. *APOA5* and *BUD13* were also additionally replicated in a population of over 13,000 Han Chinese individuals as mediators for serum triglyceride levels, while an East Asian-specific variant in *ALDH2* was found to be associated with MetS [49].

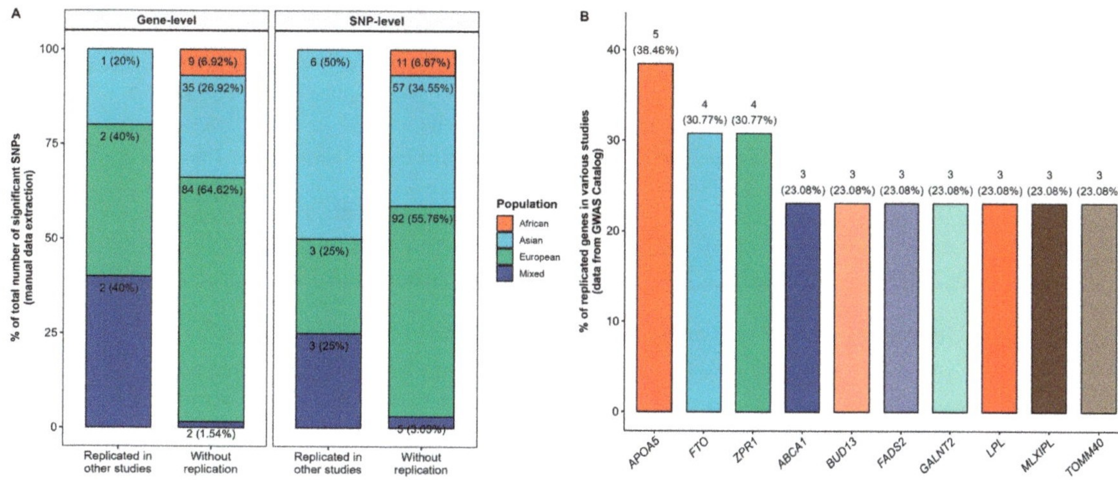

Figure 2. Summary of identified genetic risk factors associated with metabolic syndrome (MetS). (**A**) Manually extracted genes and SNPs from the largest recently published genome-wide association studies. Data are presented as numbers and percentages of genes and SNPs uniquely identified and replicated among different studies. (**B**) Available summary statistics were downloaded from the GWAS Catalog (https://www.ebi.ac.uk/gwas/, accessed on 13 January 2025). The top 10 most replicated genes are visualized with the numbers and percentages of studies in which they were found to have a significant association with MetS. Complete data used for generating these plots can be found in Supplementary Table S1.

In 2011, Avery et al. examined the integration of MetS components in a large GWAS with data from almost 20,000 European Americans and over 6000 African Americans. In this study, they analyzed six phenotypic domains connected to metabolic syndrome, including central obesity, atherogenic dyslipidemia, vascular inflammation, vascular dysfunction, a pro-thrombotic state, and elevated plasma glucose through a multivariate approach, identifying 15 loci, including three new loci near *BRAP*, *APOC1*, and *PLCG1*, with the most significant signal being at rs4420638, associated with several traits [50]. Fasil et al. found two African-ancestry-specific variants that were significantly associated with MetS—SNP rs77244975[C] in *CTNNA3* showed protection against MetS and SNP rs73989312[A], close to *CA10*, showed increased risk of the disease [51]. A GWAS by Oh et al. investigated genetic associations with lipid levels and metabolic traits in a Korean population and identified multiple SNPs significantly linked to triglycerides (TG), HDL cholesterol, and fasting blood glucose (FBG), including novel variants within the *HERPUD1*, *C2orf16*, *ZPR1*, *GCKR*, *ALDH1A2*, *LIPC*, *BUD13*, and *CETP* genes [52]. In a study by Lind from 2019, two loci, *C5orf67* and *SNX10*, were reported to have a connection to all five components of MetS [53]. However, a systematic review by Al-Homedi et al. did not find a unique genetic modifier between the Arab population and MetS, although they stated that most of the 36 studies included in their systematic review had a small population size [54]. Rana et al., in their systematic review, concluded that there is still insufficient data on the genetic predisposition of MetS, but only for certain parts of the disease [55].

6. Shared Genetic Risk Factors for T2D and MetS

Genome-wide association studies have been instrumental in identifying over 700 genetic loci associated with T2D susceptibility [56]. Most of these loci involve genes implicated in pancreatic β-cell function, insulin signaling, and glucose homeostasis, supporting the view that T2D is primarily a disease of insulin secretion rather than insulin resistance alone [56–60]. MetS encompasses heritable traits like dyslipidemia, abdominal obesity, hypertension, and fasting hyperglycemia, and though genetic factors have been linked to these traits, a shared genetic origin remains unproven [21,30,49,55,61].

Several genetic loci are shared between T2D and MetS, reflecting their overlapping pathophysiology. For example, variants in *TCF7L2* and *FTO* are implicated in insulin resistance as a hallmark of T2D, and obesity, hypertension, and dyslipidemia as hallmarks of MetS. Biological pathways that are interconnected in T2D and MetS are insulin secretion and pancreatic β-cell function, adipogenesis and lipid metabolism, inflammation and immune response, and the renin–angiotensin system and blood pressure regulation. For the purpose of this review, some of the most common genes that are replicated in several independent studies, and which are found to be shared between T2D and MetS, are summarized in Table 1 (based on our manual data extraction from the largest recently published GWA studies). A full list of all genes and SNPs can be found in Supplementary Table S1. Additionally, in Figure 3, we have summarized the top replicated and shared genes between T2D and MetS based on information obtained from available GWAS summary statistics from the GWAS Catalog. Overall, when examining the functional enrichment of these shared susceptibility genes for T2D and MetS in various ontologies and pathway databases, key terms that are highlighted are diabetes, adipogenesis, and lipid metabolism. Overall, all the identified genes for T2D and MetS are part of a large and highly interconnected network, which emphasizes the polygenic and multifactorial nature of these diseases (summarized in Figure 4, where genes shared between T2D and MetS are highlighted in yellow, MetS genes in blue, and T2D genes in green).

Table 1. Some of the identified shared genetic risk factors for T2D and MetS.

Gene Symbol *	Gene Name	Description **
CMIP	C-Maf-inducing protein	Plays a role in the T-cell signaling pathway.
FTO	Alpha-ketoglutarate-dependent dioxygenase	RNA demethylase mediates oxidative demethylation of different RNA species and acts as a regulator of fat mass, adipogenesis, and energy homeostasis.
HNF1A	Hepatocyte nuclear factor 1-alpha	Transcriptional activator that regulates the tissue-specific expression of multiple genes, especially in pancreatic islet cells and in the liver.
HNF4A	Hepatocyte nuclear factor 4-alpha	Transcriptional regulator which controls the expression of hepatic genes during the transition of endodermal cells to hepatic progenitor cells, facilitating the recruitment of RNA pol II to the promoters of target genes.
LPL	Lipoprotein lipase	Key enzyme in triglyceride metabolism, which catalyzes the hydrolysis of triglycerides from circulating chylomicrons and very low-density lipoproteins (VLDLs), and plays an important role in lipid clearance from the bloodstream and lipid utilization and storage.

Table 1. *Cont.*

Gene Symbol *	Gene Name	Description **
MBNL1	Muscleblind-like protein 1	Acts either as an activator or repressor of splicing on specific pre-mRNA targets and inhibits cardiac troponin-T (TNNT2) pre-mRNA exon inclusion but induces insulin receptor (IR) pre-mRNA exon inclusion in muscle.
MTNR1B	Melatonin receptor type 1B	Likely to mediate the reproductive and circadian actions of melatonin.
PEPD	Xaa-Pro dipeptidase	Splits dipeptides with a prolyl or hydroxyprolyl residue in the C-terminal position and plays an important role in collagen metabolism because of the high level of imino acids in collagen.
PURG	Purine-rich element-binding protein gamma	The exact function of this gene is not known; however, its encoded product is highly similar to purine-rich element binding protein A.
SUGP1	SURP and G-patch domain-containing protein 1	Member of the SURP family of splicing factors, which plays a role in pre-mRNA splicing.
VEGFA	Vascular endothelial growth factor A	Growth factor active in angiogenesis, vasculogenesis, and endothelial cell growth.

* Respective references of studies where these genes were identified as significantly associated with T2D and MetS are provided in Supplementary Table S1. ** Gene Description was retrieved from StringDB (https://string-db.org/, accessed on 21 October 2024).

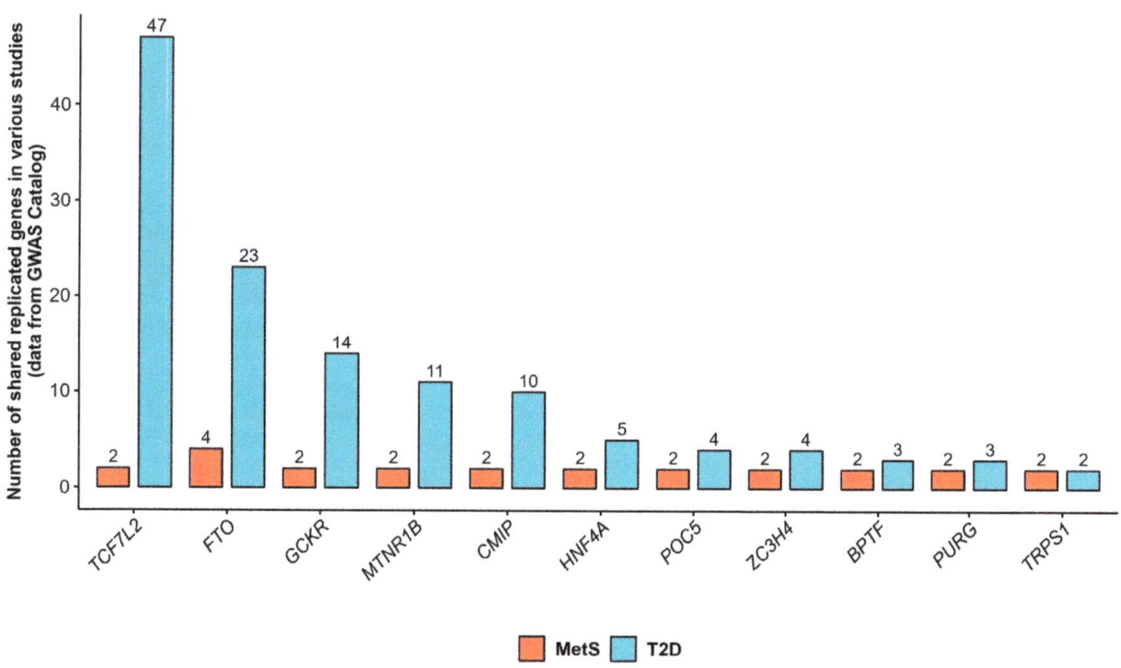

Figure 3. Summary of identified genetic risk factors that are found to be associated with both type 2 diabetes (T2D) and metabolic syndrome (MetS), based on available summary statistics downloaded from GWAS Catalog (https://www.ebi.ac.uk/gwas/, accessed on 13 January 2025.). Only genes replicated in at least two T2D and MetS GWAS are used and visualized, with the number of studies in which they were found to have a significant association with T2D or MetS indicated. Complete data used for generating this plot can be found in Supplementary Table S1.

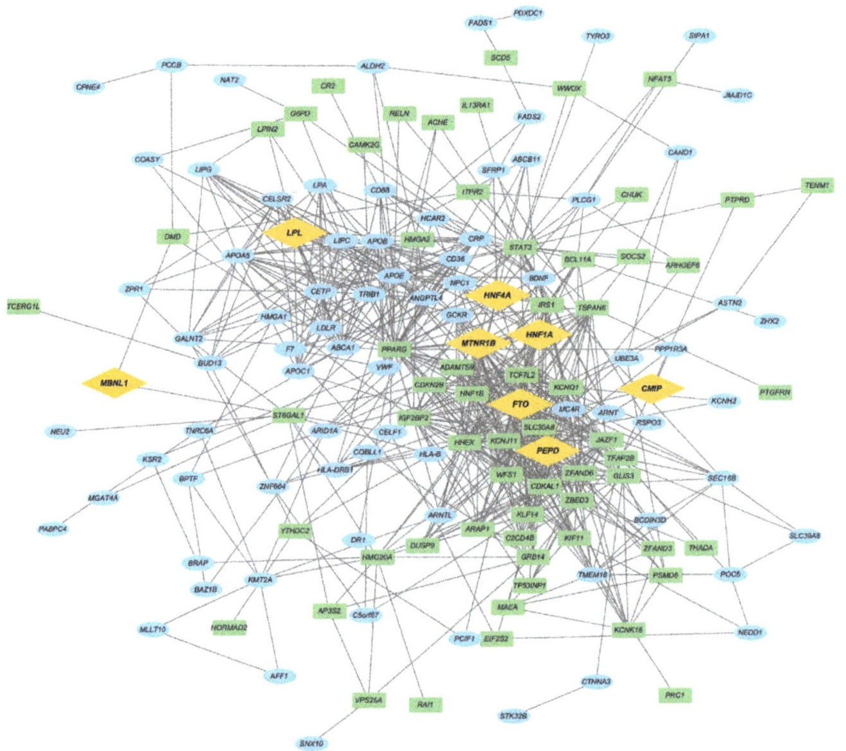

Figure 4. Network of identified genetic risk factors for type 2 diabetes (T2D; green round rectangles), metabolic syndrome (MetS; blue ellipses), and risk factors shared between both conditions (yellow diamonds). Gene interactions were retrieved from StringDB (https://string-db.org/, accessed on 21 October 2024), and the network was created in Cytoscape v3.7.1 (https://cytoscape.org/, accessed on 21 October 2024).

In addition to shared genetic loci, pathways like insulin signaling and lipid metabolism are pivotal in the development of both diseases. Disrupted insulin signaling contributes to glucose imbalance, insulin resistance, and MetS features such as obesity and hypertension, while altered lipid metabolism, including abnormal triglyceride and cholesterol processing, further connects their pathophysiology. In the state of insulin resistance, lipolysis is inhibited, and there is an increase in free fatty acids (FFAs) in the bloodstream, creating a positive loop of worsening insulin resistance by affecting the insulin signaling cascade, driving T2D through glucose imbalance and beta-cell dysfunction, while in MetS, it contributes to obesity, dyslipidemia, and hypertension by disrupting metabolic and vascular processes [24,25,62]. Nevertheless, disrupted lipid metabolism has a central role in the pathogenesis of T2D and MetS by driving abnormal triglyceride and cholesterol levels, promoting the development of insulin resistance, ectopic fat deposition, and systemic inflammation, which collectively contribute to obesity, dyslipidemia, and heightened cardiovascular risk [24,25,62]. Adipokines from adipose tissue include hormones, inflammatory cytokines, and peptides that all play a big role in the development of insulin resistance and MetS, with leptin levels being proportional to body fat percentage and the patient's obesity [25,62]. In patients with MetS, inflammatory markers such as C-reactive protein, IL-6, and TNFα, among others, remain elevated and have a big role in the development of insulin resistance via pathophysiologic mechanisms [63]. Patients with MetS experience higher oxidative stress damage and lower levels of antioxidant activity, often enhanced by vitamin and mineral deficiencies [64].

By leveraging information on key genetic variants, in combination with traditional clinical and lifestyle risk factors, individuals carrying risk alleles (those with a high genetic predisposition) for T2D and MetS could be identified. Then, tailored personalized intervention, lifestyle modifications, and pharmacological treatments can be implemented earlier and in a more targeted manner to slow down disease progression.

6.1. *FTO*

The *FTO* (fat mass and obesity-associated) gene has been identified as a key obesity-susceptibility gene, thus indirectly linked to an increased risk for T2D and MetS. Located on chromosome 16q12.2, the *FTO* gene is broadly expressed across central and peripheral tissues, including the hypothalamus, adipose tissue, and pancreas [65].

As a member of the dioxygenase superfamily, *FTO* has been shown in vitro to catalyze the demethylation of 3-methylthymine in single-stranded DNA. Bioinformatics analyses and functional studies suggest that *FTO* plays a crucial role in post-translational modifications, gene transcription, apoptosis, and metabolic processes. Furthermore, studies have demonstrated that single nucleotide polymorphisms in the first intron of the *FTO* gene are associated with an increased body mass index in Caucasian populations [65,66].

Obesity is a major risk factor for insulin resistance and β-cell dysfunction, both of which contribute to the development of T2D. Studies have demonstrated that *FTO* gene polymorphisms increase the risk of T2D, with this association being partially mediated by BMI. Notably, several studies have also shown that the *FTO* gene is independently linked to diabetes risk even after adjusting for BMI. Recent findings suggest that the *FTO* gene undergoes rapid turnover in pancreatic β-cells and plays a role in regulating insulin secretion in response to glucose stimulation. However, the precise functional role of *FTO* in pancreatic β-cells and its underlying molecular mechanisms remain unclear [66].

6.2. *HNF1A and HNF4A*

HNF1A and *HNF4A* are also notable genes. These genes encode transcription factors crucial for the development and function of the pancreas and liver. Mutations in these genes have been directly associated with Maturity-Onset Diabetes of the Young (MODY) and an increased risk of T2D [67,68].

Studies in rodent models have revealed a transcriptional hierarchy during liver development, where *HNF4A* positively regulates *HNF1A* expression. Conversely, in differentiated pancreatic cells, *HNF1A* directly binds to the P2 promoter of *HNF4A*, modulating its expression. Furthermore, *HNF1A* plays a key role in regulating *PDX1*, a gene essential for pancreatic development and beta cell function, through cooperative interactions with *PDX1* in rodent beta cells. The interplay between *HNF1A* and *HNF4A* has been shown to be critical for the differentiation of human induced pluripotent stem cells into beta cells, underscoring the importance of the *HNF1A–HNF4A* axis in pancreatic development [68].

Recent findings highlight that mutations in *HNF1A* are linked to an increased alpha cell population in human pancreatic islets and promote the differentiation of stem cell-derived beta cells toward alpha cells. However, the molecular mechanisms underlying *HNF1A*-associated abnormalities in insulin secretion and its pathophysiological role in diabetes remain to be fully elucidated [67,68].

7. Challenges and Future Perspectives

Genome-wide association studies have been shown to be of great value in identifying novel genetic loci that drive the susceptibility of various human diseases. However, one should be aware of the limitations of GWAS. While GWAS have identified numerous risk loci, their application in clinical practice remains challenging. Environmental influences like poor diet and physical inactivity, combined with genetic predisposition, add complexity to T2D and MetS, and while a portion of the risk is definitely attributable to genetics, no definitive DNA biomarkers are yet available for translation into clinical settings, and this poses the key methodological challenge [56,69]. In addition, there are several limitations to the current GWAS. There is limited population diversity since most of the studies are biased toward populations of European ancestry, which limits the generalizability of risk predictions to other populations. Underrepresentation of other ethnic groups can lead to inconsistent and variable genetic effects on disease susceptibility in other diverse populations. One such example of a clinically important variant discovered in underrepresented populations of African ancestry was in the gene *G6PD*, which is relevant for diabetes diagnosis [70].

Even though numerous genetic loci have been identified, these often have small to modest effect sizes, which means that most of them are common variants with minor allele frequencies higher than 1% in the population. Using this approach, we might not identify meaningful rare genetic variants and their polygenic nature with additive and non-additive effects. GWAS identifies associations, and it does not imply causation; because of this, there is no clear functional understanding of how these variants mechanistically influence disease risk, meaning that extensive functional studies are needed. In addition, GWAS usually focus on protein-coding genes, often ignoring epigenetic and regulatory elements, whereas in reality, many significant variants lie in these non-coding regions. Also, there is a lack of studies investigating the complex gene–gene and gene–environment interactions [56,69]. Finally, GWAS should be integrated with other molecular layers, such as transcriptomics, proteomics, epigenomics, and metabolomics, to provide a pathophysiological understanding of the disease at the system level. Only by integrating various omics data with machine learning modeling can novel insights be generated to shed light on the complex interplay of the numerous genetic variants, their functional consequences (at the transcriptome, proteome, and metabolome levels), and environmental risk factors influencing the development and progression of T2D and MetS [71,72].

To achieve a fully personalized medical approach to T2D and MetS and to enhance predictive models, integration of genetic, environmental, and clinical data is needed. To move away from association studies toward understanding causality and predictive power, there has been an increase in studies utilizing polygenic risk scores and the Mendelian randomization approach in recent years. Polygenic risk scores (PRSs) are developed from GWAS to predict an individual's genetic predisposition to multifactorial diseases such as T2D and MetS. This score quantifies an individual's genetic predisposition to disease by summing the effects of multiple genetic risk variants [73]. The predictive power of PRs decreases when used on a diverse population, in comparison to the population the model was trained on, which is, in most cases, of European origin [70]. Mendelian randomization is a statistical method that uses genetic variants as instrumental variables to infer causal relationships between diverse risk factors and disease outcomes, minimizing confounding variables and implying causality [74].

Even though such novel genetic risk predictions are still very limited in clinical settings when compared to traditional risk factors, combining genetic data from GWAS with clinical data may provide a more accurate assessment of disease risk and help guide personalized prevention and treatment strategies. In addition, ongoing studies of gene–environment interactions will further improve our understanding of how lifestyle changes might reduce genetic risk. Some of the strategies for future studies include the following: (1) inclusion of populations with diverse genetic backgrounds, (2) implementation of causal modeling with the Mendelian randomization approach to understand the interconnectedness between genetic variants and other risk factors on disease risk, (3) integration of PRSs with traditional risk factors, (4) in-depth exploration of gene–gene and gene–environment interactions, (5) investigation of functional consequences of genetic variants to help translate genetic findings into potential therapeutic targets, and (6) combination of genetic data with other omics to gain deeper insights into complex biological pathways and molecular networks. All of the above strategies would lead to more personalized preventive and therapeutic strategies, potentially reducing the burden of T2D and MetS [56,69,75–77].

There are several limitations to this review. First and foremost, this is a narrative review, which allows for more flexibility in terms of broader scope and exploratory nature, enabling us to provide an overview of known and replicated genetic loci associated with both T2D and MetS susceptibility. To overcome the potential bias of conducting a narrative review, a significant step forward would be to conduct a systematic review. However, taking into consideration the vast majority of literature on genetic susceptibility to T2D and MetS, a systematic review should be of much narrower scope, thus limiting the potential of exploring shared genetic loci between T2D and MetS. Here, we opted to additionally include available GWAS summary statistics obtained from the GWAS Catalog in order to provide a more in-depth overview of identified and shared genetic loci for T2D and MetS. Another limitation of this review is that we opted to include only large genome-wide association studies. Although GWA studies have more power, traditional case–control genetic studies should also be considered. Finally, other layers of molecular data (transcriptomics, epigenomics, proteomics, metabolomics) were out of scope in this review; however, future studies should investigate other omics data individually as well as their integrated effect on T2D and MetS susceptibility in order to understand these diseases at a systems level.

8. Conclusions

In conclusion, advances in GWAS have significantly enhanced our understanding of the genetic basis of T2D and MetS. Key genes such as TCF7L2, FTO, and HNF4A have emerged as important contributors to disease risk, affecting pathways involved in insulin secretion, adipogenesis, lipid metabolism, and blood pressure regulation. While the translation of these findings into clinical practice remains limited and challenging, ongoing research into polygenic risk scores and gene–environment interactions holds promise for improving disease prediction, prevention, and management, moving towards tailored individualized strategies.

Supplementary Materials: The following supporting information can be downloaded at: https://www.mdpi.com/article/10.3390/diabetology6020011/s1, Table S1: Identified genetic risk factors associated with T2D and MetS.

Author Contributions: Conceptualization, A.G.; formal analysis, V.E., M.D. and A.G.; investigation, V.E. and M.D.; data curation, V.E., M.D. and A.G.; writing—original draft preparation, V.E., M.D. and A.G.; writing—review and editing, A.G.; visualization, A.G.; supervision, A.G. All authors have read and agreed to the published version of the manuscript.

Funding: This research received no external funding.

Institutional Review Board Statement: Not applicable.

Informed Consent Statement: Not applicable.

Data Availability Statement: No new data were created in this study. Data used for this narrative review are appropriately referenced.

Conflicts of Interest: The authors declare no conflicts of interest.

References

1. Chew, N.W.S.; Ng, C.H.; Tan, D.J.H.; Kong, G.; Lin, C.; Chin, Y.H.; Lim, W.H.; Huang, D.Q.; Quek, J.; Fu, C.E.; et al. The global burden of metabolic disease: Data from 2000 to 2019. *Cell Metab.* **2023**, *35*, 414–428.e3. [CrossRef] [PubMed]
2. Xue, A.; Wu, Y.; Zhu, Z.; Zhang, F.; Kemper, K.E.; Zheng, Z.; Yengo, L.; Lloyd-Jones, L.R.; Sidorenko, J.; Wu, Y.; et al. Genome-wide association analyses identify 143 risk variants and putative regulatory mechanisms for type 2 diabetes. *Nat. Commun.* **2018**, *9*, 2941. [CrossRef] [PubMed]
3. McCarthy, M.I. Painting a new picture of personalised medicine for diabetes. *Diabetologia* **2017**, *60*, 793–799. [CrossRef] [PubMed]
4. Udler, M.S.; Kim, J.; von Grotthuss, M.; Bonàs-Guarch, S.; Cole, J.B.; Chiou, J.; Boehnke, M.; Laakso, M.; Atzmon, G.; Glaser, B.; et al. Type 2 diabetes genetic loci informed by multi-trait associations point to disease mechanisms and subtypes: A soft clustering analysis. *PLoS Med.* **2018**, *15*, e1002654. [CrossRef] [PubMed]
5. Liane Ong, K.; Stafford, L.K.; McLaughlin, S.A.; Boyko, E.J.; Emil Vollset, S.; Smith, A.E.; Dalton, B.E.; Duprey, J.; Cruz, J.A.; Hagins, H.; et al. Global, regional, and national burden of diabetes from 1990 to 2021, with projections of prevalence to 2050: A systematic analysis for the Global Burden of Disease Study 2021. *Lancet* **2023**, *402*, 203–234. [CrossRef]
6. Ma, C.X.; Ma, X.N.; Guan, C.H.; Li, Y.D.; Mauricio, D.; Fu, S.B. Cardiovascular disease in type 2 diabetes mellitus: Progress toward personalized management. *Cardiovasc. Diabetol.* **2022**, *21*, 74. [CrossRef]
7. Mahajan, A.; Wessel, J.; Willems, S.M.; Zhao, W.; Robertson, N.R.; Chu, A.Y.; Gan, W.; Kitajima, H.; Taliun, D.; Rayner, N.W.; et al. Refining the accuracy of validated target identification through coding variant fine-mapping in type 2 diabetes article. *Nat. Genet.* **2018**, *50*, 559–571. [CrossRef]
8. Newsholme, P.; Keane, D.; Welters, H.J.; Morgan, N.G. Life and death decisions of the pancreatic β-cell: The role of fatty acids. *Clin. Sci.* **2007**, *112*, 27–42. [CrossRef]
9. Kruit, J.K.; Brunham, L.R.; Verchere, C.B.; Hayden, M.R. HDL and LDL cholesterol significantly influence β-cell function in type 2 diabetes mellitus. *Curr. Opin. Lipidol.* **2010**, *21*, 178–185. [CrossRef]
10. Javeed, N.; Matveyenko, A.V. Circadian etiology of type 2 diabetes mellitus. *Physiology* **2018**, *33*, 138–150. [CrossRef]
11. Hicks, C.W.; Selvin, E. Epidemiology of Peripheral Neuropathy and Lower Extremity Disease in Diabetes. *Curr. Diab. Rep.* **2019**, *19*, 1–8. [CrossRef] [PubMed]
12. Harding, J.L.; Pavkov, M.E.; Magliano, D.J.; Shaw, J.E.; Gregg, E.W. Global trends in diabetes complications: A review of current evidence. *Diabetologia* **2019**, *62*, 3–16. [CrossRef]
13. Chen, L.; Magliano, D.J.; Zimmet, P.Z. The worldwide epidemiology of type 2 diabetes mellitus—Present and future perspectives. *Nat. Rev. Endocrinol.* **2012**, *8*, 228–236. [CrossRef]
14. Leitner, D.R.; Frühbeck, G.; Yumuk, V.; Schindler, K.; Micic, D.; Woodward, E.; Toplak, H. Obesity and type 2 diabetes: Two diseases with a need for combined treatment strategies—EASO can lead the way. *Obes. Facts* **2017**, *10*, 483–492. [CrossRef]
15. Grundy, S.M.; Brewer, H.B.; Cleeman, J.I.; Smith, S.C.; Lenfant, C. Definition of Metabolic Syndrome: Report of the National Heart, Lung, and Blood Institute/American Heart Association Conference on Scientific Issues Related to Definition. In Proceedings of the Circulation, Hampton, VA, USA, 16–17 March 2004.
16. National Cholesterol Education Program (US). Third Report of the National Cholesterol Education Program (NCEP) Expert Panel on Detection, Evaluation, and Treatment of High Blood Cholesterol in Adults (Adult Treatment Panel III) final report. In *Circulation*; National Cholesterol Education Program (US): Bethesda, MD, USA, 2002. [CrossRef]
17. Vgontzas, A.N.; Bixler, E.O.; Chrousos, G.P. Sleep apnea is a manifestation of the metabolic syndrome. *Sleep Med. Rev.* **2005**, *9*, 211–224. [CrossRef] [PubMed]
18. Esposito, K.; Chiodini, P.; Colao, A.; Lenzi, A.; Giugliano, D. Metabolic syndrome and risk of cancer: A systematic review and meta-analysis. *Diabetes Care* **2012**, *35*, 2402–2411. [CrossRef] [PubMed]
19. Kotronen, A.; Yki-Järvinen, H. Fatty liver: A novel component of the metabolic syndrome. *Arterioscler. Thromb. Vasc. Biol.* **2008**, *28*, 27–38. [CrossRef] [PubMed]
20. Eckel, R.H.; Grundy, S.M.; Zimmet, P.Z. The metabolic syndrome. *Lancet* **2005**, *365*, 1415–1428. [CrossRef]
21. Fathi Dizaji, B. The investigations of genetic determinants of the metabolic syndrome. *Diabetes Metab. Syndr. Clin. Res. Rev.* **2018**, *12*, 783–789. [CrossRef] [PubMed]
22. Pekgor, S.; Duran, C.; Berberoglu, U.; Eryilmaz, M.A. The role of visceral adiposity index levels in predicting the presence of metabolic syndrome and insulin resistance in overweight and obese patients. *Metab. Syndr. Relat. Disord.* **2019**, *17*, 296–302. [CrossRef] [PubMed]
23. Matsuzawa, Y.; Funahashi, T.; Nakamura, T. The concept of metabolic syndrome: Contribution of visceral fat accumulation and its molecular mechanism. *J. Atheroscler. Thromb.* **2011**, *18*, 629–639. [CrossRef]
24. Griffin, M.E.; Marcucci, M.J.; Cline, G.W.; Bell, K.; Barucci, N.; Lee, D.; Goodyear, L.J.; Kraegen, E.W.; White, M.F.; Shulman, G.I. Free fatty acid-induced insulin resistance is associated with activation of protein kinase C θ and alterations in the insulin signaling cascade. *Diabetes* **2000**, *48*, 1270–1274. [CrossRef]

25. Boden, G.; Shulman, G.I. Free fatty acids in obesity and type 2 diabetes: Defining their role in the development of insulin resistance and β-cell dysfunction. *Eur. J. Clin. Investig.* **2002**, *32*, 14–23. [CrossRef] [PubMed]
26. Ioannidis, J.P.A.; Trikalinos, T.A.; Khoury, M.J. Implications of Small Effect Sizes of Individual Genetic Variants on the Design and Interpretation of Genetic Association Studies of Complex Diseases. *Am. J. Epidemiol.* **2006**, *164*, 609–614. [CrossRef] [PubMed]
27. Stringer, S.; Wray, N.R.; Kahn, R.S.; Derks, E.M. Underestimated Effect Sizes in GWAS: Fundamental Limitations of Single SNP Analysis for Dichotomous Phenotypes. *PLoS ONE* **2011**, *6*, e27964. [CrossRef]
28. Feng, Y.; Li, X.; Mao, Z.; Huo, W.; Hou, J.; Wang, C.; Li, W.; Yu, S. Heritability Estimation and Environmental Risk Assessment for Type 2 Diabetes Mellitus in a Rural Region in Henan, China: Family-Based and Case-Control Studies. *Front. Public Health* **2021**, *9*, 690889. [CrossRef] [PubMed]
29. Van Dongen, J.; Willemsen, G.; Chen, W.M.; De Geus, E.J.C.; Boomsma, D.I. Heritability of metabolic syndrome traits in a large population-based sample. *J. Lipid Res.* **2013**, *54*, 2914. [CrossRef]
30. Fall, T.; Ingelsson, E. Genome-wide association studies of obesity and metabolic syndrome. *Mol. Cell. Endocrinol.* **2014**, *382*, 740–757. [CrossRef] [PubMed]
31. Del Bosque-Plata, L.; Martínez-Martínez, E.; Espinoza-Camacho, M.Á.; Gragnoli, C. The Role of TCF7L2 in Type 2 Diabetes. *Diabetes* **2021**, *70*, 1220–1228. [CrossRef] [PubMed]
32. Brunetti, A.; Chiefari, E.; Foti, D. Recent advances in the molecular genetics of type 2 diabetes mellitus. *World J. Diabetes* **2014**, *5*, 128. [CrossRef] [PubMed]
33. O'hare, E.A.; Yerges-Armstrong, L.M.; Perry, J.A.; Shuldiner, A.R.; Zaghloul, N.A. Assignment of Functional Relevance to Genes at Type 2 Diabetes-Associated Loci Through Investigation of-Cell Mass Deficits. *Mol. Endocrinol.* **2016**, *30*, 429–445. [CrossRef] [PubMed]
34. Ding, Q.; Tan, A.L.M.; Parra, E.J.; Cruz, M.; Sim, X.; Teo, Y.Y.; Long, J.; Alsafar, H.; Petretto, E.; Tai, E.S.; et al. Genome-wide meta-analysis associates GPSM1 with type 2 diabetes, a plausible gene involved in skeletal muscle function. *J. Hum. Genet.* **2020**, *65*, 411–420. [CrossRef] [PubMed]
35. Vujkovic, M.; Keaton, J.M.; Lynch, J.A.; Miller, D.R.; Zhou, J.; Tcheandjieu, C.; Huffman, J.E.; Assimes, T.L.; Lorenz, K.; Zhu, X.; et al. Discovery of 318 new risk loci for type 2 diabetes and related vascular outcomes among 1.4 million participants in a multi-ancestry meta-analysis. *Nat. Genet.* **2020**, *52*, 680–691. [CrossRef] [PubMed]
36. Noordam, R.; Läll, K.; Smit, R.A.J.; Laisk, T.; Loos, R.J.F.; Mägi, R.; van Dijk, K.W.; van Heemst, D. Stratification of Type 2 Diabetes by Age of Diagnosis in the UK Biobank Reveals Subgroup-Specific Genetic Associations and Causal Risk Profiles. *Diabetes* **2021**, *70*, 1816–1825. [CrossRef] [PubMed]
37. Christiansen, C.E.; Arathimos, R.; Pain, O.; Molokhia, M.; Bell, J.T.; Lewis, C.M. Stratified genome-wide association analysis of type 2 diabetes reveals subgroups with genetic and environmental heterogeneity. *Hum. Mol. Genet.* **2023**, *32*, 2638–2645. [CrossRef]
38. Suzuki, K.; Hatzikotoulas, K.; Southam, L.; Taylor, H.J.; Yin, X.; Lorenz, K.M.; Mandla, R.; Huerta-Chagoya, A.; Melloni, G.E.M.; Kanoni, S.; et al. Genetic drivers of heterogeneity in type 2 diabetes pathophysiology. *Nature* **2024**, *627*, 347–357. [CrossRef] [PubMed]
39. Elashi, A.A.; Toor, S.M.; Umlai, U.K.I.; Al-Sarraj, Y.A.; Taheri, S.; Suhre, K.; Abou-Samra, A.B.; Albagha, O.M.E. Genome-wide association study and trans-ethnic meta-analysis identify novel susceptibility loci for type 2 diabetes mellitus. *BMC Med. Genomics* **2024**, *17*, 115.
40. Travers, M.E.; Mackay, D.J.G.; Nitert, M.D.; Morris, A.P.; Lindgren, C.M.; Berry, A.; Johnson, P.R.; Hanley, N.; Groop, L.C.; McCarthy, M.I.; et al. Insights into the molecular mechanism for type 2 diabetes susceptibility at the KCNQ1 locus from temporal changes in imprinting status in human islets. *Diabetes* **2013**, *62*, 987–992. [CrossRef]
41. Kasuga, M. KCNQ1, a susceptibility gene for type 2 diabetes. *J. Diabetes Investig.* **2011**, *2*, 413. [CrossRef] [PubMed]
42. Kissebah, A.H.; Sonnenberg, G.E.; Myklebust, J.; Goldstein, M.; Broman, K.; James, R.G.; Marks, J.A.; Krakower, G.R.; Jacob, H.J.; Weber, J.; et al. Quantitative trait loci on chromosomes 3 and 17 influence phenotypes of the metabolic syndrome. *Proc. Natl. Acad. Sci. USA* **2000**, *97*, 14478–14483. [CrossRef]
43. Lehman, D.M.; Arya, R.; Blangero, J.; Almasy, L.; Puppala, S.; Dyer, T.D.; Leach, R.J.; O'Connell, P.; Stern, M.P.; Duggirala, R. Bivariate linkage analysis of the insulin resistance syndrome phenotypes on chromosome 7q. *Hum. Biol.* **2005**, *77*, 231–246. [CrossRef] [PubMed]
44. Chasman, D.I.; Paré, G.; Mora, S.; Hopewell, J.C.; Peloso, G.; Clarke, R.; Cupples, L.A.; Hamsten, A.; Kathiresan, S.; Mälarstig, A.; et al. Forty-three loci associated with plasma lipoprotein size, concentration, and cholesterol content in genome-wide analysis. *PLoS Genet.* **2009**, *5*, e1000730. [CrossRef] [PubMed]
45. Zabaneh, D.; Balding, D.J. A genome-wide association study of the metabolic syndrome in Indian Asian men. *PLoS ONE* **2010**, *5*, e11961. [CrossRef] [PubMed]

46. Prasad, G.; Bandesh, K.; Giri, A.K.; Kauser, Y.; Chanda, P.; Parekatt, V.; Mathur, S.; Madhu, S.V.; Venkatesh, P.; Bhansali, A.; et al. Genome-wide association study of metabolic syndrome reveals primary genetic variants at CETP locus in Indians. *Biomolecules* **2019**, *9*, 321. [CrossRef]
47. Kraja, A.T.; Vaidya, D.; Pankow, J.S.; Goodarzi, M.O.; Assimes, T.L.; Kullo, I.J.; Sovio, U.; Mathias, R.A.; Sun, Y.V.; Franceschini, N.; et al. A bivariate genome-wide approach to metabolic syndrome: STAMPEED Consortium. *Diabetes* **2011**. [CrossRef] [PubMed]
48. Park, Y.J.; Moon, S.; Choi, J.; Kim, J.; Kim, H.J.; Son, H.Y.; Im, S.W.; Kim, J. Il Genome-wide association study for metabolic syndrome reveals APOA5 single nucleotide polymorphisms with multilayered effects in Koreans. *Lipids Health Dis.* **2024**, *23*, 1–12. [CrossRef] [PubMed]
49. Zhu, Y.; Zhang, D.; Zhou, D.; Li, Z.; Li, Z.; Fang, L.; Yang, M.; Shan, Z.; Li, H.; Chen, J.; et al. Susceptibility loci for metabolic syndrome and metabolic components identified in Han Chinese: A multi-stage genome-wide association study. *J. Cell. Mol. Med.* **2017**, *21*, 1106–1116. [CrossRef] [PubMed]
50. Avery, C.L.; He, Q.; North, K.E.; Ambite, J.L.; Boerwinkle, E.; Fornage, M.; Hindorff, L.A.; Kooperberg, C.; Meigs, J.B.; Pankow, J.S.; et al. A phenomics-based strategy identifies loci on APOC1, BRAP, and PLCG1 associated with metabolic syndrome phenotype domains. *PLoS Genet.* **2011**, *7*, e1002322. [CrossRef] [PubMed]
51. Tekola-Ayele, F.; Doumatey, A.P.; Shriner, D.; Bentley, A.R.; Chen, G.; Zhou, J.; Fasanmade, O.; Johnson, T.; Oli, J.; Okafor, G.; et al. Genome-wide association study identifies African-ancestry specific variants for metabolic syndrome. *Mol. Genet. Metab.* **2015**, *116*, 305–313. [CrossRef]
52. Oh, S.W.; Lee, J.E.; Shin, E.; Kwon, H.; Choe, E.K.; Choi, S.Y.; Rhee, H.; Choi, S.H. Genome-wide association study of metabolic syndrome in Korean populations. *PLoS ONE* **2020**, *15*, e0227357. [CrossRef] [PubMed]
53. Lind, L. Genome-Wide Association Study of the Metabolic Syndrome in UK Biobank. *Metab. Syndr. Relat. Disord.* **2019**, *17*, 505–511. [CrossRef]
54. Al-Homedi, Z.; Afify, N.; Memon, M.; Alsafar, H.; Tay, G.; Jelinek, H.F.; Mousa, M.; Abu-Samra, N.; Osman, W. Genetic Studies of Metabolic Syndrome in Arab Populations: A Systematic Review and Meta-Analysis. *Front. Genet.* **2021**, *12*, 733746. [CrossRef] [PubMed]
55. Rana, S.; Ali, S.; Wani, H.A.; Mushtaq, Q.D.; Sharma, S.; Rehman, M.U. Metabolic syndrome and underlying genetic determinants-A systematic review. *J. Diabetes Metab. Disord.* **2022**, *21*, 1095–1104. [CrossRef] [PubMed]
56. Imamura, M.; Maeda, S. Perspectives on genetic studies of type 2 diabetes from the genome-wide association studies era to precision medicine. *J. Diabetes Investig.* **2024**, *15*, 410–422. [CrossRef] [PubMed]
57. Abuhendi, N.; Qush, A.; Naji, F.; Abunada, H.; Al Buainain, R.; Shi, Z.; Zayed, H. Genetic polymorphisms associated with type 2 diabetes in the Arab world: A systematic review and meta-analysis. *Diabetes Res. Clin. Pract.* **2019**, *151*, 198–208. [CrossRef] [PubMed]
58. Kodama, S.; Fujihara, K.; Ishiguro, H.; Horikawa, C.; Ohara, N.; Yachi, Y.; Tanaka, S.; Shimano, H.; Kato, K.; Hanyu, O.; et al. Quantitative Relationship Between Cumulative Risk Alleles Based on Genome-Wide Association Studies and Type 2 Diabetes Mellitus: A Systematic Review and Meta-analysis. *J. Epidemiol.* **2018**, *28*, 3–18. [CrossRef]
59. Vohra, M.; Sharma, A.R.; Prabhu, B.N.; Rai, P.S. SNPs in Sites for DNA Methylation, Transcription Factor Binding, and miRNA Targets Leading to Allele-Specific Gene Expression and Contributing to Complex Disease Risk: A Systematic Review. *Public Health Genom.* **2021**, *23*, 155–170. [CrossRef]
60. Xia, W.; Chen, N.; Peng, W.; Jia, X.; Yu, Y.; Wu, X.; Gao, H. Systematic Meta-analysis Revealed an Association of PGC-1α rs8192678 Polymorphism in Type 2 Diabetes Mellitus. *Dis. Markers* **2019**, *2019*, 2970401. [CrossRef] [PubMed]
61. Ziki, M.D.A.; Mani, A. Metabolic syndrome: Genetic insights into disease pathogenesis. *Curr. Opin. Lipidol.* **2016**, *27*, 142–149.
62. Trayhurn, P. Adipokines: Inflammation and the pleiotropic role of white adipose tissue. *Br. J. Nutr.* **2022**, *128*, 312–325. [CrossRef]
63. Considine, R.V.; Sinha, M.K.; Heiman, M.L.; Kriauciunas, A.; Stephens, T.W.; Nyce, M.R.; Ohannesian, J.P.; Marco, C.C.; McKee, L.J.; Bauer, T.L.; et al. Serum Immunoreactive-Leptin Concentrations in Normal-Weight and Obese Humans. *N. Engl. J. Med.* **1996**, *334*, 292–295. [CrossRef]
64. Manna, P.; Jain, S.K. Obesity, Oxidative Stress, Adipose Tissue Dysfunction, and the Associated Health Risks: Causes and Therapeutic Strategies. *Metab. Syndr. Relat. Disord.* **2015**, *13*, 423–444. [CrossRef] [PubMed]
65. Fan, H.Q.; He, W.; Xu, K.F.; Wang, Z.X.; Xu, X.Y.; Chen, H. FTO Inhibits Insulin Secretion and Promotes NF-κB Activation through Positively Regulating ROS Production in Pancreatic β cells. *PLoS ONE* **2015**, *10*, e0127705. [CrossRef] [PubMed]
66. Frayling, T.M.; Timpson, N.J.; Weedon, M.N.; Zeggini, E.; Freathy, R.M.; Lindgren, C.M.; Perry, J.R.B.; Elliott, K.S.; Lango, H.; Rayner, N.W.; et al. A common variant in the FTO gene is associated with body mass index and predisposes to childhood and adult obesity. *Science* **2007**, *316*, 889–894. [CrossRef]
67. Ng, N.H.J.; Ghosh, S.; Bok, C.M.; Ching, C.; Low, B.S.J.; Chen, J.T.; Lim, E.; Miserendino, M.C.; Tan, Y.S.; Hoon, S.; et al. HNF4A and HNF1A exhibit tissue specific target gene regulation in pancreatic beta cells and hepatocytes. *Nat. Commun.* **2024**, *15*, 4288. [CrossRef]

68. Miyachi, Y.; Miyazawa, T.; Ogawa, Y. HNF1A Mutations and Beta Cell Dysfunction in Diabetes. *Int. J. Mol. Sci.* **2022**, *23*, 3222. [CrossRef]
69. Tam, V.; Patel, N.; Turcotte, M.; Bossé, Y.; Paré, G.; Meyre, D. Benefits and limitations of genome-wide association studies. *Nat. Rev. Genet.* **2019**, *20*, 467–484. [CrossRef] [PubMed]
70. Fatumo, S.; Chikowore, T.; Choudhury, A.; Ayub, M.; Martin, A.R.; Kuchenbaecker, K. Diversity in Genomic Studies: A Roadmap to Address the Imbalance. *Nat. Med.* **2022**, *28*, 243. [CrossRef] [PubMed]
71. Hu, C.; Jia, W. Multi-omics profiling: The way toward precision medicine in metabolic diseases. *J. Mol. Cell Biol.* **2021**, *13*, 576–593. [CrossRef] [PubMed]
72. Mandla, R.; Lorenz, K.; Yin, X.; Bocher, O.; Huerta-Chagoya, A.; Arruda, A.L.; Piron, A.; Horn, S.; Suzuki, K.; Hatzikotoulas, K.; et al. Multi-omics characterization of type 2 diabetes associated genetic variation. *medRxiv* **2024**. [CrossRef]
73. Adeyemo, A.; Balaconis, M.K.; Darnes, D.R.; Fatumo, S.; Granados Moreno, P.; Hodonsky, C.J.; Inouye, M.; Kanai, M.; Kato, K.; Knoppers, B.M.; et al. Responsible use of polygenic risk scores in the clinic: Potential benefits, risks and gaps. *Nat. Med.* **2021**, *27*, 1876–1884. [CrossRef]
74. Richmond, R.C.; Smith, G.D. Mendelian Randomization: Concepts and Scope. *Cold Spring Harb. Perspect. Med.* **2022**, *12*, a040501. [CrossRef]
75. Sanghera, D.K.; Blackett, P.R. Type 2 Diabetes Genetics: Beyond GWAS. *J. Diabetes Metab.* **2012**, *3*, 123–135. [CrossRef]
76. Ishigaki, K. Beyond GWAS: From simple associations to functional insights. *Semin. Immunopathol.* **2022**, *44*, 3–14. [CrossRef] [PubMed]
77. Harris, L.; McDonagh, E.M.; Zhang, X.; Fawcett, K.; Foreman, A.; Daneck, P.; Sergouniotis, P.I.; Parkinson, H.; Mazzarotto, F.; Inouye, M.; et al. Genome-wide association testing beyond SNPs. *Nat. Rev. Genet.* **2024**, *25*, 607–625. [CrossRef]

diabetology MDPI

Review

Exosome-Derived microRNAs: Bridging the Gap Between Obesity and Type 2 Diabetes in Diagnosis and Treatment

Iva Vukelić [1,†], Branislav Šuša [2,†], Sanja Klobučar [3,4,*], Sunčica Buljević [1], Ana-Marija Liberati Piršo [4,5,6], Andrej Belančić [7], Dario Rahelić [8,9,10] and Dijana Detel [1]

1 Department of Medical Chemistry, Biochemistry and Clinical Chemistry, Faculty of Medicine, University of Rijeka, Braće Branchetta 20, 51000 Rijeka, Croatia; iva.vukelic@uniri.hr (I.V.); suncica.buljevic@uniri.hr (S.B.); dijana.detel@uniri.hr (D.D.)
2 Department of Internal Medicine, General Hospital Pula, Santoriova 24a, 52100 Pula, Croatia; drbranislav.susa@gmail.com
3 Department of Endocrinology, Diabetes and Metabolic Diseases, Clinical Hospital Centre Rijeka, Krešimirova 42, 51000 Rijeka, Croatia
4 Department of Internal Medicine, Faculty of Medicine, University of Rijeka, Braće Branchetta 20, 51000 Rijeka, Croatia; anamarijaliberati@gmail.com
5 Faculty of Food Technology and Biotechnology, University of Zagreb, Pierottijeva 6, 10000 Zagreb, Croatia
6 Department of Endocrinology and Diabetology, University Hospital "Sveti Duh", Sveti Duh 64, 10000 Zagreb, Croatia
7 Department of Basic and Clinical Pharmacology with Toxicology, Faculty of Medicine, University of Rijeka, Braće Branchetta 20, 51000 Rijeka, Croatia; a.belancic93@gmail.com
8 Endocrinology and Metabolic Diseases, Vuk Vrhovac University Clinic for Diabetes, Merkur University Hospital, Dugi dol 4, 10000 Zagreb, Croatia; dario.rahelic@gmail.com
9 Faculty of Medicine, J.J. Strossmayer University Osijek, 31000 Osijek, Croatia
10 School of Medicine, Catholic University of Croatia, 10000 Zagreb, Croatia
* Correspondence: sanja.klobucar@uniri.hr
† These authors contributed equally to this work.

Abstract: Obesity and type 2 diabetes represent global public health challenges that are continuously growing at an alarming rate. The etiology of obesity is complex and multifactorial, with a substantial interplay between behavioral, biological, and environmental factors. Dysregulation of immunometabolism through chronic low-intensity inflammation in obesity has long been recognized as the main driver of insulin resistance and the development of type 2 diabetes. However, the intricate mechanisms underlying these alterations have yet to be fully elucidated. Exosomes are extracellular vesicles that carry biomolecules including various types of RNA molecules. Of particular importance are microRNAs (miRNAs), known as modulators of gene expression whose altered expression is observed in various pathophysiological conditions. Recent research suggests that exosome-derived miRNAs, such as miR-155, miR-27a, and miR-29, play an essential role in the regulation of inflammatory processes, while miR-122 and miR-192 are associated with metabolic dysfunction. These and many other miRNAs influence signaling pathways that are critical for maintaining insulin sensitivity, thereby contributing to the development of insulin resistance in individuals with obesity. Hence, there is a growing interest in the potential of exosomes and miRNAs as biomarkers for the early detection of insulin resistance and other obesity-related complications, as well as promising therapeutic targets or next-generation drug delivery carriers. This review provides a comprehensive overview of the interplay between exosome-derived miRNA, obesity, and type 2 diabetes and summarizes the latest findings in exosome biology.

Keywords: obesity; type 2 diabetes; exosomes; microRNA; biomarkers; therapy; insulin resistance

1. Introduction—Obesity and Type 2 Diabetes

1.1. Obesity as the Beginning of Diabetes

Obesity and type 2 diabetes (T2D) represent global public health challenges that are continuously growing at an alarming rate. According to recent data, it is estimated that more than 650 million people worldwide are obese, while the most devastating data are on the number of children and adolescents with obesity [1]. The World Health Organization rates obesity as a prominent health problem that is easily recognized but often overlooked, undiagnosed, and untreated. Obesity substantially increases the risk of metabolic diseases, and there is no doubt that obesity is a major driver for the development of T2D. However, despite the shared genetic and environmental features, the mechanisms linking these two conditions remain unclear. In line, reports show that 86% of adults with T2D are overweight or obese; 52% are classified as obese, and 8.1% have morbid obesity.

Over the last hundred years or more, information as well as knowledge addressing obesity has been harvested from a wealth of research, although a single primary cause has yet to be identified. Instead, several factors—including behavioral, biological, and environmental influences—are widely recognized as contributors. Foremost, among these are dietary habits, particularly the increasing consumption of high-calorie, processed foods rich in sugar and fat, along with a sedentary lifestyle and insufficient exercise. In addition, psychological factors such as emotional stress, depression, and other mental health issues can also lead to overeating or unhealthy eating patterns. While lifestyle changes are essential, they alone have not been sufficient to halt the growing obesity epidemic. This underscores the importance of biological factors, including genetic susceptibility and, metabolic and immune factors, in the development of obesity. While monogenic causes of obesity are rare and cannot explain the scale of the obesity pandemic, numerous mutations in genes encoding molecules such as leptin, adiponectin, and glucose transporters 2 and 4 as well as the large number of genes identified by genome-wide association studies can influence caloric intake and, metabolism, including food processing, fat storage, and body-fat distribution. However, the strength of genetic influence on weight disorders varies significantly among individuals. Research indicates that genes account for about 25% of the predisposition to being overweight in some people, while the genetic influence in others is 70% to 80% [2].

Nowadays, it is known that persistent fat-positive balance leads to weight gain, white adipose tissue (WAT) enlargement, and low-grade inflammation which may underlie the development of tissue dysfunction, insulin resistance, and metabolic comorbidities such as cardiovascular disease, diabetes, and cancer [3]. As discussed later, enlarged adipose tissue, particularly visceral tissue, is a main source of chronic inflammation while being the most important cog in the complex developmental mechanism. Therefore, it is important to determine the size and distribution of adipose tissue, and body mass index has been used as a non-invasive measure of adiposity for more than a century [4]. Although widely used, it has significant limitations as it does not distinguish between fat and muscle mass and may not accurately reflect the distribution of body fat or the risk of developing obesity-associated comorbidities [4].

Low-grade inflammation is characterized by elevated levels of circulating pro-inflammatory cytokines, which have deleterious effects on the central nervous system and disrupt the function of organs involved in maintaining immune responses and metabolic processes [5]. Furthermore, the metabolic disturbance that occurs in obesity leads to an up- or down-regulation of metabolic pathways that influence the differentiation, phenotype, and functions of immune cells as well as the further production of cytokines and chemokines. In line with this, studies have shown that obesity increases intracellular lipid metabolism and glucose uptake in macrophages, which can trigger their M1 polarization [6]. In addition, inflammation can interfere with insulin signaling, glucose metabolism, and lipid homeostasis, contributing to insulin resistance. Each of the above factors can interact with the others, making obesity a complex disease with multiple interrelated elements. To integrate all these findings, the concept of dysregulated immunometabolism in obesity has been postulated. A step forward in understanding the dysregulation of immunometabolism underlying obesity is the increasing evidence that the above-mentioned interactions are also driven and regulated by the microbiome–gut–brain axis. Despite lifestyle changes and the best available medical and surgical treatments for obesity and T2D, gaps in pathophysiology and clinical management remain. Since their discovery in 1993, evidence and understanding of the physiological significance of microRNAs (miRNAs) have steadily grown. Distinct miRNA profiles have been identified in patients with metabolic disorders, such as obesity and T2D [7], compared to healthy individuals, positioning them as potential new biomarkers. Additionally, the recognition that miRNAs are transported within extracellular vesicles [8] has opened a new perspective, suggesting that they act as an endocrine factor involved in maintaining communication between organs. This insight could also open new avenues for understanding the mechanisms behind obesity-related complications in various organs and pave the way for the development of improved treatments.

1.2. Adipose Tissue—A Critical Player in the Disturbance of Immunometabolism

Adipose tissue is an important player in controlling metabolism, and it is divided into two main classes: WAT, where lipids, in the form of triglycerides, are mainly stored in a single droplet within the adipocytes, and brown adipose tissue, predominantly located in the neck, supraclavicular, perirenal/adrenal, and vertebral fat depots. Compared to WAT, brown adipose tissue stores lipids in multiple lipid droplets, maintains body temperature, and is less involved in immunometabolic control. WAT is found at various locations in the human body. Based on its anatomical location, functional characteristics, and impact on obesity development, it is classified into two main types: subcutaneous and visceral adipose tissue. Besides storage function and contrary to earlier perceptions, nowadays it is well established that adipose tissue is an active endocrine organ that releases numerous pro-inflammatory and anti-inflammatory molecules, known as adipocytokines, including tumor necrosis factor-α (TNF-α), interleukin (IL) 6, resistin, leptin, and adiponectin, which have several local, peripheral, and central effects [9]. Thus, adipose tissue regulates the metabolism of various tissues both directly and indirectly through the production of bioactive molecules, having a tremendous impact on metabolic homeostasis.

Total body fat is mainly stored in subcutaneous adipose tissue since it is the preferred site for storage of excess fat, while visceral adipose tissue stores 5–20% of the total body fat. Although adipose tissue is highly adaptable and can increase its mass by more than twofold, the storage capacity of adipose tissue varies among individuals. Storing lipids in WAT protects the rest of the body from the expansion of visceral adipose tissue, ectopic lipid accumulation, and lipotoxicity. In obesity, prolonged lipid overload leads to changes in adipose tissue features, including size, function, inflammatory state, and adipokine secretion of adipocytes resulting in metabolic disturbance and rise in insulin resistance [10].

Fundamentally, the excessive fat accumulation and expansion of WAT are also related to inflammatory cell activation. It has been shown that metabolic stress in hypertrophic and/or hyperplasia adipocytes induces the surface expression of ligands for stress receptor Ncr1 [11]. After ligand binding, the signal initiates the recruitment of NK cells but also the polarization of tissue-resident macrophage from phenotype M2 to M1 (Figure 1) [12]. This results in a shift from anti-inflammatory cytokine production [13] to pro-inflammatory cytokine production mediated by TNF-α, IL6, and IL1β [12,14–17]. This production is mediated by the activation of toll-like receptors 2 and 4 stimulated by the elevation of saturated fatty acids [18]. This is regulated through the activation of nuclear factor kappa B/c-Jun N-terminal kinases (NF-κB/JNK) pathways [19]. Consequently, the macrophage shift induces activation and influx of other adipose-resident immune cells, such as Th1 and Th 17 CD4+ T cells, cytotoxic CD8+ T cells, B cells, and NK cells, which in turn produce cytokines that further amplify the inflammation [20]. Concomitantly, the cytokines and cells contribute to a chronic low-grade pro-inflammatory state, thereby contributing to systemic inflammation, impaired insulin signaling, and insufficient insulin production by β-cells in the pancreas, which are critical factors and main drivers in the development of metabolic diseases, particularly in the development of T2D.

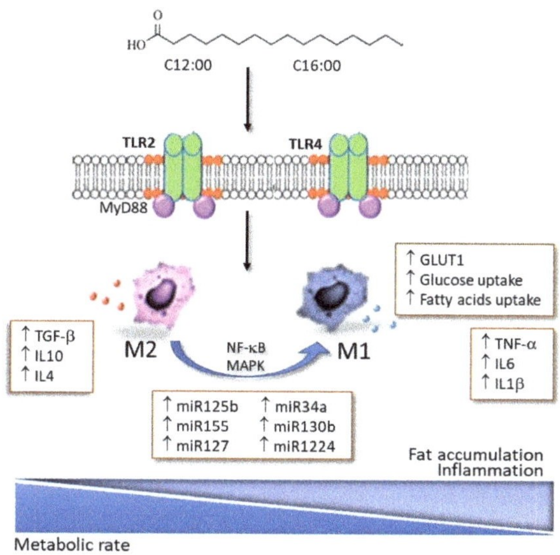

Figure 1. The interplay between fat accumulation and adipose tissue-derived exosomal miRNAs in macro-phage activation and polarization. The polarization of macrophages from the M2 to the M1 phenotype leads to a shift from the production of anti-inflammatory cytokines to pro-inflammatory cytokines, including TNF-α, IL6, and IL1β. This pro-inflammatory cytokine production is driven by the activation of TLR 2 and 4, which are stimulated by elevated levels of saturated fatty acids. TLR, toll-like receptor; GLUT1, glucose transporter type 1; TNF, tumor necrosis factor; TGF, transforming growth factor; IL, interleukin; miR, microRNA; ↑, up-regulation.

The expansion of adipose tissue creates a low-oxygen microenvironment, leading to angiogenesis, reduced vascular density, decreased production of vascular growth factor A, and activation of hypoxia-inducible factor 1A. These changes promote the activation of pro-fibrotic pathways and the NF-κB signaling pathway, which together accelerate pro-inflammatory conditions, drive alterations in the extracellular matrix, and impair fatty acid uptake by adipocytes [10]. Although the primary function of adipose tissue is the storage of lipids, it contains a variety of non-immune and immune cells, including macrophages, T, and B cells.

Due to insulin resistance in obesity, the dysregulation of lipolysis in adipose tissue leads to an impaired, yet constant release of fatty acids into the circulation. The resulting elevated concentration of fatty acids contributes to their accumulation, initially in the liver and subsequently in other organs including skeletal muscles. It has been established that individuals with a given level of BMI, with low muscle mass and higher total body fat percentage and waist circumference, are more likely to have T2D, and face an increased risk of death, highlighting the importance of skeletal muscles. Increased muscle mass improves insulin sensitivity and metabolic health, which can help mitigate some of the negative effects of obesity. Recent research has revealed that adipose tissue, along with other metabolic tissues, communicates with different tissues through small membrane-bound particles called extracellular vesicles. In obesity, these vesicles play a key role in facilitating crosstalk between macrophages, adipose tissue, and other organs. Additionally, they have been found to contain the lipid droplet-associated protein perilipin1, as well as phospholipids, neutral lipids, free cholesterol, and miRNAs [21].

1.3. Type 2 Diabetes

T2D is a long-term metabolic disorder caused by impaired insulin secretion and/or action due to partially understood pathophysiological mechanisms. These mechanisms are complex and involve interactions between chronic inflammation, abnormal lipid accumulation, endoplasmic reticulum stress, and oxidative stress. It is one of the most widespread chronic diseases in the adult population, and, therefore, it is recognized as a serious public health problem with a significant impact on human lives and healthcare costs. In many parts of the world, urbanization and economic development have led to its increased prevalence [22]. Clinical studies to date have reported a large number of young adults diagnosed with T2D, most of whom are obese [23]. One of the key pathophysiological mechanisms behind the onset and progression of T2D is insulin resistance. It is generally recognized that in the early stages of insulin resistance, β-cells overwork to increase insulin secretion in order to keep blood glucose levels stable. The ability of β-cells to compensate is largely determined by genetic factors. However, with disease progression, β-cells lose their ability to produce insulin to counteract the rise in blood glucose levels, ultimately leading to prediabetes or the development of T2D.

As mentioned above, prolonged overnutrition and an excess of metabolites lead to lipid accumulation, metabolic stress, and cellular infiltration in adipose tissue, which in turn triggers the release of pro-inflammatory factors like IL1β and TNF-α [24]. These factors disrupt insulin receptor activation and its downstream IRS1/PI3K/Akt2 signaling pathway through various mechanisms. Pioneering research by Hotamisligil et al. demonstrated elevated levels of TNF-α in the adipose tissue of obese individuals. On the other hand, it has been shown that TNF-α neutralization improves insulin sensitivity in obese rodents [25,26]. Mentioned metabolic disorders can disrupt the transcription of key genes involved in the insulin signaling pathway, leading to its down-regulation, which is the first step toward impaired glucose uptake and hyperglycemia. Additionally, they can activate alternative signaling pathways. Pro-inflammatory cytokines, such as TNF-α and IL1β, inhibit the transcription of insulin signaling molecules by activating stress-related pathways like NF-κB, JAK/STAT, and JNK. These pathways further interfere with the normal expression of genes related to insulin signaling [27]. Finally, an excessive influx of fatty acids into adipose tissue leads to incomplete oxidation of fatty acids, production of reactive oxygen species, and, as expected, accumulation of toxic metabolites, such as ceramides and diacylglycerols, that can directly interfere with the insulin signaling pathway by inhibiting Akt, activation of NF-κB, and JNK-mediated signaling [28].

Low-grade inflammation, combined with the excessive production of metabolites, triggers the phosphorylation of the IκB kinase (IKK) complex and the degradation of IκB, leading to the translocation of NF-κB into the nucleus. NF-κB can negatively affect insulin signaling and glucose homeostasis through various direct and indirect mechanisms. One well-known pathway involves the activation of inducible nitric oxide synthase (iNOS) and the subsequent production of nitric oxide. Furthermore, a component of the activated IKK complex can directly phosphorylate insulin receptor substrate (IRS) 1 on serine residues, thereby inhibiting its activation. In addition to its role in the insulin signaling pathway, according to available data, NF-κB plays a significant role in the development of diabetes complications. Its activation leads to the aggravation of kidney fibrosis [29] and promotes apoptosis of human endothelial cells by enhancing caspase-3 activity, which also delays wound healing in diabetic foot ulcerations [30]. As previously mentioned, inflammatory factors such as IL6 and interferon (INF)-γ can inhibit the IRS1 signaling cascade by activating JAK2/STAT3, which in turn up-regulates the expression of suppressor of cytokine signaling 3. JAK/STAT3 is also found to promote the NF-κB cascade [31]. Like NF-κB, increased phosphorylation of STAT3, as a result of increased IL6 synthesis, impairs immune cell activation, recruitment, and survival, leading to delayed wound healing.

As JNK activity is increased in obesity as well as diabetes and responds to various cellular stress signals activated by pro-inflammatory cytokines, free fatty acids, and hyperglycemia, it is considered one of the key mediators in the transition between obesity and T2D [32]. JNK plays a broad role across various tissues and serves as a key effector in the intricate MAPK signaling pathway, and it is the last kinase to be activated within the MAPK/JNK pathway.

It has been established that JNK1 knockout mice are protected from high-fat diet induced inflammation, obesity, and insulin resistance, likely due to JNK's effect on hypothalamic inflammation, which influences the central regulation of energy balance by insulin and leptin. Initially, these effects were linked to a reduction in serine-307 phosphorylation of IRS1, which impairs proper activation of the insulin signaling pathway However, later studies showed that a serine-to-alanine mutation at residue 307 (S307A) on IRS1, which prevents JNK1-mediated phosphorylation, does not protect mice from HFD-induced insulin resistance. This led to the suggestion that JNK1, as a Ser/Thr kinase, likely phosphorylates multiple sites on IRS1/2 [32,33]. Interestingly, several miRNAs have been shown to regulate the NF-κB and JNK signaling pathway, either by targeting key components of the pathway or by modulating upstream or downstream signaling elements. Therefore, we will further discuss its crosstalk.

2. Exosomes and miRNAs

2.1. Biogenesis and Composition of Exosomes

Exosomes are small, 30 to 150 nm bilayered extracellular vesicles secreted from all cell types [34]. Although they were primarily considered cellular waste, exosomes were found to be a novel mechanism of intercellular communication [35]. Released from the parental cells into the extracellular space, exosomes exert local effects, or they enter circulation causing distal systemic effects. However, a significant number of studies have shown that exosomes act not only as messengers of information between cells but also as a relevant biomarker of a certain physiological status and pathophysiological changes [34,35]. As they are naturally produced in the human body, they are able to evade recognition by the immune system and subsequent removal. Furthermore, exosomes are recognized as vehicles for the efficient delivery of drugs to the target cells, a characteristic for which it was shown to increase bioavailability and reduce side effects [35]. Therefore, according to all the above advantages, it is clear why interest in a more detailed study of the biology and mechanisms of exosomes is constantly growing.

Exosomes are generated in a complex process by an endosomal route [35,36]. This process is under the regulation of several proteins of endosomal sorting complexes required for transport (ESCRT) protein family, which act together with certain accessory proteins, such as Alix, TSG101, HSC70, and HSP90β. Along with membrane-bound tetraspanins CD63, CD81, and CD9, these proteins are considered markers of exosomes as they are present as the main constituents of the exosomes regardless of the type of cells from which the exosomes originate [35]. In addition to proteins, exosomes contain other bioactive molecules, such as lipids (sphingolipids, cholesterol, phosphatidylserine, saturated fatty acids, and ceramides), DNA (genomic DNA, mitochondrial DNA), and various types of RNA [37–40], among which miRNA has been receiving the most attention lately [41]. An illustration of the structure and components of exosomes, including proteins, lipids, and nucleic acids, is shown in Figure 2.

2.2. Exosomal miRNAs and Their Role in Physiological and Pathophysiological Conditions

miRNAs are noncoding RNA molecules of ~22 nucleotides synthesized in a tightly regulated multiple-step process that includes DGCR8/DROSHA, Dicer, Exportin-5, and RISC molecular complexes [42,43]. Although several miRNAs are expressed in a tissue or developmental stage-specific manner, thus contributing to tissue-specific mRNA and protein expression profiles, most of them are widely expressed [18,44]. The main function of these small RNAs is to modulate gene expression through translation inhibition, thereby affecting the stability of the mRNA. Accordingly, one single miRNA can target multiple mRNAs, but one mRNA can also be targeted by several miRNAs [45]. As such, miRNAs regulate a wide range of cellular physiological processes (proliferation, differentiation, development, homeostasis, and apoptosis); however, changes in their expression have been reported in many pathophysiological conditions (inflammation, neurodegeneration, tumorigenesis) making them potential novel biomarkers, not only of physiological status but also of various pathophysiological changes and diseases [41,46]. Therefore, the study of exosome-derived miRNAs gives a better insight into the etiology of diseases, but also opens up the possibility of using them as a new therapeutic strategy by modulating their expression.

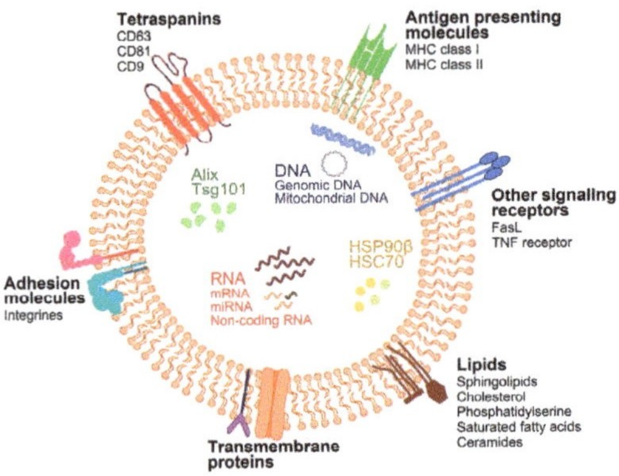

Figure 2. The structure and content of an exosome. Alix, ALG-2-interacting protein X; Tsg101, tumor susceptibility gene 101; HSP, heat shock protein; HSC, heat shock cognate; FasL, fas ligand; TNF, tumor necrosis factor; mRNA, messenger RNA; miR, microRNA.

2.3. Exosomal miRNA as Biomarkers in Obesity and Type 2 Diabetes

There is a growing interest in the research on the biomarker potential of exosomal miRNAs, which could indicate changes at the organ level and thus help in the early diagnosis as well as monitoring of diseases. Significantly, miRNA sequencing studies showed that exosomes collected from blood and conditioned media of specific cell types contain hundreds of different miRNAs [47,48], and changes in the profile of those miRNAs are a reliable indicator of the physiological responses to the development of metabolic diseases, including obesity and T2D [41,49]. So far, a difference in the expression profile of exosomal miRNAs of adipose tissue or plasma between lean and obese subjects has already been demonstrated, indicating their involvement in the induction and promotion of obesity [49–51]. In addition, miRNA from exosomes derived from the adipose tissue of obese individuals, either adipocyte or adipose tissue macrophages, have been specifically shown to be involved in promoting glucose intolerance and insulin resistance, stimulating lipogenesis and adipocyte hypertrophy, as well as enhancing inflammation [49,50]. All of the above indicates the use of miRNAs as biomarkers of obesity, although detailed molecular mechanisms of their involvement need further investigation.

A significant role of exosomal miRNA has been already shown in the development and progression of T2D and its complications. Based on numerous research, exosomal miRNAs have a strong relationship with β-cell damage and dysfunction, as well as the development of insulin resistance [52]. Furthermore, they are also involved in the development of T2D-related complications, such as diabetic nephropathy, diabetic foot ulcer, diabetic peripheral neuropathy, and diabetic cardiomyopathy [52]. Therefore, exosomal miRNAs can be used as very relevant biomarkers for the early detection of insulin resistance and diabetes, as well as related chronic complications [53].

2.4. Therapeutic Challenges of Exosomal miRNAs in Obesity and Type 2 Diabetes

Due to the deep correlation between epidemiology and pathogenesis, therapeutic management of both, obesity and T2D, includes lifestyle changes and adjustments, pharmacotherapy, and newer treatment methods such as bariatric surgery [54]. Moreover, it was shown that available pharmacotherapeutic treatments recommended for either obesity or T2D have a mutual effect on each other, meaning that anti-obesity drugs can be anti-diabetic to some extent and vice versa [54]. However, although effective in reducing body weight and regulating blood glucose levels, these therapeutics have a significant number of disadvantages, such as side effects due to the necessary long-term use, dose adjustments, or even high costs [54]. Therefore, there is a growing need for the development of a new therapy that, in addition to effectiveness, would prevent or at least reduce the development of side effects, as well as the cost of treatment. Profiling analysis showed a strong correlation between the dysregulation in the expression of miRNAs and the development of metabolic diseases, including obesity and T2D [43]. This expression disturbance refers not only to the endogenous miRNAs that are tissue- or cell-specific and involved in adipogenesis, insulin resistance, lipid and glucose metabolism, or induction of inflammation, but also to the exogenous miRNAs that circulate through the biological fluids packed in exosomes and act as systemic signaling molecules in distant tissues [55–58]. Although of great potential, the use of miRNAs in general in the treatment of metabolic disorders has not been sufficiently investigated [59]. On the other hand, they have been investigated in terms of therapy for various other diseases, including autoimmune diseases, metabolic syndrome, neurocognitive disorders, and cancer, and some miRNA-based therapeutics are already in clinical trials for certain diseases [60]. When it comes to metabolic disorders, only two miRNAs, miR-103 and miR-107, have entered clinical trials in the treatment of T2D, NAFLD, and NASH, although the therapeutic potential of a much larger number has been demonstrated by research in animal models [60]. These studies showed the anti-obesity action of miRNA, as well as the role of exosomal miRNA in the prevention of glucose intolerance and insulin resistance [60]. Overall, exosomal miRNAs hold great potential as therapeutic agents for treating metabolic disorders, and further research should delve into their mechanisms of action. There are several advantages to utilizing exosomal miRNAs in therapy, particularly circulating miRNAs, as they can be easily isolated and detected through non-invasive methods.

2.5. Circulating miRNAs as Biomarkers and Therapeutic Targets of Insulin Resistance—Challenges and Limitations

Insulin resistance is the underlying factor in the etiology of T2D, and the presence of excessive adipose tissue mass may contribute to mechanisms that trigger its development. On the other hand, obesity and insulin resistance must also be viewed as a two-way street: the possibility that insulin resistance promotes the development of obesity should also be considered. As obesity represents a significant health risk with severe consequences, and its association with insulin resistance has been confirmed, the need for its rapid, effective, and simple diagnosis has become a global priority since current tools are not sufficient for prompt diagnoses. Based on the described dysregulation in the expression of circulating miRNAs in insulin resistance and liquid biopsy as a new minimally invasive technique, these molecules have been proposed as potential biomarkers [41] although certain limitations in their use still need to be explored. The first issue that could pose a technical problem is their stability. miRNAs are generally stable in serum or plasma samples as they are encapsulated in exosomes or bound to proteins and lipoproteins, which protects them from degradation [61]. Surprisingly, miRNAs have been shown to remain stable over long periods, even under storage conditions well above −80 °C, and are not affected by the patient's food intake status [62]. Despite their shown stability, variability in miRNA levels could be a consequence of different factors, such as sample collection, processing, and storage conditions, so each test should be optimized separately as the observed variability can affect the reproducibility and reliability of miRNA-based diagnostics. The next issue is standardization or the lack of standardized protocols in miRNA manipulation. Sample preparation procedures, methods for their analysis, and approaches to standardize results differ greatly [63], and this lack of global standardization can lead to inconsistent results across different studies and clinical settings with very little comparability. Moreover, the detection and quantification of miRNAs requires the use of sensitive and specific techniques (real-time PCR and next-generation sequencing) that can be affected by technical variations and require rigorous validation, making them a serious analytical challenge.

There are several advantages of using exosomal miRNAs as therapeutic agents, but this also poses some challenges in terms of their targeting. The delivery of miRNA-based therapeutics to specific tissues or cells remains a major challenge because an effective delivery system must protect the highly sensitive content from degradation, ensure uptake into cells, and release the miRNAs in a controlled manner [64]. To overcome these issues and optimize the process, different delivery vehicles, such as viral vectors, nanoparticles, and exosomes, are currently being investigated. Each of these carriers has its advantages and limitations, including potential immunogenicity, toxicity, and scalability [65]. Since miRNAs can target multiple mRNAs, their application can lead to several off-target effects, causing unintended and potentially dangerous biological consequences, including toxicity, a major concern in the use of miRNA therapeutics [64]. Therefore, the specificity of miRNA-based therapies needs to be thoroughly reviewed as a crucial step in minimizing the possibility of such effects. Strategies aiming to improve specificity and reduce toxicity in miRNA-based treatments are, therefore, being actively researched [66]. Furthermore, to achieve the desired therapeutic effect by administration of miRNA inhibitors or mimics that typically show moderate efficacy, the required dose is very high, consequently increasing the risk of unwanted side effects. Finally, the functional complexity of miRNAs, molecules that participate in multiple signaling pathways and interact with various targets, introduces an additional challenge in developing effective and safe miRNA-based therapies [64].

2.6. Future Perspectives for miRNA-Based Therapies and Biomarker Development

Recently, numerous clinical trials have been designed to investigate the use of miRNA mimics as a replacement for tumor-suppressive miRNAs as well as miRNA inhibitors to inhibit oncogenic miRNAs in cancer therapy but also lipid metabolism, inflammation, and fibrosis in liver diseases [67]. For example, the role of a liposomal mimic of miR-34a, MRX34, was evaluated in patients with refractory solid tumors. Treatment with dexamethasone premedication and MX34 demonstrated a manageable toxicity profile and some clinical activity in the majority of patients [68]. A study analyzing miR-122 revealed significantly differential expression of that particular miRNA between cancer and healthy patients, and the overall survival rate predictions in hepatocellular carcinoma as well as other types of cancer varied significantly. The authors concluded that miR-122 may serve as an indispensable biomarker for the diagnosis, prognostic evaluation, and targeted therapy in pan-cancer [69]. Certain miRNAs (i.e., microR (miR)-22, miR-122, and miR-132) can exacerbate or attenuate fibrotic and carcinogenic processes in hepatic cells linked to metabolic dysfunction-associated steatotic liver disease, its progression to metabolic dysfunction-associated steatohepatitis and hepatocellular carcinoma. The authors conclude that modulating these miRNAs, either by synthetic mimics or inhibitors, represents a promising therapeutic strategy that could be maintained since preclinical models demonstrate that miRNA-based therapies can attenuate liver inflammation, reduce fibrosis, and inhibit tumorigenesis [70].

The incorporation of miRNA-based therapy and the development of novel non-invasive molecular biomarkers through the use of liquid biopsy techniques in blood and other body fluids is an emerging approach in T2D management. Some of the recognized circulating miRNAs could serve as a non-invasive diagnostic tool for predicting the development of T2D, especially in the elderly population. New miRNA molecular marker candidates are also being investigated as effectors in monitoring metabolic responses of prescribed anti-diabetic drugs to help predict and track the development of chronic complications in T2D [71]. Studies are exploring their stability in plasma and serum, as well as their correlation with disease states to deepen the understanding of possible etiological pathways to disease onset [72]. The search for new blood-based or urinary biomarkers for T2D is being conducted using advanced "omics" technologies, encompassing specific gene variations and metabolites associated with glucose intolerance and other related traits. Although reports associate numerous biomarkers with the risk of developing T2D, the utility of most of them for clinical prediction is still largely unknown. A separate ongoing research line focuses on the validation of these biomarkers in clinical settings to improve the accuracy of T2D diagnosis and treatment [71].

When it comes to the use of miRNA-based therapies or biomarkers, issues of stability, standardized protocols for collection and processing, effective delivery, and minimization of off-target effects are crucial. By overcoming these challenges and leveraging ongoing research, miRNA-based therapies and biomarkers hold great promise for improving the diagnosis and treatment of T2D and other diseases. Continued advancements in this field are expected to lead to more effective and personalized medical interventions.

3. Obesity-Derived Exosomal miRNAs: Bridging the Gap Between Insulin Resistance and Type 2 Diabetes

3.1. miRNAs as New Messengers in Intercellular Communication

As previously described, miRNAs act as mediators of gene expression, and any dysregulation in their expression is associated with the development of many diseases including diabetes, cardiovascular disease, kidney disease, and cancer [73]. Except for local action in the cell, miRNAs can be released in the extracellular space and, more importantly, in extracellular fluids either packaged in extracellular vesicles, mainly exosomes, associated with high-density lipoprotein or RNA-binding protein nucleophosmin or they are in a complex with proteins, especially Argonaute 2 [74–76]. As such, miRNAs are protected from degradation by ribonucleases present in body fluids. Moreover, the level of extracellular or circulating miRNA expression in the body fluids is constant, and any alteration can indicate the development of a certain disease [76]. Therefore, circulating miRNAs are shown to be useful as potential biomarkers of disease [77–79]. More importantly, it was shown that circulating miRNAs act as messengers in intercellular communication under physiological but also pathophysiological conditions, thus contributing to the development and progression of a wide variety of human diseases, such as cardiovascular, autoimmune, neurodegenerative, liver, and inflammatory diseases, as well as cancer [77,80–85]. These are mostly miRNAs that are packaged in exosomes, by which miRNAs are transferred between cells either locally or to distant sites.

3.2. The Role of Circulating miRNA in Obesity, Insulin Resistance and Type 2 Diabetes

Obesity is characterized by a chronic low-grade inflammation developing in adipose tissue, which is considered to have a pivotal role in the development of insulin resistance, thus increasing the risk and contributing to the development of T2D [86]. Although many studies have focused on explaining the relationship between obesity and T2D, the whole mechanism is still not fully understood. So far, a significant correlation between changes in the expression of circulating miRNAs and the development of obesity and insulin resistance, as well as related metabolic disorders has been shown [87]. However, despite numerous research, either the origin or relationship with adipose tissue, as well as the detailed mechanism of action of many circulating miRNAs in the induction of insulin resistance and T2D, have not yet been fully or at all investigated (Figure 3). An increased expression of miR144 in whole blood of patients with T2D was shown to be associated with the development of T2D through a negative modulation of the expression of IRS1, a key molecule in insulin signaling [88,89]. Furthermore, an increased level of miR-144 in obesity was in association with reduced expression of immune-responsive gene 1 (*Irg1*), which was restored after miR-144 silencing in vitro and in vivo, demonstrating that miR-144 can impair intracellular liver metabolism and nuclear factor E2-related factor 2 (NRF2) activity [90]. miR-122 was shown to be robustly elevated in the blood of obese patients with a tendency to increase with the degree of obesity [91], while it was shown to be reduced in response to diet-induced weight loss [92]. Besides the involvement in obesity, an increase in the level of circulating miR-122 was shown to be related to the development of insulin resistance, metabolic syndrome, and T2D [93]. Following this, an increase in the circulating miR-122 correlated with the obtained homeostatic model assessment for insulin resistance (HOMA-IR) data, indicating its involvement in insulin resistance. Furthermore, a positive correlation with the increase in lipid subspecies containing saturated and monounsaturated fatty acids demonstrated an association with the development of metabolic syndrome and T2D, and a significant reduction in miR-122 was shown in vitro and in vivo after statin treatment, which confirmed the involvement of miR-122 in lipid metabolism. In a study by Parrizas et al. [94], miR-192 and miR-193b are described as biomarkers for prediabetes due to their significantly increased expression in the serum of prediabetic subjects but not in T2D patients, and the same effect was shown in an animal model of glucose tolerance caused by high-fat diet. Although the mechanism of action of miR-192 in obesity and insulin resistance has not been investigated, miR-193b-3p has been shown to affect glucose metabolism by directly targeting YWHAZ/14-3-3ζ and up-regulating the transcription factor Forkhead box O (FOXO) 1 downstream of the PI3K-Akt pathway in T2D [95]. Contrary to the described down-regulation of miR-192 in diabetes compared to the condition that precedes it, the study by Jaeger et al. has shown an elevation of miR-192 together with miR-194 in the serum of patients with the presence of both T2D and T1D, as well as a correlation of increased expression of both miRNAs with blood parameters of insulin resistance [96]. Additionally, miR-194 has previously been shown to be differentially regulated through different stages of insulin resistance until the onset of T2D as an adaptive response to facilitate tissue glucose uptake and metabolism and is involved in multiple aspects of glucose metabolism in skeletal muscle, potentially through mechanisms that include Akt, glycogen synthase kinase-3, and oxidative phosphorylation [97].

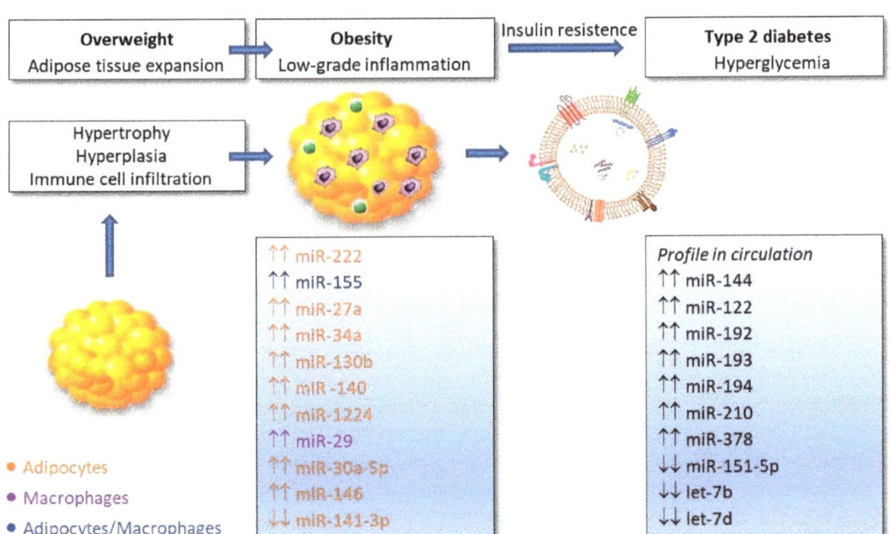

Figure 3. The involvement of adipose tissue-derived exosomal miRNAs in the development of obesity-induced insulin resistance and the subsequent progression of T2D. The figure illustrates miRNAs originating from exosomes of altered adipose tissue that contribute to enhanced inflammation in obesity and the induction of insulin resistance through studied mechanisms. Additionally, another list of miRNAs highlights those with altered expression in the plasma of obese and/or T2D patients, with or without an explained mechanism and origin. miR, microRNA; ↑↑, up-regulation; ↓↓, down-regulation.

A detailed study by Jones et al. showed a correlation between circulating plasma miRNA levels and obesity with a phenotype of insulin sensitivity, insulin resistance, or T2D in human individuals, as well as the origin of those miRNAs in a mouse model of obesity [98]. However, apart from the circulating miRNAs that have already been shown to be related to obesity and associated metabolic disorders, like miR-144, authors also demonstrated the involvement of other miRNAs, such as miR-23b, miR-26a, miR-28-5p, miR-30-3p, miR-374b, miR-365, and miR-32, in the development of these diseases without defined plasma levels or role in obesity. This indicates the need for a more detailed investigation of the involvement as well as a molecular mechanism of dysregulated exosomal miRNA in causing insulin resistance and associated T2D. Moreover, this opens the possibility of the usage of circulating miRNAs as relevant biomarkers of obesity and insulin resistance phenotypes in obesity and T2D. However, since obesity is known to be a trigger for the development of insulin resistance and consequently T2D, it is of great importance to determine the origin of circulating miRNAs and, more importantly, their relationship with abnormal adipose tissue, as well as a mechanism of their action in the target tissue. Therefore, this review aims to present and emphasize the significance of circulatory exosomal-derived miRNAs originating from obesity-changed adipose tissue in the development of insulin resistance, a key mechanism that leads to the development of T2D.

3.3. The Involvement of Adipose Tissue-Derived Exosomal miRNAs in Adipose Tissue Inflammation During Obesity

Exosomal miRNAs are significantly involved in the initiation and prolongation of inflammation associated with the expansion of adipose tissue in obesity, which is mediated by the activation of immune cells, mainly macrophages (Table 1). Infiltration of macrophages into adipose tissue is a crucial factor that induces dysfunction of adipose tissue, thus contributing to the induction of inflammation and related metabolic disorders [99].

The most investigated exosomal miRNA involved in the induction of adipose tissue inflammation is miR-155, whose increased expression is shown in circulation and adipose tissue in obesity, more so in adipose tissue macrophages than in adipocytes [100]. Adipocyte-derived exosomal miR-155 can be transferred to adipose tissue macrophages, where it triggers inflammation by promoting the inflammatory STAT1 signaling pathway and suppressing the anti-inflammatory STAT6 pathway through the activation of the pro-inflammatory M1 macrophages [51,58]. Moreover, the expression of miR-155 in a significantly increased number of adipose tissue macrophages may be the first sign of the upcoming development of systematic inflammation, as it was shown that the increase in the expression of this miRNA is present despite the increase in adipocyte markers of inflammation such as IL6, C-reactive protein, and TNF-α [100]. Besides M1 macrophage activation, miRNAs affect the polarization of anti-inflammatory M2 macrophages. An increased level of adipocyte-derived exosomal miRNAs, such as miR-34a, miR-130b, or miR-1224, inhibit anti-inflammatory M2 macrophages activation by suppressing Krüppel-like factor 4 (KLF4), peroxisome proliferator-activated receptor (PPAR-γ), or Wnt/β-catenin signaling pathways, respectively, thus contributing to the exacerbation of obesity-induced adipose tissue inflammation [101–103]. However, Pan et al. showed that adipose tissue-specific deletion of miR-34a reduced local and systemic inflammation through enhanced polarization of macrophages from M1 to M2 phenotype [102]. Besides adipose tissue inflammation, increased expression of the same miR-34a also induces metabolic inflammation and insulin resistance, effects that are shown to be reversed by specific ablation of miR-34a [102]. The polarization of macrophages from M1 to M2 phenotype is also regulated by modulation of PPAR-γ activation, which is ultimately mediated by a change in miR-130b expression [103]. Accordingly, it can be concluded that exosomal miRNAs originating from adipocytes significantly contribute to the development of inflammation in obesity, primarily by polarizing macrophages and modulating the activation of related signaling pathways.

3.4. The Involvement of Adipose Tissue-Derived Exosomal miRNAs in the Induction of Insulin Resistance and Type 2 Diabetes

Obesity is the most significant risk factor in the development of insulin resistance, which is a major pathological mechanism that leads to the development of T2D. Based on the published data, it can be assumed that exosomes and their cargo act as communication media in obesity-induced insulin resistance [104]. There is a growing number of evidence of the involvement of miRNAs in the induction and promotion of insulin resistance associated with obesity (Table 1). Previously mentioned adipose tissue macrophage-derived exosomal miR-155 suppresses PPAR-γ and reduces the expression of PPAR-γ target gene glucose transporter type 4 (GLUT4), thus contributing to the development of insulin resistance by inhibiting insulin signaling and glucose tolerance in adipocytes and skeletal muscle [100,105,106]. Overexpression of miR-155 derived from adipose tissue macrophages plays an important role in reducing insulin sensitivity through PPAR-γ down-regulation and suppression of Akt phosphorylation in hepatocytes [105]. However, an investigation of the impact of the complete deletion of miR-155 showed protection from high-fat-diet-induced insulin resistance and glucose tolerance in mice, not just in adipocytes, but also in other insulin-sensitive tissues. A similar effect was shown for adipose tissue-derived exosomal miR-27a. Elevated expression of miR-27a transferred by exosomes from adipocytes to skeletal muscle cells also suppresses PPAR-γ, which ultimately leads to insulin resistance and impairment of insulin-dependent glucose uptake in skeletal muscle [106,107]. In addition, overexpressed miR-29 in adipose tissue macrophage-derived exosomes can be transferred into adipocytes, myocytes, and hepatocytes, which promotes insulin resistance by targeting PPAR-δ [108]. Furthermore, adipose tissue-derived exosomal miR-222 induces insulin resistance in skeletal muscle, but also in hepatocytes, by inhibiting IRS1 [109]. Up-regulation of this miRNA was shown to reduce the expression of GLUT4 and, therefore, glucose uptake in adipocytes [110].

In addition to modulating metabolism in adipocytes and skeletal muscle, exosomal miRNAs derived from adipose tissue also modulate liver metabolism. In contrast to the previously mentioned reduction in insulin sensitivity by overexpression of adipose tissue macrophage-derived exosomal miR-155, it has been shown that a decreased expression of miR-141-3p in adipocyte-derived exosomes transferred to hepatocytes contributes to the development of insulin resistance and reduced glucose uptake by hepatocytes [111], as seen in the case of miR-141-3p. The molecular mechanism involves the inhibition of Akt phosphorylation through the activation of phosphatase and tensin homolog deleted on chromosome ten (PTEN), mediated by a decrease in the expression of miR-141-3p in adipocyte-derived exosomes during obesity.

3.5. The Effect of Adipose Tissue-Derived Exosomal miRNAs on the Homeostasis of Pancreatic β-Cells

Adipose tissue-derived exosomal miRNAs affect pancreatic β-cells, although direct crosstalk between adipocytes and pancreatic β-cells mediated by exosomes and their cargo remains unclear. In general, adipose tissue-derived extracellular vesicles have a positive or negative effect on the survival, proliferation, and function of pancreatic β-cells and human pancreatic islets, depending on the state of obesity [112]. The change in the miRNA profile in adipocytes related to obesity induces local, but also systemic inflammation and the development of insulin resistance, and this effect can impact β-cells homeostasis [112]. For example, in vitro analysis demonstrated that the up-regulation of miR-155 in adipocyte-derived vesicles treated with inflammatory cytokines has a significant role in glucose and lipid metabolism, as well as β-cell function. In addition, an increased level of miR-30a-5p in cytokine-treated adipocyte-derived vesicles was shown to be related to β-cell dysfunction, while miR-146 was shown to be related to the induction of apoptosis of β-cells.

Table 1. Role of key miRNAs associated with obesity, insulin resistance, and T2D.

miRNA	Target Molecules	Signaling Pathways	Role in Obesity, Insulin Resistance and T2D	Reference
miR-27a	PPAR-γ	PPAR	Increased insulin resistance and impairment of insulin-dependent glucose uptake in skeletal muscle	[106] [107]
miR-29a	PPAR-δ	PPAR	Promotes insulin resistance in adipocytes, myocytes, and hepatocytes	[108]
miR-222	IRS1, GLUT4	Insulin signaling	Induces insulin resistance in skeletal muscle and hepatocytes. Reduces glucose uptake in adipocytes	[109] [110]
miR-144	IRS1	Insulin signaling	Impairs insulin signaling A potential therapeutic target in T2D	[88] [89]
miR-378a	C/EBPα, PGC-1β	PGC-1, adipogenesis	Enhances lipid storage and reduces thermogenesis	[113]
miR-103/107	Caveolin-1	Insulin signaling	Impair insulin sensitivity and glucose homeostasis. Promote adipocyte expansion	[114]
miR-34a	KLF4	-	Inhibits M2 macrophage activation	[102]
miR-130b	PPAR-γ	PPAR	Inhibits M2 macrophage activation	[103]
miR-1224	MSI2	Wnt/β-catenin	Inhibits M2 macrophage activation	[101]
miR-155	STAT1, STAT6, PPAR-γ/GLUT4	JAK/STAT, PPAR	Regulates inflammation in obesity. Modulates insulin signaling and glucose tolerance	[51] [58] [105] [100]

Abbreviations: T2D, type 2 diabetes; PPAR, peroxisome proliferator-activated receptor; IRS1, insulin receptor substrate 1; GLUT4, glucose transporter type 4; C/EBP, CCAAT-enhancer-binding proteins; PGC, peroxisome proliferator-activated receptor-gamma coactivator; KLF, Krüppel-like factor; MSI2, Musashi RNA binding protein; STAT, signal transducer and activator of transcription; JAK, Janus kinase; miR, microRNA.

4. Conclusions and Future Directions

In conclusion, there is an undeniable link between obesity and T2D, with insulin resistance serving as the bridge between the two conditions, alongside altered expression of various miRNAs. miRNAs play a crucial role, as they are transported by exosomes—small extracellular vesicles—not only to nearby tissues but also systemically to distant ones, where they exert their effects. Since exosome-derived miRNAs are found in nearly all body fluids, including plasma and serum, they have potential as easily accessible biomarkers for different stages of the disease and could serve as therapeutic targets by modulating their expression to influence disease progression. However, several challenges such as stability, reproducibility, efficient delivery carriers, and minimization of off-target effects and toxicity need to be addressed to uncover their full potential in clinical use. Continuous research and technological advancements are, therefore, essential to overcome these issues and utilize the diagnostic and therapeutic properties of miRNAs.

Given the significant advancements in research on exosome-derived miRNAs in obesity and T2D, adipocyte-derived exosomal miRNAs associated with insulin resistance may be reliable biomarkers of insulin resistance and the development of T2D. Additionally, they hold promise for therapeutic applications. Some studies have already shown that administering miRNA mimics or anti-miRNAs has potential in the treatment of T2D [115]. However, further research is necessary due to the large number of dysregulated miRNAs involved in insulin resistance, as well as uncertainties around the concentration and delivery of such therapies to the target tissues through circulation. Finally, one thing is certain: the awarding of the Nobel Prize in 2024 for the discovery of miRNA will reignite interest and bring miRNA research into focus. How we manage and apply the knowledge that has accumulated over the years remains to be seen.

Author Contributions: Conceptualization and design of the article, B.Š., I.V., S.K. and D.D.; literature research, I.V., B.Š., S.B., A.-M.L.P. and A.B.; writing—original draft preparation, I.V., B.Š., D.D. and S.B.; supervision, S.K., A.B., D.R. and D.D.; writing—review and editing, all authors. All authors have read and agreed to the published version of the manuscript.

Funding: The review relates to projects funded by the University of Rijeka, Croatia; project No. uniri-biomed-23-285, uniri-biomed-23-243, and uniri-biomed-23-54.

Data Availability Statement: No new data were created or analyzed in this study. Data sharing is not applicable to this article.

Conflicts of Interest: The authors declare no conflicts of interest.

References

1. Phelps, N.H.; Singleton, R.K.; Zhou, B.; Heap, R.A.; Mishra, A.; Bennett, J.E.; Paciorek, C.J.; Lhoste, V.P.; Carrillo-Larco, R.M.; Stevens, G.A.; et al. Worldwide Trends in Underweight and Obesity from 1990 to 2022: A Pooled Analysis of 3663 Population-Representative Studies with 222 Million Children, Adolescents, and Adults. *Lancet* **2024**, *403*, 1027–1050. [CrossRef] [PubMed]
2. Loos, R.J.F.; Yeo, G.S.H. The Genetics of Obesity: From Discovery to Biology. *Nat. Rev. Genet.* **2022**, *23*, 120–133. [CrossRef]
3. Adams, K.F.; Schatzkin, A.; Harris, T.B.; Kipnis, V.; Mouw, T.; Ballard-Barbash, R.; Hollenbeck, A.; Leitzmann, M.F. Overweight, Obesity, and Mortality in a Large Prospective Cohort of Persons 50 to 71 Years Old. *N. Engl. J. Med.* **2006**, *355*, 763–778. [CrossRef]
4. Bray, G.A. Obesity: A 100 Year Perspective. *Int. J. Obes.* **2024**. [CrossRef]
5. Deehan, E.C.; Mocanu, V.; Madsen, K.L. Effects of Dietary Fibre on Metabolic Health and Obesity. *Nat. Rev. Gastroenterol. Hepatol.* **2024**, *21*, 301–318. [CrossRef]
6. Hu, T.; Liu, C.-H.; Lei, M.; Zeng, Q.; Li, L.; Tang, H.; Zhang, N. Metabolic Regulation of the Immune System in Health and Diseases: Mechanisms and Interventions. *Signal Transduct. Target. Ther.* **2024**, *9*, 268. [CrossRef]
7. Pescador, N.; Pérez-Barba, M.; Ibarra, J.M.; Corbatón, A.; Martínez-Larrad, M.T.; Serrano-Ríos, M. Serum Circulating microRNA Profiling for Identification of Potential Type 2 Diabetes and Obesity Biomarkers. *PLoS ONE* **2013**, *8*, e77251. [CrossRef]
8. Fabbri, M. MicroRNAs and miRceptors: A New Mechanism of Action for Intercellular Communication. *Philos. Trans. R. Soc. B* **2018**, *373*, 20160486. [CrossRef]
9. Jung, S.H.; Park, H.S.; Kim, K.-S.; Choi, W.H.; Ahn, C.W.; Kim, B.T.; Kim, S.M.; Lee, S.Y.; Ahn, S.M.; Kim, Y.K.; et al. Effect of Weight Loss on Some Serum Cytokines in Human Obesity: Increase in IL-10 after Weight Loss. *J. Nutr. Biochem.* **2008**, *19*, 371–375. [CrossRef] [PubMed]
10. Hagberg, C.E.; Spalding, K.L. White Adipocyte Dysfunction and Obesity-Associated Pathologies in Humans. *Nat. Rev. Mol. Cell Biol.* **2024**, *25*, 270–289. [CrossRef]
11. Wensveen, F.M.; Jelenčić, V.; Valentić, S.; Šestan, M.; Wensveen, T.T.; Theurich, S.; Glasner, A.; Mendrila, D.; Štimac, D.; Wunderlich, F.T.; et al. NK Cells Link Obesity-Induced Adipose Stress to Inflammation and Insulin Resistance. *Nat. Immunol.* **2015**, *16*, 376–385. [CrossRef] [PubMed]
12. Mosser, D.M.; Edwards, J.P. Exploring the Full Spectrum of Macrophage Activation. *Nat. Rev. Immunol.* **2008**, *8*, 958–969. [CrossRef] [PubMed]
13. Gordon, S.; Martinez, F.O. Alternative Activation of Macrophages: Mechanism and Functions. *Immunity* **2010**, *32*, 593–604. [CrossRef] [PubMed]
14. Hotamisligil, G.S.; Arner, P.; Caro, J.F.; Atkinson, R.L.; Spiegelman, B.M. Increased Adipose Tissue Expression of Tumor Necrosis Factor-Alpha in Human Obesity and Insulin Resistance. *J. Clin. Investig.* **1995**, *95*, 2409–2415. [CrossRef]
15. Fink, L.N.; Costford, S.R.; Lee, Y.S.; Jensen, T.E.; Bilan, P.J.; Oberbach, A.; Blüher, M.; Olefsky, J.M.; Sams, A.; Klip, A. Pro-Inflammatory Macrophages Increase in Skeletal Muscle of High fat-Fed Mice and Correlate with Metabolic Risk Markers in Humans. *Obesity* **2014**, *22*, 747–757. [CrossRef]
16. Lumeng, C.N.; Bodzin, J.L.; Saltiel, A.R. Obesity Induces a Phenotypic Switch in Adipose Tissue Macrophage Polarization. *J. Clin. Investig.* **2007**, *117*, 175–184. [CrossRef] [PubMed]
17. Morinaga, H.; Mayoral, R.; Heinrichsdorff, J.; Osborn, O.; Franck, N.; Hah, N.; Walenta, E.; Bandyopadhyay, G.; Pessentheiner, A.R.; Chi, T.J.; et al. Characterization of Distinct Subpopulations of Hepatic Macrophages in HFD/Obese Mice. *Diabetes* **2015**, *64*, 1120–1130. [CrossRef]

18. Ivey, K.N.; Srivastava, D. microRNAs as Developmental Regulators. *Cold Spring Harb. Perspect. Biol.* **2015**, *7*, a008144. [CrossRef]
19. McKernan, K.; Varghese, M.; Patel, R.; Singer, K. Role of TLR4 in the Induction of Inflammatory Changes in Adipocytes and Macrophages. *Adipocyte* **2020**, *9*, 212–222. [CrossRef]
20. Mukherjee, S.; Skrede, S.; Haugstøyl, M.; López, M.; Fernø, J. Peripheral and Central Macrophages in Obesity. *Front. Endocrinol.* **2023**, *14*, 1232171. [CrossRef]
21. Margolis, L.; Sadovsky, Y. The Biology of Extracellular Vesicles: The Known Unknowns. *PLoS Biol.* **2019**, *17*, e3000363. [CrossRef] [PubMed]
22. Onyango, E.M.; Onyango, B.M. The Rise of Noncommunicable Diseases in Kenya: An Examination of the Time Trends and Contribution of the Changes in Diet and Physical Inactivity. *J. Epidemiol. Glob. Health* **2018**, *8*, 1–7. [CrossRef] [PubMed]
23. Kadiki, O.A.; Reddy, M.R.S.; Marzouk, A.A. Incidence of Insulin-Dependent Diabetes (IDDM) and Non-Insulin-Dependent Diabetes (NIDDM) (0–34 Years at Onset) in Benghazi, Libya. *Diabetes Res. Clin. Pract.* **1996**, *32*, 165–173. [CrossRef] [PubMed]
24. Glass, C.K.; Olefsky, J.M. Inflammation and Lipid Signaling in the Etiology of Insulin Resistance. *Cell Metab.* **2012**, *15*, 635–645. [CrossRef] [PubMed]
25. Hotamisligil, G.S.; Shargill, N.S.; Spiegelman, B.M. Adipose Expression of Tumor Necrosis Factor-α: Direct Role in Obesity-Linked Insulin Resistance. *Science* **1993**, *259*, 87–91. [CrossRef]
26. Hotamisligil, G.S.; Peraldi, P.; Budavari, A.; Ellis, R.; White, M.F.; Spiegelman, B.M. IRS-1-Mediated Inhibition of Insulin Receptor Tyrosine Kinase Activity in TNF-α- and Obesity-Induced Insulin Resistance. *Science* **1996**, *271*, 665–670. [CrossRef] [PubMed]
27. Lu, X.; Xie, Q.; Pan, X.; Zhang, R.; Zhang, X.; Peng, G.; Zhang, Y.; Shen, S.; Tong, N. Type 2 Diabetes Mellitus in Adults: Pathogenesis, Prevention and Therapy. *Signal Transduct. Target. Ther.* **2024**, *9*, 262. [CrossRef] [PubMed]
28. Merrill, A.H. De Novo Sphingolipid Biosynthesis: A Necessary, but Dangerous, Pathway. *J. Biol. Chem.* **2002**, *277*, 25843–25846. [CrossRef] [PubMed]
29. Matoba, K.; Takeda, Y.; Nagai, Y.; Kawanami, D.; Utsunomiya, K.; Nishimura, R. Unraveling the Role of Inflammation in the Pathogenesis of Diabetic Kidney Disease. *Int. J. Mol. Sci.* **2019**, *20*, 3393. [CrossRef]
30. Sheu, M.L.; Ho, F.M.; Yang, R.S.; Chao, K.F.; Lin, W.W.; Lin-Shiau, S.Y.; Liu, S.-H. High Glucose Induces Human Endothelial Cell Apoptosis Through a Phosphoinositide 3-Kinase–Regulated Cyclooxygenase-2 Pathway. *Arter. Thromb. Vasc. Biol.* **2005**, *25*, 539–545. [CrossRef] [PubMed]
31. Tian, S.; Zhao, H.; Song, H. Shared Signaling Pathways and Targeted Therapy by Natural Bioactive Compounds for Obesity and Type 2 Diabetes. *Crit. Rev. Food Sci. Nutr.* **2024**, *64*, 5039–5056. [CrossRef] [PubMed]
32. Yung, J.H.M.; Giacca, A. Role of C-Jun N-Terminal Kinase (JNK) in Obesity and Type 2 Diabetes. *Cells* **2020**, *9*, 706. [CrossRef]
33. Solinas, G.; Becattini, B. JNK at the Crossroad of Obesity, Insulin Resistance, and Cell Stress Response. *Mol. Metab.* **2017**, *6*, 174–184. [CrossRef] [PubMed]
34. Chen, Y.-F.; Luh, F.; Ho, Y.-S.; Yen, Y. Exosomes: A Review of Biologic Function, Diagnostic and Targeted Therapy Applications, and Clinical Trials. *J. Biomed. Sci.* **2024**, *31*, 67. [CrossRef] [PubMed]
35. Zhang, Y.; Liu, Y.; Liu, H.; Tang, W.H. Exosomes: Biogenesis, Biologic Function and Clinical Potential. *Cell Biosci.* **2019**, *9*, 19. [CrossRef]
36. Larios, J.; Mercier, V.; Roux, A.; Gruenberg, J. ALIX- and ESCRT-III–Dependent Sorting of Tetraspanins to Exosomes. *J. Cell Biol.* **2020**, *219*, e201904113. [CrossRef] [PubMed]
37. Murphy, D.E.; De Jong, O.G.; Brouwer, M.; Wood, M.J.; Lavieu, G.; Schiffelers, R.M.; Vader, P. Extracellular Vesicle-Based Therapeutics: Natural versus Engineered Targeting and Trafficking. *Exp. Mol. Med.* **2019**, *51*, 32. [CrossRef] [PubMed]
38. Trajkovic, K.; Hsu, C.; Chiantia, S.; Rajendran, L.; Wenzel, D.; Wieland, F.; Schwille, P.; Brügger, B.; Simons, M. Ceramide Triggers Budding of Exosome Vesicles into Multivesicular Endosomes. *Science* **2008**, *319*, 1244–1247. [CrossRef] [PubMed]
39. Skotland, T.; Sagini, K.; Sandvig, K.; Llorente, A. An Emerging Focus on Lipids in Extracellular Vesicles. *Adv. Drug Deliv. Rev.* **2020**, *159*, 308–321. [CrossRef]
40. O'Brien, K.; Breyne, K.; Ughetto, S.; Laurent, L.C.; Breakefield, X.O. RNA Delivery by Extracellular Vesicles in Mammalian Cells and Its Applications. *Nat. Rev. Mol. Cell Biol.* **2020**, *21*, 585–606. [CrossRef]
41. Mori, M.A.; Ludwig, R.G.; Garcia-Martin, R.; Brandão, B.B.; Kahn, C.R. Extracellular miRNAs: From Biomarkers to Mediators of Physiology and Disease. *Cell Metab.* **2019**, *30*, 656–673. [CrossRef] [PubMed]
42. Shang, R.; Lee, S.; Senavirathne, G.; Lai, E.C. microRNAs in Action: Biogenesis, Function and Regulation. *Nat. Rev. Genet.* **2023**, *24*, 816–833. [CrossRef] [PubMed]
43. Landrier, J.-F.; Derghal, A.; Mounien, L. MicroRNAs in Obesity and Related Metabolic Disorders. *Cells* **2019**, *8*, 859. [CrossRef] [PubMed]
44. Ludwig, N.; Leidinger, P.; Becker, K.; Backes, C.; Fehlmann, T.; Pallasch, C.; Rheinheimer, S.; Meder, B.; Stähler, C.; Meese, E.; et al. Distribution of miRNA Expression across Human Tissues. *Nucleic Acids Res.* **2016**, *44*, 3865–3877. [CrossRef] [PubMed]
45. Correia De Sousa, M.; Gjorgjieva, M.; Dolicka, D.; Sobolewski, C.; Foti, M. Deciphering miRNAs' Action through miRNA Editing. *Int. J. Mol. Sci.* **2019**, *20*, 6249. [CrossRef] [PubMed]
46. Saliminejad, K.; Khorram Khorshid, H.R.; Soleymani Fard, S.; Ghaffari, S.H. An Overview of microRNAs: Biology, Functions, Therapeutics, and Analysis Methods. *J. Cell. Physiol.* **2019**, *234*, 5451–5465. [CrossRef]
47. Bhome, R.; Del Vecchio, F.; Lee, G.-H.; Bullock, M.D.; Primrose, J.N.; Sayan, A.E.; Mirnezami, A.H. Exosomal microRNAs (exomiRs): Small Molecules with a Big Role in Cancer. *Cancer Lett.* **2018**, *420*, 228–235. [CrossRef]

48. Van den Brande, S.; Gijbels, M.; Wynant, N.; Santos, D.; Mingels, L.; Gansemans, Y.; Van Nieuwerburgh, F.; Vanden Broeck, J. The Presence of Extracellular microRNAs in the Media of Cultured Drosophila Cells. *Sci. Rep.* **2018**, *8*, 17312. [CrossRef] [PubMed]
49. Isaac, R.; Reis, F.C.G.; Ying, W.; Olefsky, J.M. Exosomes as Mediators of Intercellular Crosstalk in Metabolism. *Cell Metab.* **2021**, *33*, 1744–1762. [CrossRef]
50. Castaño, C.; Kalko, S.; Novials, A.; Párrizas, M. Obesity-Associated Exosomal miRNAs Modulate Glucose and Lipid Metabolism in Mice. *Proc. Natl. Acad. Sci. USA* **2018**, *115*, 12158–12163. [CrossRef]
51. Kwan, H.Y.; Chen, M.; Xu, K.; Chen, B. The Impact of Obesity on Adipocyte-Derived Extracellular Vesicles. *Cell. Mol. Life Sci.* **2021**, *78*, 7275–7288. [CrossRef]
52. He, X.; Kuang, G.; Wu, Y.; Ou, C. Emerging Roles of Exosomal miRNAs in Diabetes Mellitus. *Clin. Transl. Med.* **2021**, *11*, e468. [CrossRef]
53. Lange, T.; Stracke, S.; Rettig, R.; Lendeckel, U.; Kuhn, J.; Schlüter, R.; Rippe, V.; Endlich, K.; Endlich, N. Identification of miR-16 as an Endogenous Reference Gene for the Normalization of Urinary Exosomal miRNA Expression Data from CKD Patients. *PLoS ONE* **2017**, *12*, e0183435. [CrossRef]
54. Ruze, R.; Liu, T.; Zou, X.; Song, J.; Chen, Y.; Xu, R.; Yin, X.; Xu, Q. Obesity and Type 2 Diabetes Mellitus: Connections in Epidemiology, Pathogenesis, and Treatments. *Front. Endocrinol.* **2023**, *14*, 1161521. [CrossRef]
55. Benavides-Aguilar, J.A.; Torres-Copado, A.; Isidoro-Sánchez, J.; Pathak, S.; Duttaroy, A.K.; Banerjee, A.; Paul, S. The Regulatory Role of MicroRNAs in Obesity and Obesity-Derived Ailments. *Genes* **2023**, *14*, 2070. [CrossRef]
56. Heyn, G.S.; Corrêa, L.H.; Magalhães, K.G. The Impact of Adipose Tissue–Derived miRNAs in Metabolic Syndrome, Obesity, and Cancer. *Front. Endocrinol.* **2020**, *11*, 563816. [CrossRef] [PubMed]
57. Tonyan, Z.N.; Barbitoff, Y.A.; Nasykhova, Y.A.; Danilova, M.M.; Kozyulina, P.Y.; Mikhailova, A.A.; Bulgakova, O.L.; Vlasova, M.E.; Golovkin, N.V.; Glotov, A.S. Plasma microRNA Profiling in Type 2 Diabetes Mellitus: A Pilot Study. *Int. J. Mol. Sci.* **2023**, *24*, 17406. [CrossRef] [PubMed]
58. Brandao, B.B.; Lino, M.; Kahn, C.R. Extracellular miRNAs as Mediators of Obesity-Associated Disease. *J. Physiol.* **2022**, *600*, 1155–1169. [CrossRef] [PubMed]
59. Lino, M.; Garcia-Martin, R.; Muñoz, V.R.; Ruiz, G.P.; Nawaz, A.; Brandão, B.B.; Dreyfus, J.; Pan, H.; Kahn, C.R. Multi-Step Regulation of microRNA Expression and Secretion into Small Extracellular Vesicles by Insulin. *Cell Rep.* **2024**, *43*, 114491. [CrossRef]
60. Ji, C.; Guo, X. The Clinical Potential of Circulating microRNAs in Obesity. *Nat. Rev. Endocrinol.* **2019**, *15*, 731–743. [CrossRef]
61. Grasedieck, S.; Sorrentino, A.; Langer, C.; Buske, C.; Döhner, H.; Mertens, D.; Kuchenbauer, F. Circulating microRNAs in Hematological Diseases: Principles, Challenges, and Perspectives. *Blood* **2013**, *121*, 4977–4984. [CrossRef] [PubMed]
62. Kupec, T.; Bleilevens, A.; Iborra, S.; Najjari, L.; Wittenborn, J.; Maurer, J.; Stickeler, E. Stability of Circulating microRNAs in Serum. *PLoS ONE* **2022**, *17*, e0268958. [CrossRef]
63. Gareev, I.; Beylerli, O.; Yang, G.; Sun, J.; Pavlov, V.; Izmailov, A.; Shi, H.; Zhao, S. The Current State of MiRNAs as Biomarkers and Therapeutic Tools. *Clin. Exp. Med.* **2020**, *20*, 349–359. [CrossRef] [PubMed]
64. Momin, M.Y.; Gaddam, R.R.; Kravitz, M.; Gupta, A.; Vikram, A. The Challenges and Opportunities in the Development of MicroRNA Therapeutics: A Multidisciplinary Viewpoint. *Cells* **2021**, *10*, 3097. [CrossRef] [PubMed]
65. Pagoni, M.; Cava, C.; Sideris, D.C.; Avgeris, M.; Zoumpourlis, V.; Michalopoulos, I.; Drakoulis, N. miRNA-Based Technologies in Cancer Therapy. *J. Pers. Med.* **2023**, *13*, 1586. [CrossRef] [PubMed]
66. Segal, M.; Slack, F.J. Challenges Identifying Efficacious miRNA Therapeutics for Cancer. *Expert Opin. Drug Discov.* **2020**, *15*, 987–991. [CrossRef]
67. Grillone, K.; Caridà, G.; Luciano, F.; Cordua, A.; Di Martino, M.T.; Tagliaferri, P.; Tassone, P. A Systematic Review of Non-Coding RNA Therapeutics in Early Clinical Trials: A New Perspective against Cancer. *J. Transl. Med.* **2024**, *22*, 731. [CrossRef] [PubMed]
68. Hong, D.S.; Kang, Y.-K.; Borad, M.; Sachdev, J.; Ejadi, S.; Lim, H.Y.; Brenner, A.J.; Park, K.; Lee, J.-L.; Kim, T.-Y.; et al. Phase 1 Study of MRX34, a Liposomal miR-34a Mimic, in Patients with Advanced Solid Tumours. *Br. J. Cancer* **2020**, *122*, 1630–1637. [CrossRef]
69. Dai, M.; Li, L.; Qin, X. Clinical Value of miRNA-122 in the Diagnosis and Prognosis of Various Types of Cancer. *Oncol. Lett.* **2019**, *17*, 3919–3929. [CrossRef]
70. Carpi, S.; Daniele, S.; De Almeida, J.F.M.; Gabbia, D. Recent Advances in miRNA-Based Therapy for MASLD/MASH and MASH-Associated HCC. *Int. J. Mol. Sci.* **2024**, *25*, 12229. [CrossRef] [PubMed]
71. Mandal, S. New Molecular Biomarkers in Precise Diagnosis and Therapy of Type 2 Diabetes. *Health Technol.* **2020**, *10*, 601–608. [CrossRef]
72. Abbasi, A.; Sahlqvist, A.-S.; Lotta, L.; Brosnan, J.M.; Vollenweider, P.; Giabbanelli, P.; Nunez, D.J.; Waterworth, D.; Scott, R.A.; Langenberg, C.; et al. A Systematic Review of Biomarkers and Risk of Incident Type 2 Diabetes: An Overview of Epidemiological, Prediction and Aetiological Research Literature. *PLoS ONE* **2016**, *11*, e0163721. [CrossRef] [PubMed]
73. Paul, P.; Chakraborty, A.; Sarkar, D.; Langthasa, M.; Rahman, M.; Bari, M.; Singha, R.S.; Malakar, A.K.; Chakraborty, S. Interplay between miRNAs and Human Diseases. *J. Cell. Physiol.* **2018**, *233*, 2007–2018. [CrossRef]
74. Turchinovich, A.; Weiz, L.; Langheinz, A.; Burwinkel, B. Characterization of Extracellular Circulating microRNA. *Nucleic Acids Res.* **2011**, *39*, 7223–7233. [CrossRef] [PubMed]
75. O'Brien, J.; Hayder, H.; Zayed, Y.; Peng, C. Overview of MicroRNA Biogenesis, Mechanisms of Actions, and Circulation. *Front. Endocrinol.* **2018**, *9*, 402. [CrossRef]

76. Gayosso-Gómez, L.V.; Ortiz-Quintero, B. Circulating MicroRNAs in Blood and Other Body Fluids as Biomarkers for Diagnosis, Prognosis, and Therapy Response in Lung Cancer. *Diagnostics* **2021**, *11*, 421. [CrossRef]
77. Wang, F.; Chen, C.; Wang, D. Circulating microRNAs in Cardiovascular Diseases: From Biomarkers to Therapeutic Targets. *Front. Med.* **2014**, *8*, 404–418. [CrossRef] [PubMed]
78. Kumar, A.; Su, Y.; Sharma, M.; Singh, S.; Kim, S.; Peavey, J.J.; Suerken, C.K.; Lockhart, S.N.; Whitlow, C.T.; Craft, S.; et al. MicroRNA Expression in Extracellular Vesicles as a Novel Blood-based Biomarker for Alzheimer's Disease. *Alzheimer's Dement.* **2023**, *19*, 4952–4966. [CrossRef] [PubMed]
79. Zeng, L.; Cui, J.; Wu, H.; Lu, Q. The Emerging Role of Circulating microRNAs as Biomarkers in Autoimmune Diseases. *Autoimmunity* **2014**, *47*, 419–429. [CrossRef]
80. Zhang, L.; Wu, H.; Zhao, M.; Chang, C.; Lu, Q. Clinical Significance of miRNAs in Autoimmunity. *J. Autoimmun.* **2020**, *109*, 102438. [CrossRef] [PubMed]
81. Wang, X.; He, Y.; Mackowiak, B.; Gao, B. MicroRNAs as Regulators, Biomarkers and Therapeutic Targets in Liver Diseases. *Gut* **2021**, *70*, 784–795. [CrossRef]
82. Liu, X.; Pan, Q.; Cao, H.; Xin, F.; Zhao, Z.; Yang, R.; Zeng, J.; Zhou, H.; Fan, J. Lipotoxic Hepatocyte-Derived Exosomal MicroRNA 192-5p Activates Macrophages Through Rictor/Akt/Forkhead Box Transcription Factor O1 Signaling in Nonalcoholic Fatty Liver Disease. *Hepatology* **2020**, *72*, 454–469. [CrossRef] [PubMed]
83. Das, K.; Rao, L.V.M. The Role of microRNAs in Inflammation. *Int. J. Mol. Sci.* **2022**, *23*, 15479. [CrossRef]
84. Conti, I.; Varano, G.; Simioni, C.; Laface, I.; Milani, D.; Rimondi, E.; Neri, L.M. miRNAs as Influencers of Cell–Cell Communication in Tumor Microenvironment. *Cells* **2020**, *9*, 220. [CrossRef]
85. Sepúlveda, F.; Mayorga-Lobos, C.; Guzmán, K.; Durán-Jara, E.; Lobos-González, L. EV-miRNA-Mediated Intercellular Communication in the Breast Tumor Microenvironment. *Int. J. Mol. Sci.* **2023**, *24*, 13085. [CrossRef]
86. Zatterale, F.; Longo, M.; Naderi, J.; Raciti, G.A.; Desiderio, A.; Miele, C.; Beguinot, F. Chronic Adipose Tissue Inflammation Linking Obesity to Insulin Resistance and Type 2 Diabetes. *Front. Physiol.* **2020**, *10*, 1607. [CrossRef] [PubMed]
87. Chao, Y.; Gu, T.; Zhang, Z.; Wu, T.; Wang, J.; Bi, Y. The Role of MIRNAS Carried by Extracellular Vesicles in Type 2 Diabetes and Its Complications. *J. Diabetes* **2023**, *15*, 838–852. [CrossRef] [PubMed]
88. Karolina, D.S.; Armugam, A.; Tavintharan, S.; Wong, M.T.K.; Lim, S.C.; Sum, C.F.; Jeyaseelan, K. MicroRNA 144 Impairs Insulin Signaling by Inhibiting the Expression of Insulin Receptor Substrate 1 in Type 2 Diabetes Mellitus. *PLoS ONE* **2011**, *6*, e22839. [CrossRef]
89. Karolina, D.S.; Armugam, A.; Tavintharan, S.; Wong, M.T.K.; Lim, S.C.; Sum, C.F.; Jeyaseelan, K. Correction: MicroRNA 144 Impairs Insulin Signaling by Inhibiting the Expression of Insulin Receptor Substrate 1 in Type 2 Diabetes Mellitus. *PLoS ONE* **2011**, *6*. [CrossRef]
90. Azzimato, V.; Chen, P.; Barreby, E.; Morgantini, C.; Levi, L.; Vankova, A.; Jager, J.; Sulen, A.; Diotallevi, M.; Shen, J.X.; et al. Hepatic miR-144 Drives Fumarase Activity Preventing NRF2 Activation During Obesity. *Gastroenterology* **2021**, *161*, 1982–1997.e11. [CrossRef] [PubMed]
91. Wang, R.; Hong, J.; Cao, Y.; Shi, J.; Gu, W.; Ning, G.; Zhang, Y.; Wang, W. Elevated Circulating microRNA-122 Is Associated with Obesity and Insulin Resistance in Young Adults. *Eur. J. Endocrinol.* **2015**, *172*, 291–300. [CrossRef] [PubMed]
92. Hess, A.L.; Larsen, L.H.; Udesen, P.B.; Sanz, Y.; Larsen, T.M.; Dalgaard, L.T. Levels of Circulating miR-122 Are Associated with Weight Loss and Metabolic Syndrome. *Obesity* **2020**, *28*, 493–501. [CrossRef] [PubMed]
93. Willeit, P.; Skroblin, P.; Moschen, A.R.; Yin, X.; Kaudewitz, D.; Zampetaki, A.; Barwari, T.; Whitehead, M.; Ramírez, C.M.; Goedeke, L.; et al. Circulating MicroRNA-122 Is Associated With the Risk of New-Onset Metabolic Syndrome and Type 2 Diabetes. *Diabetes* **2017**, *66*, 347–357. [CrossRef]
94. Párrizas, M.; Brugnara, L.; Esteban, Y.; González-Franquesa, A.; Canivell, S.; Murillo, S.; Gordillo-Bastidas, E.; Cussó, R.; Cadefau, J.A.; García-Roves, P.M.; et al. Circulating miR-192 and miR-193b Are Markers of Prediabetes and Are Modulated by an Exercise Intervention. *J. Clin. Endocrinol. Metab.* **2015**, *100*, E407–E415. [CrossRef] [PubMed]
95. Hu, H.; Zhao, M.; Li, Z.; Nie, H.; He, J.; Chen, Z.; Yuan, J.; Guo, H.; Zhang, X.; Yang, H.; et al. Plasma miR-193b-3p Is Elevated in Type 2 Diabetes and Could Impair Glucose Metabolism. *Front. Endocrinol.* **2022**, *13*, 814347. [CrossRef] [PubMed]
96. Jaeger, A.; Zollinger, L.; Saely, C.H.; Muendlein, A.; Evangelakos, I.; Nasias, D.; Charizopoulou, N.; Schofield, J.D.; Othman, A.; Soran, H.; et al. Circulating microRNAs -192 and -194 Are Associated with the Presence and Incidence of Diabetes Mellitus. *Sci. Rep.* **2018**, *8*, 14274. [CrossRef]
97. Latouche, C.; Natoli, A.; Reddy-Luthmoodoo, M.; Heywood, S.E.; Armitage, J.A.; Kingwell, B.A. MicroRNA-194 Modulates Glucose Metabolism and Its Skeletal Muscle Expression Is Reduced in Diabetes. *PLoS ONE* **2016**, *11*, e0155108. [CrossRef]
98. Jones, A.; Danielson, K.M.; Benton, M.C.; Ziegler, O.; Shah, R.; Stubbs, R.S.; Das, S.; Macartney-Coxson, D. miRNA Signatures of Insulin Resistance in Obesity. *Obesity* **2017**, *25*, 1734–1744. [CrossRef] [PubMed]
99. Li, X.; Ren, Y.; Chang, K.; Wu, W.; Griffiths, H.R.; Lu, S.; Gao, D. Adipose Tissue Macrophages as Potential Targets for Obesity and Metabolic Diseases. *Front. Immunol.* **2023**, *14*, 1153915. [CrossRef]
100. Tryggestad, J.B.; Teague, A.M.; Sparling, D.P.; Jiang, S.; Chernausek, S.D. Macrophage-Derived microRNA-155 Increases in Obesity and Influences Adipocyte Metabolism by Targeting Peroxisome Proliferator-Activated Receptor Gamma. *Obesity* **2019**, *27*, 1856–1864. [CrossRef] [PubMed]

101. Zhang, D.; Yao, X.; Teng, Y.; Zhao, T.; Lin, L.; Li, Y.; Shang, H.; Jin, Y.; Jin, Q. Adipocytes-Derived Exosomal microRNA-1224 Inhibits M2 Macrophage Polarization in Obesity-Induced Adipose Tissue Inflammation via MSI2-Mediated Wnt/β-Catenin Axis. *Mol. Nutr. Food Res.* **2022**, *66*, 2100889. [CrossRef]
102. Pan, Y.; Hui, X.; Hoo, R.L.C.; Ye, D.; Chan, C.Y.C.; Feng, T.; Wang, Y.; Lam, K.S.L.; Xu, A. Adipocyte-Secreted Exosomal microRNA-34a Inhibits M2 Macrophage Polarization to Promote Obesity-Induced Adipose Inflammation. *J. Clin. Investig.* **2019**, *129*, 834–849. [CrossRef]
103. Zhang, M.; Zhou, Z.; Wang, J.; Li, S. MiR-130b Promotes Obesity Associated Adipose Tissue Inflammation and Insulin Resistance in Diabetes Mice through Alleviating M2 Macrophage Polarization via Repression of PPAR-γ. *Immunol. Lett.* **2016**, *180*, 1–8. [CrossRef] [PubMed]
104. Lei, L.-M.; Lin, X.; Xu, F.; Shan, S.-K.; Guo, B.; Li, F.-X.-Z.; Zheng, M.-H.; Wang, Y.; Xu, Q.-S.; Yuan, L.-Q. Exosomes and Obesity-Related Insulin Resistance. *Front. Cell Dev. Biol.* **2021**, *9*, 651996. [CrossRef] [PubMed]
105. Ying, W.; Riopel, M.; Bandyopadhyay, G.; Dong, Y.; Birmingham, A.; Seo, J.B.; Ofrecio, J.M.; Wollam, J.; Hernandez-Carretero, A.; Fu, W.; et al. Adipose Tissue Macrophage-Derived Exosomal miRNAs Can Modulate In Vivo and In Vitro Insulin Sensitivity. *Cell* **2017**, *171*, 372–384.e12. [CrossRef] [PubMed]
106. Payet, T.; Gabinaud, E.; Landrier, J.; Mounien, L. Role of micro-RNAs Associated with Adipose-derived Extracellular Vesicles in Metabolic Disorders. *Obes. Rev.* **2024**, *25*, e13755. [CrossRef] [PubMed]
107. Yu, Y.; Du, H.; Wei, S.; Feng, L.; Li, J.; Yao, F.; Zhang, M.; Hatch, G.M.; Chen, L. Adipocyte-Derived Exosomal MiR-27a Induces Insulin Resistance in Skeletal Muscle Through Repression of PPARγ. *Theranostics* **2018**, *8*, 2171–2188. [CrossRef] [PubMed]
108. Liu, T.; Sun, Y.-C.; Cheng, P.; Shao, H.-G. Adipose Tissue Macrophage-Derived Exosomal miR-29a Regulates Obesity-Associated Insulin Resistance. *Biochem. Biophys. Res. Commun.* **2019**, *515*, 352–358. [CrossRef] [PubMed]
109. Li, D.; Song, H.; Shuo, L.; Wang, L.; Xie, P.; Li, W.; Liu, J.; Tong, Y.; Zhang, C.-Y.; Jiang, X.; et al. Gonadal White Adipose Tissue-Derived Exosomal MiR-222 Promotes Obesity-Associated Insulin Resistance. *Aging* **2020**, *12*, 22719–22743. [CrossRef]
110. Shi, Z.; Zhao, C.; Guo, X.; Ding, H.; Cui, Y.; Shen, R.; Liu, J. Differential Expression of MicroRNAs in Omental Adipose Tissue From Gestational Diabetes Mellitus Subjects Reveals miR-222 as a Regulator of ERα Expression in Estrogen-Induced Insulin Resistance. *Endocrinology* **2014**, *155*, 1982–1990. [CrossRef]
111. Dang, S.-Y.; Leng, Y.; Wang, Z.-X.; Xiao, X.; Zhang, X.; Wen, T.; Gong, H.-Z.; Hong, A.; Ma, Y. Exosomal Transfer of Obesity Adipose Tissue for Decreased miR-141-3p Mediate Insulin Resistance of Hepatocytes. *Int. J. Biol. Sci.* **2019**, *15*, 351–368. [CrossRef] [PubMed]
112. Gesmundo, I.; Pardini, B.; Gargantini, E.; Gamba, G.; Birolo, G.; Fanciulli, A.; Banfi, D.; Congiusta, N.; Favaro, E.; Deregibus, M.C.; et al. Adipocyte-Derived Extracellular Vesicles Regulate Survival and Function of Pancreatic β Cells. *JCI Insight* **2021**, *6*, e141962. [CrossRef] [PubMed]
113. Machado, I.F.; Teodoro, J.S.; Palmeira, C.M.; Rolo, A.P. miR-378a: A New Emerging microRNA in Metabolism. *Cell. Mol. Life Sci.* **2020**, *77*, 1947–1958. [CrossRef] [PubMed]
114. Trajkovski, M.; Hausser, J.; Soutschek, J.; Bhat, B.; Akin, A.; Zavolan, M.; Heim, M.H.; Stoffel, M. MicroRNAs 103 and 107 Regulate Insulin Sensitivity. *Nature* **2011**, *474*, 649–653. [CrossRef]
115. Palihaderu, P.; Mendis, B.; Premarathne, J.; Dias, W.; Yeap, S.K.; Ho, W.Y.; Dissanayake, A.; Rajapakse, I.; Karunanayake, P.; Senarath, U.; et al. Therapeutic Potential of miRNAs for Type 2 Diabetes Mellitus: An Overview. *Genet. Epigenet.* **2022**, *15*, 25168657221130041. [CrossRef] [PubMed]

diabetology

MDPI

Review

Metabolic Syndrome Drug Therapy: The Potential Interplay of Pharmacogenetics and Pharmacokinetic Interactions in Clinical Practice: A Narrative Review

Sandra Knežević [1,†], Francesca Filippi-Arriaga [2,3,†], Andrej Belančić [1,4,*], Tamara Božina [5], Jasenka Mršić-Pelčić [1] and Dinko Vitezić [1,4]

1 Department of Basic and Clinical Pharmacology with Toxicology, Faculty of Medicine, University of Rijeka, 51000 Rijeka, Croatia; sandra.knezevic@uniri.hr (S.K.); jasenka.mrsic.pelcic@uniri.hr (J.M.-P.); dinko.vitezic@uniri.hr (D.V.)

2 Centre Investigació Medicaments (CIM), Institut de Recerca Sant Pau (IR-Sant Pau), 08041 Barcelona, Spain; mfilippi@santpau.cat

3 Diabetes and Metabolism Research Unit, Vall d'Hebron Institut de Recerca (VHIR), 08035 Barcelona, Spain

4 Department of Clinical Pharmacology, Clinical Hospital Centre Rijeka, 51000 Rijeka, Croatia

5 Department of Medical Chemistry, Biochemistry and Clinical Chemistry, University of Zagreb School of Medicine, 10000 Zagreb, Croatia; tamara.bozina@mef.hr

* Correspondence: a.belancic93@gmail.com

† These authors contributed equally to this work.

Abstract: Metabolic syndrome (MetS) presents a significant global health challenge, characterized by a cluster of metabolic alterations including obesity, hypertension, insulin resistance/dysglycemia, and atherogenic dyslipidemia. Advances in understanding and pharmacotherapy have added complexity to MetS management, particularly concerning drug interactions and pharmacogenetic variations. Limited literature exists on drug–drug–gene interactions (DDGIs) and drug–drug–transporter gene interactions (DDTGIs), which can significantly impact pharmacokinetics and pharmacodynamics, affecting treatment outcomes. This narrative review aims to address the following three key objectives: firstly, shedding a light on the PK metabolism, transport, and the pharmacogenetics (PGx) of medicines most commonly used in the MetS setting (relevant lipid-lowering drugs, antihypertensives and antihyperglycemics agents); secondly, exemplifying potential clinically relevant pharmacokinetic drug interactions, including drug–drug interactions, DDGIs, and DDTGIs; and, thirdly, describing and discussing their potential roles in clinical practice. This narrative review includes relevant information found with the use of interaction checkers, pharmacogenetic databases, clinical pharmacogenetic practice guidelines, and literature sources, guided by evidence-based medicine principles.

Keywords: metabolic syndrome; pharmacogenetics; pharmacokinetics; drug–drug–transporter gene interactions; drug–drug-gene interactions; lipid-lowering agents; antihypertensives; antihyperglycemics; clinical decision making

1. Introduction

Metabolic syndrome (MetS) is an escalating global public-health problem most commonly defined as the cluster of several metabolic alterations, including visceral obesity, elevation of arterial blood pressure, insulin resistance/dysglycemia, and atherogenic dyslipidemia [1].

Due to substantial progress in the understanding of the latter metabolic entities and pharmacotherapy armamentarium, the management of MetS has become even more complex. Besides bearing in mind the anorexigenic potential of medicines and the impact on major adverse cardiac events (MACEs), in the current era of polytherapy it is increasingly important to consider potential drug–drug interactions (DDIs). The management of MetS is becoming even more demanding in cases of pharmacogenetic variations leading to substantial drug–drug–gene interactions which are influencing pharmacokinetics (PK) and/or pharmacodynamics (PD) [2].

In general, the body of literature on DDGIs as well as drug–drug–transporter genes interactions (DDTGIs) is quite scarce. Inhibitory and induction interactions may substantially affect PK conditions and thus increase or decrease drug concentrations, respectively. Since MetS is a complex phenomenon, both clinically and pharmacologically speaking, it is important to decrease the rate of adverse drug reactions (ADRs) and improve treatment outcomes in the setting of increasing multi-morbidity and polytherapy [3].

The aim of the present narrative review is to (i) shed the light on the PK metabolism, transport, and pharmacogenetics (PGx) of medicines most commonly used in the MetS setting (relevant lipid-lowering drugs, antihypertensive, and antihyperglycemic agents), (ii) to exemplify potential clinically relevant pharmacokinetic DD, DDG, and DDTG interactions that may arise, and (iii) to describe and discuss their potential role in clinical practice.

2. Methodology

To conduct this narrative review, current clinical practice guidelines were consulted to identify relevant lipid-lowering drugs as well as antihypertensive and hypoglycemic drug therapies. Drug labels were reviewed to compile the most relevant pharmacokinetic and pharmacogenetic information for each identified drug group. The Lexicomp Drug Interactions tool [4] was used to identify potential drug–drug interactions, and the PharmGKB [5] database and DrugBank [6] database were utilized to further explore relevant pharmacogenetic data and to identify relevant drug transporters or enzymes. Finally, we examined existing recommendations within pharmacogenetic guidelines, including those from the Clinical Pharmacogenetics Implementation Consortium (CPIC) [7] and the Dutch Pharmacogenetics Working Group (DPWG) [8].

3. Pharmacogenetics of Lipid-Lowering Drug Drugs

Dyslipidemias are disorders of lipoprotein metabolism (cholesterol, low-density lipoprotein cholesterol (LDL-C), triglycerides, and high-density lipoprotein cholesterol (HDL-C)) and represent an important risk factor for atherosclerotic cardiovascular disease (ASCVD) [9,10]. Different drugs are used for its treatment [11]. Recent data on the PGx and PK of statins, fibrates, and ezetimibe will be presented.

3.1. 3-Hydroxy-3-Methylglutaryl-Coenzyme A Reductase (HMG-CoA Reductase) Inhibitors

Statins are HMG-CoA reductase inhibitors and belong to the most prescribed drugs in the world, being used to reduce cholesterol and prevent cardiovascular diseases. Although they are considered safe drugs, 5–10% of the patients develop statin intolerance, most often due to statin-associated musculoskeletal symptoms (SAMSs) that affect adherence and, ultimately, treatment outcomes. PGx studies have identified several biomarkers that impact statin PK, modulating drug exposure and ADRs. These biomarkers are often called ADME genes because they have an impact on absorption, distribution, metabolism, and excretion. Some of them have been included in the guidelines for personalized treatment [12] while, for others, it is still necessary to collect additional evidence on their relevance for clinical practice.

According to their PK, statins are administered orally and absorbed into systemic circulation via intestinal cells through both passive diffusion and active transport facilitated by ABC and SLC gene family transporters. The liver and, to a lesser extent, the kidney are the primary sites of metabolism and elimination. Metabolism is catalyzed by CYP and UGT gene family enzymes, and the predominant elimination pathway is biliary excretion mediated by ABC transporters [5].

Organic anion-transporting polypeptide 1B1 (OATP1B1), coded by the *SLCO1B1* gene, has a vital role in transporting statins into the liver for hepatic clearance. ABCG2 (BCRP) is an efflux transporter involved in absorption and disposition and CYP2C9 is involved in the metabolism of some statins (fluvastatin, rosuvastatin). All of these biomarkers are polymorphic, and gene variants can modulate the PK of statins (i.e., simvastatin, atorvastatin, rosuvastatin, fluvastatin, pravastatin, pitavastatin, lovastatin), representing a genetic predisposition to an increased risk of SAMSs.

Due to genetic variability or drug inhibition, decreased functioning of OATP1B1/*SLCO1B1* can result in significantly increased systemic exposure to statins, resulting in higher risk for SAMSs [13]. The most studied variant, *SLCO1B1* c.521T>C (rs4149056, p.V174A), contained within *SLCO1B1**5 and *15 haplotypes, causes nearly total loss of OATP1B1 function and raises systemic exposure to statins and ADRs risk [14–16].

From the data obtained in vitro, decreased transport function has been associated with the minor C allele at c.521T>C, while increased systemic exposure to several drugs has been observed in vivo. A recent study reported that a *SLCO1B1* variant with increased activity (c.388A>G, rs2306283) has a significant impact on atorvastatin PK, also finding that the area under the curve (AUC) (0–∞) was 41% smaller compared to individuals with a normal function genotype [17].

Differences in allele frequencies have been observed across populations and races. The variant allele *SLCO1B1* 521C is more common in European (15%) populations than in Asian (14%) and African (1%) populations [18].

Besides statins, OATP1B1 is responsible for the uptake of mainly weakly acidic drugs like valsartan, bosentan, enalapril, methotrexate, rifampicin, SN-38 (the active metabolite of irinotecan), and HIV protease inhibitors, as well as some endogenous compounds (bilirubin, bile acids (taurocholic acid), conjugated steroids, and leukotriene C4, into the liver [19–21].

ABCG2 gene encodes the membrane transporter adenosine triphosphate (ATP)–binding cassette G2 (also known as breast cancer resistance protein, BCRP). It is expressed in many tissues, including the intestine, liver, blood–brain barrier, and kidney [5,22].

As an efflux transporter on the cell membrane, it limits the entry of drugs and other xenobiotics into the cell. Its primary role is in the enterocyte membrane, where it limits the entry of xenobiotics from the gastrointestinal system into circulation. It acts as a canalicular efflux pump on the hepatocyte membrane, transporting substrates from hepatocytes into the bile, while, in the brain, microvascular endothelial cells limit the entry of substrates into the CNS. Acting in renal proximal tubular cells additionally contributes to the modulation of drug exposure. Therefore, genetically determined variable ABCG2 activity may have an impact on absorption, distribution, and elimination of drugs, as well as on tissue protection against xenobiotic exposure [23].

In addition to xenobiotics, ABCG2 also has endogenous substrates. Its important role is in renal and extrarenal urate secretion, and reduced function ABCG2 variants are linked to the risk for developing hyperuricemia and gout [5,24].

Clinically relevant drug substrates of ABCG2 other than lipid-lowering drugs (rosuvastatin, atorvastatin, fluvastatin, ezetimibe, fibrates) are cytostatics, such as camptothecin analogs (diflomotecan, irinotecan, topotecan), mitoxantrone, methotrexate, tyrosine kinase inhibitors (TKIs, e.g., erlotinib, gefitinib, imatinib, nilotinib), proton pump inhibitors (PPIs, e.g., pantoprazole), cimetidine, anticoagulants (apixaban, rivaroxaban), cyclosporine, prazosin, sulfasalazine, etc. [22,25–30].

ABCG2 is considered an important factor in drug interactions because it can be inhibited by drugs and other xenobiotics [29,31,32]. A number of ABCG2 inhibitors have been identified [22] and many convincing data point to ABCG2 as an important mediator of DDGIs in humans [21,33,34].

The common, most extensively studied *ABCG2* variant is c.421C>A (rs2231142 p.Q141K). The minor A allele is associated with 30–40% reduced protein expression compared with the C allele and increased plasma levels of drug substrates have been observed. Many studies have highlighted the *ABCG2* c.421C>A variant as a determinant of the PK variability, efficacy, and toxicity of different drugs [28,32,35,36].

In populations of European descent, the frequency of the *ABCG2* variant allele is estimated at around 10–15% [37]. The highest frequency was recorded in the Asian population (30%) and the lowest was recorded in the African population (2%) [32,35,37]. Although a

CPIC guideline has only been issued for rosuvastatin, some study results found an ABCG2 variant associated with the PK and PD of other statins. The AUC of inactive simvastatin lactone was 111% higher, and, for fluvastatin, 97% higher in subjects with *ABCG2* 421 A/A genotype compared to concentrations in the carriers of 421 C/C genotype. This increase is likely due to decreased efflux transporter function [38]. The Keskitalo group reported that *ABCG2* 421 A/A genotype carriers had a 72% greater atorvastatin AUC and a 144% greater rosuvastatin AUC compared to the *ABCG2* 421 C/C genotype [35]. Similar results were obtained for atorvastatin in the Japanese population [39].

The prolonged bioavailability of statins in carriers of variant *ABCG2* allele represents a risk for the development of ADRs, as was confirmed in a case–control study for rosuvastatin, atorvastatin, and fluvastatin [40–42].

ABCG2 transporter has been recognized as one of the key drug transporters involved in clinically relevant drug disposition [36,43,44]. A study in hypertensive breastfeeding women found that concentrations of nifedipine in breast milk in *ABCG2* c.421 C/A genotype carriers were approximately three times greater than in the 421 C/C genotype [45].

The CYP2C9 enzyme participates in the metabolism of many clinically important drugs such as coumarin anticoagulants, antidiabetics, sartans, fluvastatin, antiepileptics, and nonsteroidal anti-inflammatory drugs, most of which have a narrow therapeutic range [46]. People with poor or no activity of the CYP2C9 enzyme may experience toxic side effects (phenytoin, diclofenac) or life-threatening bleeding (warfarin). The *CYP2C9* gene belongs to the *CYP2C* gene cluster (2C8-2C9-2C19-2C18) located on chromosome 10q24. More than 70 different alleles of the CYP2C9 enzyme are known, and the most important are alleles *2 (rs1799853, p.R144C) and *3 (rs1057910, p.I359L) due to their association with a reduced drug-substrate metabolism of ~30–40% and 80%, respectively, resulting in increased systemic drug exposure. The frequency of allele *2 in the Caucasian population is ~12% and allele *3~8%.

Among the first pieces of evidence of the association of the CYP2C9 polymorphism with the side effects of statins was a case–control study in renal transplant patients taking fluvastatin [42]. Results showed that *CYP2C9* homozygous and heterozygous variant allele (*2 or *3) carriers had 2.5 times greater odds of developing adverse effects ($p = 0.037$). Besides patients who were carriers of at least one variant *CYP2C9* allele (*2 or *3) and who were receiving CYP2C9 inhibitors, had more than six times greater odds of having adverse effects than those without the inhibitor ($p = 0.027$). Besides that, patients with *ABCG2* 421CA or AA (taken together) had almost four times greater odds of developing adverse effects than those with the *ABCG2* 421CC genotype ($p = 0.013$; OR: 3.81; 95% CI: 1.27–11.45).

Given that patients with MetS are most often on polytherapy with drugs that may be substrates of CYP2C9 and/or ABCG2, they may have an increased risk of ADRs due to DDIs and/or genetic variability.

The most recent CPIC guidelines for statins [12], published in January 2022, replace the original 2012 guidelines and the updates from 2014 [47,48]. In addition to previous gene-based guidelines prescribing simvastatin based on *SLCO1B1* genotype, recommendations based on the *SLCO1B1* (simvastatin, rosuvastatin, atorvastatin, pravastatin, pitavastatin, fluvastatin, and lovastatin), *CYP2C9* (fluvastatin), and *ABCG2* (rosuvastatin) genotypes were added. The guidelines are specifically used in cases when the results of PGx tests are available to achieve the best possible clinical results with the most suitable statin in its optimal dose [12].

There are other relevant genetic polymorphisms for hypolopidemic theraphy that are not yet in the guidelines. The published literature includes studies that have investigated other enzymes involved in statin metabolism, such as CYP3A4/5 [49–51]. Because of insufficient evidence to support clinical implementation, there are still no recommendations for their application in practice.

Although not covered by the guidelines for statins, *CYP3A4/5* gene polymorphisms could be relevant, especially in concomitant therapy with drugs that are CYP3A substrates.

Given that nearly 50% of drugs are metabolized by CYP3A enzymes which show significant interindividual variability in activity, DDGIs in the treatment of MetS may be relevant.

The *CYP3A* gene cluster is located on chromosome 7q22. Important substrates of the CYP3A besides statins are antibiotics, antivirals, antiepileptics, antidepressants, anticoagulants, antipsychotics, immunosuppressants, tyrosine kinase inhibitors, etc. CYP3A4/5 enzymes are expressed in the liver and intestines, whereby CYP3A5 predominates in extrahepatic tissues. Both enzymes mostly share substrates and show very high variability in activity [52]. In the Caucasian population, only 3–15% of people have an active enzyme CYP3A5 (carriers of the allele *1, (expressers), while the most common variant *CYP3A5*3*, substitution 6986A>G in the intron 3 (nonexpressers) results in the synthesis of an inactive enzyme [46]. The *CYP3A5* expression may overcome/prevent drug interactions at the CYP3A4 level.

Several polymorphisms affect CYP3A4 expression and function [53]. The polymorphism *CYP3A4*22* (rs35599367, c.522-191C>T), an intronic variant with a frequency of 5–7% in the Caucasian population, determines a significantly reduced activity of the enzyme. *CYP3A4*22* can change hepatic CYP3A4 enzyme expression by 2–6 times. The *CYP3A4*20* in/del variant results in a complete loss of function [54]. However, according to the Genome Aggregation Database, the frequency in the European population is only 0.04%. The *CYP3A4*6* variant also results in very low enzyme activity and a low frequency in the Caucasian population. According to the Ensembl genome database, a variant with enhanced CYP3A4 function, *CYP3A4*18*, has been described in Asians but has not been detected in the European population. Studies indicate a possible role of *CYP3A* polymorphisms in PK modulation and dosing of some drug-substrates such as statins, tacrolimus, cyclosporin, and DOACs [55]. The *CYP3A4*22* variant may increase the cholesterol-lowering efficacy of atorvastatin [56].

In a study of a Finish group [49] of individuals with the intermediate metabolizer *CYP3A4* genotype (*CYP3A4*2* or *CYP3A4*22* heterozygotes), 33% ($p = 0.022$) had larger atorvastatin AUC0–∞ compared to those with a normal metabolizer genotype. The same authors reported the results of a genome-wide association study (GWAS) of atorvastatin PK. Besides the relevance of the well-known variant *SLCO1B1* c.521T>C (rs4149056) for the increased AUC0–∞ of atorvastatin (140%), an intronic LPP variant, rs1975991 was found to be associated with reduced atorvastatin lactone; three *UGT1A* variants linked with *UGT1A3*2* were associated with increased 2-hydroxy atorvastatin lactone, and increased function *SLCO1B1* variants were associated with 41% smaller AUC0–∞. These data suggest that genetic variations in *SLCO1B1*, *UGT1A3*, *LPP*, and *CYP3A4* affect atorvastatin PK. The relevance of these newly discovered correlations for efficacy and side effects remains to be examined.

In addition to genetic predisposition, *CYP3A* variability is strongly influenced by environmental factors such as food, smoking, and other concurrently administered drugs, such as some azole compounds, antibiotics, antiepileptics. Citrus fruits, especially grapefruit juice, have considerable inhibitory effects on CYP3A4 already at the intestinal level, but they also have effects on the drug transporter, P-glycoprotein, which can result in increased bioavailability of drug-substrates [57].

Of phase II polymorphic enzymes, *UGT1A3*2* is relevant for statin therapy, which increases UGT1A3 enzyme expression and the lactonization of atorvastatin [58].

As for the transporters, polymorphisms of P-gp/ABCB1 and ABCG2 has been found to modulate PK of some statins [38,59,60].

3.2. Fibrates

In addition to statins, fibrates (gemfibrozil, fenofibric acid) and ezetimibe are often prescribed for MetS. Risk of myopathy increases if fibrates are given with statins [61].

Although the results of PGx research on these drugs are insufficient and there are no relevant guidelines, it is important to consider the pathways of metabolism and transport and the potential interactions in MetS polytherapy (Table 1). Drug interactions can additionally be complex and significant for the development of side effects in patients carrying inactivating ADME gene variants involved in the PK of drugs in use (drug–drug–gene interactions).

Table 1. Enzymes and transporters of metabolic syndrome drugs.

Group	Drug	ABCB1	ABCG2	CYP2C8	CYP2C9	CYP2C19	CYP2D6	CYP3A4/5	UGT1A	UGT1A9	UGT2B4	UGT2B7	SLC2A2	SLC22A/OCT	SLC47A1	SLC47A2	SLC5A2	SLCO1B1/OATP1B1	SLC29A4/PMAT	SLC47A1/MATE1	SLC47A2/MATE2	SP1
HMG-CoA Reductase Inhibitors	Simvastatin	+	+				+	+	+	+		+						+				
	Atorvastatin	+	+	+				+	+	+		+						+				
	Lovastatin	+				+		+	+	+		+						+				
	Pitavastatin	+	+	+	+			+	+			+						+				
	Fluvastatin	+	+	+	+													+				
	Rosuvastatin		+		+	+												+				
	Pravastatin	+	+															+				
Fibrates	Fenofibrate									+												
	Gemfibrozil	+																+				
SCAI	Ezetimibe	+	+															+				
BB	Atenolol						+											+				
	Bisoprolol	+					+	+														
	Carvedilol	+			+	+	+	+	+			+										
	Metoprolol						+	+						+								
	Nebivolol					+	+	+														
	Propranolol	+			+	+	+	+														
ARBs	Losartan	+			+	+		+	+			+										
CCBs	Amlodipine	+	+					+														
	Lacidipine		+					+														
	Lercanidipine		+					+														
	Diltiazem	+				+	+	+														
	Verapamil	+		+	+	+		+														
Biguanides	Metformin												+	+	+	+			+	+	+	+
Glitazones	Pioglitazone	+		+	+			+										+				
Sulphonylureas	Gliclazide				+	+																
	Glimepiride				+																	
	Glibenclamide		+		+	+		+														
SGLT2i	Empagliflozin	+	+						+	+		+					+	+				
	Ertugliflozin	+	+						+	+		+										
	Dapagliflozin	+			+		+	+		+	+	+										
	Canagliflozin	+			+			+		+	+											
GLP1-RA	Exenatide																					+
DPP4-inhibitors	Sitagliptin							+														
	Saxagliptin							+														

CCBs: calcium channel blockers, ARBs: angiotensin receptor blockers, BB: beta-blockers, GLP1-RA: glucagon-like peptide-1 receptor agonists, HMG-CoA reductase inhibitors: 3-hydroxy-3-methylglutaryl-coenzyme A reductase inhibitors, SCAI: selective cholesterol absorption inhibitors, SGLT2i: sodium glucose co-transporter-2 inhibitors, DPP4-inhibitors: dipeptidyl peptidase-4 inhibitors.

Gemfibrozil undergoes hydroxylation and O-glucuronidation to form gemfibrozil 1-beta glucuronide, an inhibitor of CYP2C8 [62]. Glucuronidation is primarily mediated by UGT2B7 and several UGT1A enzymes. The metabolism of fenofibric acid is also mediated primarily by glucuronidation and excretion in urine.

As fibrates can inhibit some CYPs and UGTs [62] this can have important implications for the mechanism of the clinical interaction observed between gemfibrozil and CYP2C8 substrates such as cerivastatin (withdrawn from market), repaglinide, rosiglitazone, and pioglitazone.

Physiologically based PK models for prediction of complex CYP2C8 and OATP1B1 (*SLCO1B1*) drug–drug–gene interactions have been proposed for several drugs, including gemfibrozil, repaglinide and pioglitazone [63].

3.3. *Selective Cholesterol Absorption Inhibitors*

Ezetimibe, a selective cholesterol absorption inhibitor, is primarily metabolized in the liver and small intestine by glucuronide conjugation (UGT1A) with subsequent renal and biliary excretion [64]. It is also the substrate of several transporters (*ABCB1, ABCC2, ABCG2, SLCO1B1*) [65,66]. Various genetic polymorphisms seem to influence the PK of ezetimibe with different effects [67]. Ezetimibe also has the potential to interact (by inhibition) at the level of drug metabolism and transport. These interactions can be clinically significant, especially in patients with a PGx predisposition, i.e., with a low metabolic and/or transport capacity [68]. Relevant genetic polymorphisms for lipid-lowering drug therapy are not yet contemplated in guidelines.

3.4. *Novel Lipid-Lowering Drugs*

3.4.1. Proprotein Convertase Subtilisin/Kexin Type 9 (PCSK9) Inhibitors

PCSK9 inhibitors, alirocumab, and evolocumab are fully humanized monoclonal antibodies that target PCSK9, a serine protease primarily produced in the liver. PCSK9 binds to LDL receptors (LDL-Rs) on hepatocytes, leading to the degradation of LDL-Rs and elevated plasma LDL-C levels. By inhibiting this binding, these antibodies increase the expression of LDL-Rs on the hepatocyte surface and reduce plasma LDL-C levels [69]. They are given as subcutaneous injections, administered every 2 to 4 weeks, with flexibility to adjust the interval based on clinical judgment and patient outcomes. Evolocumab and alirocumab are composed solely of amino acids and carbohydrates, functioning as natural immunoglobulins. Consequently, they are unlikely to be metabolized via hepatic pathways. Instead, their metabolism and clearance are anticipated to follow the typical routes for immunoglobulins, leading to their degradation into smaller peptides and individual amino acids. Genetic variations in PCSK9 and LDLR genes may affect drug response, but significant pharmacogenetic insights are still lacking. Despite their efficacy, the pharmacogenetic landscape of PCSK9 inhibitors is still under development [69,70].

3.4.2. Inclisiran

Inclisiran, a small interfering RNA that inhibits PCSK9 synthesis, provides an even more efficient mechanism of action compared to monoclonal antibodies. It offers the advantage of less frequent dosing (as the initial dose is followed by a second dose after 3 months and the dosing regimen subsides to a 6-month interval), making it an efficient option for long-term management of hypercholesterolemia in metabolic syndrome [71].

Inclisiran is not a substrate for common drug transporters and, although in vitro studies have not been performed, it is not expected to be a cytochrome P450 substrate; therefore, it is not expected to have clinically significant interactions with other drugs. Although inclisiran's clinical efficacy and safety profile have been demonstrated, its pharmacogenetic implications need further investigation [70,71].

4. Pharmacogenetics of Antihypertensive Drugs

Arterial hypertension is a widespread global health issue affecting millions of people worldwide. Its prevalence varies across different populations and is influenced by factors such as age, gender, ethnicity, lifestyle, and genetics [72–74]. Clinicians frequently rely on a "trial-and-error" approach or a combination approach to identify the most suitable drug treatment for patients. However, hypertension PGx aims to discover genetic markers that predict individual drug responses. As new data emerge and evidence accumulates, there is potential for this field to reach a point where the evidence supports its clinical implementation [75,76].

Recent data on PGx and PK of beta-blockers (BBs), calcium channel blockers (CCBs), angiotensin receptor blockers (ARBs), and hydralazine and angiotensin converting enzyme inhibitors (ACEIs) will be presented.

Various antihypertensive medications, including BBs, CCBs, and ARBs, undergo hepatic metabolism primarily through CYP enzymes. This metabolism process contributes to significant interindividual variability in drug response due to differences in enzyme expression and activity levels [74]. Polymorphisms, age, hepatic dysfunction, and conditions affecting hepatic blood supply contribute to changes in biotransformation, affecting drug exposure during antihypertensive therapy and cardiovascular response [77].

The labels of hydralazine, losartan, and metoprolol mention metabolic enzymes, implying that, if these enzymes are affected, the drug concentrations may be altered [78–80]. For some antihypertensive drugs, major society guidelines are available, as DPWG published guidelines for metoprolol and carvedilol that will be mentioned in the following section [80–82].

4.1. Beta-Blockers (BB)

Beta-adrenergic receptor antagonists, commonly known as BBs, are prescribed for various cardiovascular conditions, including heart failure, hypertension, and the secondary prevention of myocardial infarction. While some beta-blockers, like atenolol and nadolol, are eliminated unchanged in urine, most undergo hepatic metabolism. Carvedilol, metoprolol, nebivolol and propranolol, as a majority of BBs, are primarily metabolized by the highly polymorphic CYP2D6 enzyme. Factors affecting CYP2D6 activity, such as age, race, smoking, and concomitant medications, influence beta-blocker PK, leading to variability in drug response [83]. Common genetic variants in CYP2D6 can result in a range of enzyme phenotypes, from increased function due to gene duplication to complete loss of function due to gene deletion or splicing defects [84,85].

Metoprolol undergoes primary metabolism via the CYP2D6 enzyme. Approximately 8% of Caucasians and 2% of other populations lack CYP2D6 activity and are categorized as "CYP2D6 poor metabolizers" [86]. A retrospective cohort study by Collet et al. that aimed to evaluate adverse effects such as bradycardia, hypotension, and syncope in patients who were expected to have absent CYP2D6 enzyme activity due to DDIs or DGIs found statistically significant differences in the incidence of bradycardia amongst poor metabolizers and phenoconverters [87]. Phenoconversion occurs due to strong inhibition, in this case, of CYP2D6, causing patients who display normal or intermediate metabolism to mimic a poor metabolizer. Certain drugs that cause strong CYP2D6 inhibition and are frequently prescribed include antidepressant drugs (fluoxetine, paroxetine, bupropion), antifungic terbinafine, and antiarrhythmic propafenone [88]. Metoprolol and propafenone are common cardiological drug entities used in the treatment of atrial fibrillation, so the DDI of these drugs is important and should be noted [89]. CYP2D6 was investigated to have potential as a predictive biomarker of beta-blocker maintenance dose in heart failure patients. Consistent with the role of CYP2D6 in the metabolism of metoprolol, the tolerated maintenance dose of metoprolol was lower in *CYP2D6*4* carriers compared to non-carriers. Conversely, with the dosage of carvedilol, the finding was also consistent, as it was higher in *CYP2D6*4* carriers compared to non-carriers [90].

As aforementioned, the DPWG published guidelines for metoprolol that offer clinical genotype-guided dosing recommendations based on CYP2D6 metabolizer status. When prescribing metoprolol to CYP2D6 poor and intermediate metabolizers, if gradual heart rate reduction is desired or symptomatic bradycardia occurs, the guideline recommends using smaller titration steps and/or prescribing no more than 25% (poor metabolizers) or 50% (intermediate metabolizers) of the standard dose. Conversely, for CYP2D6 ultra-rapid metabolizers, the guideline suggests starting with the maximum dose for the relevant indication and, if needed, increasing it up to 2.5 times the standard dose or considering an alternative drug if efficacy remains insufficient [80,81].

Reguarding carvedilol, DPWG assessed the impact of the CYP2D6 genotype on carvedilol dosing and concluded that no dose adjustments are necessary based on this gene–drug interaction. Although variations in CYP2D6 metabolism may lead to differences in carvedilol plasma concentrations, these differences have not been shown to significantly affect the drug's efficacy or side effects [8,82].

Nebivolol, on the other hand, even though it is metabolized by CYP2D6 phenotypes, does not present a significant difference between poor metabolizer and extensive metabolizer patients and does not significantly affect clinical outcomes [91].

Although some evidence supports the influence of *CYP2D6* genetic polymorphisms on the PK of beta-blockers, the overall evidence on the use of genetic information in prescribing beta-blockers is weak [7,92].

As for other BBs, atenolol is a hydrophilic molecule that primarily goes through renal elimination, where only about 5% is metabolized by the liver [93]. Key factors influencing atenolol PK include transporter genes and their variants, and potential DDI in vitro studies suggest that the organic anions transporting polypeptides—OATP1A2 and OATP2B1 coded by *SLCO1A2* and *SLCO2B1*—are responsible for atenolol intestinal uptake [91]. These transporters are located on the luminal side of small intestine enterocytes. Uptake is inhibited by orange (*SLCO1A2*) and apple juice (SLCO2B) [94,95]. Apple juice ingestion reduced the systemic exposure to atenolol in healthy Korean population; nevertheless, genetic variations in *SLCO2B1* were unlikely to contribute to PK variability of atenolol [95].

4.2. Calcium Channel Blockers (CCBs)

CCBs are classified into two major categories, either non-dihydropyridines or dihydropyridines. CCBs are found to be a first agent of choice in hypertension but are also indicated for various cardiovascular diseases such as coronary spasm, angina pectoris, supraventricular dysrhythmias, hypertrophic cardiomyopathy, and pulmonary hypertension [96]. CCBs are largely metabolized through CYP3A5, with considerable interindividual variability due to differences in enzyme expression and activity.

In Chinese population *CYP3A5*3* allele was associated with better antihypertensive responses to amlodipine therapy [97,98]. Nevertheless, connections were not found between CYP3A5 variants in Korean and African American population [99,100]. The observed discrepancies in responses to amlodipine may be attributed to various factors, including ethnicity, environmental influences and others.

Regarding treatment induced ADRs, Liang et al. showed that allele frequencies of *CYP3A5*1D* (rs15524), *CYP3A5*1E* (rs4646453) and *CYP3A5*3* (rs776746) were significantly different between cases and controls ($p < 0.05$), associated with amlodipine-induced peripheral edema in Han Chinese patients with hypertension [101].

While some beta-blockers and ARBs have few significant PK interactions, interactions with CCBs are more prevalent due to their metabolism primarily through CYP3A isoenzymes. Non-dihydropyridine CCBs, verapamil and diltiazem, are strong inhibitors of CYP3A4, so further inhibition of hepatic activity could increase the risk of hypotension and bradycardia. Such inhibition might increase statin blood concentration, owing to DDIs. There is a possible risk of adverse reactions such as acute kidney injury following the co-prescription of CYP3A4 metabolized statins and CCBs that inhibit CYP3A4 [102].

Clinically important mechanism based CYP3A4 inhibitors include antibacterials (e.g., clarithromycin, erythromycin and isoniazid), anticancer agents (e.g., tamoxifen and irinotecan), anti-HIV agents (e.g., ritonavir and delavirdine), antihypertensives (e.g., hydralazine, verapamil and diltiazem), sex steroids and their receptor modulators (e.g., gestodene and raloxifene), and several herbal constituents (e.g., bergamottin and glabridin). Grapefruit juice, a known CYP3A4 inhibitor, can significantly alter the bioavailability of certain CCBs, impacting treatment efficacy and safety [53]. However, predicting DDIs involving CYP3A4 inactivation is difficult since the clinical outcomes depend on a number of factors that are associated with drugs and patients and the clinical relevance of the interaction is unclear [53,83].

4.3. Angiotensin Receptor Blockers (ARBs)

ARBs offer significant benefits in various conditions, including diabetic nephropathy, chronic heart failure, heart failure following myocardial infarction, hypertension with left ventricular hypertrophy, and in patients with a high cardiovascular risk due to previous events or complicated diabetes. In the treatment of hypertension, ARBs can be chosen as first-line therapy or added during later stages of treatment titration [103].

Losartan is majorly metabolized by the CYP3A4, CYP2C9 and CYP2C10 isoenzymes [104]. Losartan is a prodrug, metabolized to its active carboxylic acid metabolite form E-3147 by CYP2C9, which is featured as its most important pathway [105]. The single *CYP2C9*3* variant significantly decreases losartan metabolism to its active form and its hypotensive effect [106,107]. Therefore, several studies have been conducted on the effect of CYP isoenzyme inhibitors/inducers on the concentration of losartan and E-3147. Fluconazole inhibits the metabolism of losartan to its E-3147 responsible for most of the angiotensin Il-receptor antagonism of losartan [108]; however, the percentage that would result in a relevant effect on blood pressure is unclear at this point [104].

The CKD-PGX study assessed uncontrolled hypertension (uHTN) in patients with chronic kidney conditions and concluded that variants in CYP2C9 had reduced efficacy (OR: 5.2; 95% and CI: 1.9 to 14.7). Conversely, individuals classified as intermediate metabolizers or poor metabolizers of the CYP2D6 enzyme, resulting in higher circulating concentrations of metoprolol or carvedilol, were less likely to have uHTN compared to normal metabolizers taking either agent (OR of 0.55; 95% CI of 0.3 to 0.95) [76].

4.4. Angiotensin Converting Enzyme Inhibitors (ACEIs)

ACEIs are common first choice antihypertensive drugs. These are prodrugs that undergo biotransformation upon administration. They release the active component through hydrolysis by esterases, primarily in the liver, plasma, and intestinal wall. The active metabolites of ACEIs are mainly eliminated through the kidneys, and conditions like renal failure or heart failure can prolong drug excretion. Unlike other drugs, ACEIs are not metabolized by CYP enzymes, thus reducing the variability in drug responses.

4.5. Vasodilators

Hydralazine is a direct vasodilator used as an oral agent in essential hypertension refractory to other therapeutic agents. Hydralazine undergoes phase-2 metabolism via acetylation, predominantly facilitated by N-acetyltransferase type 2 (NAT2) in the liver. Individuals classified as fast or intermediate acetylators may experience lower concentrations and reduced efficacy of hydralazine at a given dose [109].

The *NAT2*4* allele signifies the common rapid acetylator phenotype while alleles such as *NAT2*5*, **6*, and *7 indicate slow acetylators. Individuals with a combination of alleles, like *4/*5, are classified as intermediate acetylators [110]. Studies have demonstrated that rapid acetylators exhibit reduced hydralazine exposure compared to slow acetylators, potentially affecting the drug's efficacy. Notably, slow acetylators may experience greater blood pressure reduction.

However, the acetylator status has the potential to affect the risk of adverse effects. Although oral hydralazine use is sporadically associated with lupus-like symptoms, the relationship remains uncertain [111]. Indirect evidence suggests that slow acetylators may face a heightened risk of these adverse effects upon hydralazine exposure, but definitive conclusions are lacking [111,112]. Consequently, further research is necessary to establish the utility of NAT2 genotyping in predicting both the safety and effectiveness of hydralazine treatment.

5. Pharmacogenetics of Antihyperglycemic Drugs

Type 2 diabetes (T2D) is a chronic complex disease characterized by hyperglycemia due to a non-autoimmune progressive loss of adequate β-cell insulin secretion, frequently an underlying element of insulin resistance and metabolic syndrome [113]. Pharmacological therapy has changed in recent years due to new treatment strategies that, beyond improving glycemic control, take comorbidities, cardiovascular benefit, cardiorenal risk, chronic weight management, and risk of adverse events into consideration [114–116]. PGx is a promising concept for pharmacological treatment, as the response, effectiveness and safety of drug classes for T2D could depend on genetic variability [117,118]. However, data regarding PGs and potential DDIs or DDGIs in recent drug classes for T2D remain scarce. Below is described the most relevant PGx and PKs findings of main antihyperglycemics drugs according to current clinical guidelines [114–118].

5.1. Biguanides

Metformin is a biguanide hypoglycemic agent that lowers basal and postprandial plasma glucose, suppresses hepatic glucose production, decreases intestinal absorption of glucose, and improves insulin sensitivity by increasing peripheral glucose uptake and utilization. Metformin is not metabolized and is excreted unchanged in the urine and distributed in the liver and kidney via various organic cation transporters [119–122].

PGx related to metformin has been studied with heterogeneous results for genes that encode organic cation transporters (OCTs), multidrug and toxin extrusion transporters (MATEs), plasma membrane monoamine transporters (PMATs), or others [123–125]. Up to the present date, for metformin, no data have been so far identified in the CPIC guidelines, PharmGKB, and in the prescribing information or Drug Label Annotation [45]. However, there are recently published studies in the literature, meta-analyses, GWAS, and clinical notes on the PGx of metformin.

According to its PK, after metformin oral consumption, it is first absorbed into intestinal epithelial cells by PMAT/*SLC29A4* and OCT3/*SLC22A3* and then transported into the blood by OCT1/*SLC22A1*. Subsequently, metformin binds to corresponding receptors and exerts its effects on various target cells through blood circulation. It is transported to the liver by OCT1/*SLC22A1* and OCT3/*SLC22A3* and then transferred into bile by the MATE1 protein. Alternatively, metformin is eliminated through the urine pathway, in which metformin is absorbed by OCT2 in the kidney and transported into the urine by MATE1 and MATE2 [123,125–128].

A review and meta-analysis evaluated the associations between OCT genetic polymorphisms and metformin response in individuals with T2D. A total of 30 related eligible studies about OCT genes (*SLC22A1*, *SLC22A1*, and *SLC22A3*) and metformin PGx were identified, and 14, three, and six single nucleotide polymorphisms (SNPs) in *SLC22A1*, *SLC22A1*, and *SLC22A3*, respectively, were investigated. The meta-analysis showed that *SLC22A1* rs622342 was associated with a reduction in HbA1c levels ($p = 0.001$). The GG genotype of *SLC22A1* rs628031 was associated with a reduction in fast plasma glucose levels (GG vs. AA: $p = 0.007$; GG vs. AG: $p < 0.001$) [125].

A GWAS studied the association between metformin response and variants on gene *SLC22A1*, the variants R61C and 420del were genotyped in a total of 3450 patients who were incident users of metformin with T2D. In 1531 patients that were identified as metformin responders, the R61C and 420del variants did not affected the initial HbA1c reduction ($p = 0.47$ and $p = 0.92$, respectively), the chance of achieving a treatment target ($p = 0.83$ and $p = 0.36$), the average HbA1c on monotherapy up to 42 months ($p = 0.44$ and $p = 0.75$), or the hazard of monotherapy failure ($p = 0.85$ and $p = 0.56$). The researchers concluded that the *SLC22A1* loss-of-function variants, R61C and 420del, did not attenuate the HbA1c reduction achieved by metformin in patients with T2D [126].

For gene SP1 variant rs2683511, allele C was associated with decreased HbA1c levels and secretory clearance when treated with metformin in people with T2D as compared to allele T [124]. With the variant rs784888, allele G was associated with decreased severity of hyperglycemia when treated with metformin in people T2D as compared to allele C. Allele C was not associated with exposure to metformin as compared to allele G [127,128].

It is important to mention that metformin only passes through the liver by its transporters, OCTs and MATEs, which is why they are of clinical relevance regarding DDIs [129].

Recent studies have highlighted various medications that can interfere with metformin uptake and elimination pathways, although a majority of them are on in vitro models. Proton-pump inhibitors, such as omeprazole, have been found to inhibit metformin transporters OCT1, OCT2, and OCT3 in vitro [130]. Regarding literature findings, transporter-mediated interactions between metformin and certain tyrosine kinase inhibitors, such as imatinib, nilotinib, gefitinib, and erlotinib, which could impact metformin's efficacy, toxicity leading to potential state of lactic acidosis [131,132].

5.2. Thiazolidinedinones (TZDs)

Pioglitazone, a member of TZDs, belongs to a class of peripheral insulin sensitizer drug family. It is a specific activator of the peroxisome proliferator-activated receptor gamma (PPARG) and is extensively metabolized in the liver by hydroxylation and oxidation [133]. Four primary (M-I, M-II, M-IV and M-V) and two secondary metabolites (M-III and M-VI) have been described. The M-III and M-IV are the principal metabolites found in human serum after multiple dosings. The major contributors to pioglitazone metabolism are CYP2C8 and CYP3A4 [134–136]. Regarding pioglitazone transporters, *SLCO1B1* gene encodes the hepatic drug transporter OATP1B1, which may participate in transporting TZDs from the blood into the liver [118].

A study of pioglitazone PK in healthy African American volunteers found that the metabolites M-III AUC0-48 ratio was significantly lower in *CYP2C8*2* carriers than *CYP2C8*1* homozygote ($p = 0.006$). Similarly, *CYP2C8*2* carriers had a significantly lower M-III:M-IV AUC0-48 ratio than participants with the *CYP2C8 *1/*1* genotype ($p = 0.006$) [137]. In Chinese individuals, a study with 244 subjects suggested that the *CYP2C8*, *CYP3A5*, and *ABCB1* genes play no significant role in the interindividual variation of pioglitazone PK, whereas *CYP2C9 *1/*3* was significantly associated with increased metabolism of pioglitazone as compared to *CYP2C9 *1* [138].

Anther study that enrolled 30 healthy Caucasian subjects found that *CYP2C8*3* was associated with decreased pioglitazone plasma exposure AUC0, ∞ [139]. Also, after studied the effects of the co-administration of the CYP2C8 inhibitor trimethoprim and pioglitazone in 16 healthy subjects, a rise in the pioglitazone AUC 0, ∞ of 42% ($p < 0.001$) and a decreased formation rate of pioglitazone metabolites M-IV and M-III ($p < 0.001$) were observed. In the same study, during the placebo phase the *CYP2C8*3* variant was associated with a pioglitazone reduced AUC (0, ∞). Authors concluded that drug interactions and PGx affecting the CYP2C8 enzyme may change the safety of pioglitazone [140].

A study carried out in 80 T2D subjects concluded that gene ADIPOQ polymorphism rs2241766 T/G was significantly associated with pioglitazone efficacy. Patients with TG and TT genotypes had a better response to treatment measured by HbA1c decrease [141]. Also, there was an association between the CYP2C8*3 variant with less weight gain compared to the wildtype [142].

5.3. Sulphonylureas (SU)

Despite the advent of newer classes of antidiabetic medications, SU remain widely prescribed due to their efficacy and affordability. However, their use is not without controversy, particularly regarding the risk of hypoglycemia. The antihyperglycemic drug gliclazide is a first-generation SU. It binds to the β-cell sulfonylurea receptor, blocking ATP-sensitive potassium channels, enhancing insulin secretion from pancreatic beta cells. Accordingly, the PK is rapidly absorbed with peak plasma concentrations at 4–6 h after oral administration and is extensively metabolized in the liver by CYP2C9 and CYP2C19 [6,143,144]. In everyday clinical practice, the *CYP2C9* genotype may impact the likelihood of hypoglycemia events among elderly patients, but it does not seem to have the same effect across the broader population of individuals with type 2 diabetes [145].

Finding from the Go-DARTS study, involving 1073 patients treated with SU (with 80% receiving gliclazide), revealed that patients carrying two copies of the inactivating allele *CYP2C9(*2, *3)* were found to be 3.4 times more likely to achieve a treatment HbA1c level of less than 7% compared to the wild type, which resulted in a 0.5% greater reduction in HbA1c levels [146].

Pharmacokinetic studies found that CYP2C9*3/*3 carriers had only 20% clearance of glibenclamide and glimepiride compared to wild-type carriers [147]. Additionally, non-diabetic *CYP2C9*2/*3* carriers showed a significantly reduced clearance of these drugs [148]. The DPWG evaluated therapeutic dose recommendations for glimepiride based on the *CYP2C9* genotype; after the evaluation, they concluded that no clinical practice action is needed for this gene–drug interaction [79].

Glucose-6-phosphate dehydrogenase (G6PD) mediates the production of NADPH and Ribose-5-phosphate and is one of the first genes found to be associated with variable drug response. Individuals with G6PD deficiency may have increased risks of adverse reactions. However, according CPIC guidelines, there are currently no clinical recommendations for dosing of gliclazide, glimepiride, or glipizide based on the G6PD genotype [7].

5.4. Sodium Glucose Co-Transporter-2 Inhibitors (SGLT2i)

Recent clinical practice guidelines of T2D give great value to SGLT2i (ertugliflozin, dapagliflozin, canagliflozin, and empagliflozin). These reduce the renal tubular glucose reabsorption that subsequently results in reduction in plasma glucose concentrations in blood [149].

SGLT2i rely primarily on glucuronidation for their metabolism. Ertugliflozin (via UGT1A9 and UGT2B7), dapagliflozin (via UGT1A9), canagliflozin (via UGT1A9 and UGT2B4), and empagliflozin (via UGT2B7, UGT1A3, UGT1A8, and UGT1A9) are transformed into inactive glucuronide conjugates. Oxidative metabolism via the CYP450 system is a minor pathway for these drugs. For dapagliflozin or canagliflozin, CYP3A4 may play a very minor role in the metabolism. Importantly, none of the drugs demonstrate clinically significant inhibition or induction of common CYP450 enzymes.

The UGT1A9 gene encodes UDP-glucuronosyltransferase, an enzyme that transforms drugs into soluble and excretable metabolites. SGLT2i are glucuronidased by UGT enzymes, thereby polymorphisms of their genes may potentially influence their treatment response [120]. A study with 134 participants indicated that alleles *UGT1A9*3* and *UGT2B4*2* increased canagliflozin plasma exposure [150]. Another study that had the aim to understand canagliflozin PK also indicates that carriers of the *UGT1A9*3* allele had greater exposure to canagliflozin [151].

Ertugliflozin is primarily metabolized via glucuronidation by enzyme UGT1A9. A study that included data from 25 phase 1 clinical trials evaluated the effect on 3 UGT1A9 polymorphisms (*UGT1A9-2152, UGT1A9*3, UGT1A9*1b*) on ertugliflozin exposure. Overall, the mean effects of the selected UGT1A9 variants on ertugliflozin AUC were within $\pm 10\%$. These findings were considered not clinically meaningful in healthy subjects, and researchers concluded that no dose adjustments were required with the UGT1A9 variants assessed [152].

5.5. Glucagon-like Peptide-1 Receptor Agonists (GLP1-RA)

GLP1-RA bind and activate the GLP-1 receptor, the endogenous incretin hormone that potentiates glucose-dependent insulin secretion from the pancreatic beta cells. The synthetic GLP1-RA receptor agonists (exenatide, liraglutide, dulaglutide, semaglutide, lixisenatide) are variably resistant to degradation by the enzyme dipeptidyl peptidase-4 (DPP-4) and therefore have a longer half-life.

Semaglutide is extensively metabolized through proteolytic cleavage of the peptide backbone and sequential beta-oxidation of the fatty acid side chain. The enzyme neutral endopeptidase (NEP) is expected to be involved in semaglutide metabolism. Liraglutide is primarily excreted intact, while exenatide is eliminated independently of the dose by glomerular filtration [153–155].

The last approved antihyperglycemic drug, tirzepatide, is a dual GIP and GLP-1 receptor agonist. According to PK, 99% is bound to plasma albumin and is metabolized by proteolytic cleavage of the peptide backbone, beta oxidation of the C20 fatty diacid moiety, and amide hydrolysis [156]. To the best of our knowledge, through searching the literature, no relevant PGx evidence for tirzepatide was currently identified.

Although novelty drugs GLP1-RA and tirzepatide revolutionized the treatment of obesity, and therefore MetS, most of the PGx studies are based on PD rather than PK aspects.

5.6. Dipeptidyl Peptidase-4 (DPP-4) Inhibitors

DPP-4 inhibitors are a class of oral glucose-lowering agents which accomplish their glucose lowering effect by inhibiting the DPP-4 enzyme, which is responsible for the rapid degradation of incretin hormones such as GLP-1 and GIP. By inhibiting DPP-4, these drugs prolong the activity of incretin hormones, thereby enhancing glucose-dependent insulin secretion and suppressing glucagon release, which contributes to better glycemic control [114,115,157,158].

DPP-4 inhibitors generally exhibit no significant interactions with other drugs, and gliptins do not markedly alter the pharmacokinetics or exposure of co-administered medications. As a result, dosage adjustments are typically unnecessary when gliptins are used in combination with other pharmacological agents. However, important exceptions exist with sitagliptin and saxagliptin [158–161].

Sitagliptin is only minimally metabolized in the liver, with over 80% being excreted intact in urine [161]. Minor metabolic pathways are mediated mainly by CYP3A4 and to a lesser extent by CYP2C8. Still, a few case reports have suggested the possible inhibition of CYP3A4 and/or p-glycoprotein as well as sitagliptin-mediated impairments in renal function as causes of potential interactions [162–165]. Sitagliptin had no significant impact on simvastatin pharmacokinetics in one crossover study, increasing the AUC of the active simvastatin by only 1% [166]. Further studies are necessary to assess the in vivo impact of sitagliptin on the CYP3A4 enzyme system and to explore additional mechanisms that may contribute to these DDIs.

While selected, higher-risk individuals may experience a greater-than-average interaction between these agents, possibly explaining these few observed cases, it seems at least equally plausible that other factors, besides a sitagliptin–statin interaction, account for the toxicity observed in these cases.

Saxagliptin undergoes metabolism to an active metabolite via CYP3A4/5 enzymes. When co-administered with potent CYP3A4/5 inhibitors (e.g., ketoconazole, diltiazem) or inducers (e.g., rifampicin, dexamethasone), the exposure to saxagliptin and its primary metabolite is significantly altered [167]. In such cases, careful monitoring of glycemic control is essential.

6. Discussion

Metabolic syndrome represents a major global health challenge in today's world. The need to manage its risk factors and complications often leads to polypharmacy, significantly increasing the potential for undesirable outcomes such as ADRs, DDIs, DDGIs, poor treatment adherence, and medication errors. Furthermore, the financial burden of therapy rises with the number of medications prescribed, a cost that escalates further in the event of ADRs.

After a clear correlation has been established between genetic defects in drug-metabolizing enzymes and drug transporters and their impact on the efficacy and toxicity of certain drugs, some clinical guidelines for healthcare professionals have been developed and published by different working groups and organizations (CPIC, DPWG, PharmGKB). Depending on the scientific evidence, these guidelines and recommendations can be included in Patient Information Leaflets (PILs) and Summaries of Product Characteristics (SmPCs) by regulatory agencies such as the FDA and EMA. These guidelines significantly contribute to the transfer and implementation of pharmacogenetic knowledge into clinical practice.

Regarding clinical practice recommendations based on clinical pharmacogenetics, among the medications reviewed for MetS, we identified only the CPIC guideline for statins, considering the SLCO1B1, ABCG2, and CYP2C9 genotypes. This guideline provides statin recommendations (preferred intensity and dose) based on the SLCO1B1 phenotype and the risk of statin-associated muscle symptoms (SAMSs). For instance, in a patient with poor SLCO1B1 function requiring high-intensity statin therapy, simvastatin and atorvastatin are to be avoided due to their elevated SAMSs risk. Rosuvastatin (5–10 mg) or pitavastatin (2–4 mg) are recommended as safer alternatives. Recommendations for ABCG2 are specific to rosuvastatin, suggesting a starting dose of ≤20 mg for individuals with a poor ABCG2 function. If a higher dose is necessary, an alternative statin or combination therapy (e.g., statin + ezetimibe) is advised. CYP2C9 phenotype-based recommendations pertain to fluvastatin, with intermediate metabolizers avoiding doses > 40 mg and poor metabolizers avoiding doses > 20 mg. If higher doses are required, an alternative statin is recommended. If fluvastatin is necessary, combination therapy (40 mg for intermediate metabolizers, 20 mg for poor metabolizers) with a non-statin lipid-lowering agent is suggested. This guideline exemplifies an ideal approach to consider pharmacokinetics, adverse drug reactions (ADRs), and drug–drug interactions (DDIs) when prescribing. It would be beneficial to have more guidelines focused on MetS drugs in the future.

In daily MetS management, clinicians frequently prescribe overlapping regimens of lipid-lowering drugs, antihypertensives, and antihyperglycemic drugs. For this reason, it is of great relevance to identify and understand the potential DDIs and DDGIs within these regimens (Tables 1 and 2).

Table 2. Drug–drug interactions based on the Lexidrug database.

Substrate	Inhibitor	Relevant Genotype	Effect	Reference	Risk Rating
SLCO1B1-mediated					
gliclazide **glimepiride** **glipizide** **gliquidone**	gemfibrozil	*SLCO1B*	increased risk of hypoglycemia	[142]	C
atorvastatin **fluvastatin** **lovastatin** **pitavastatin** **pravastatin**	gemfibrozil	*SLCO1B*	increased risk of myopathy	[63,155,156]	X
repaglinid	gemfibrozil	*SLCO1B* *CYP2C8*	increase the serum concentration of repaglinide	[63]	X
Various cytochrome P450 (CYP) enzymes					
pioglitazone **rosiglitazone** *	gemfibrozil	*CYP2C8*	decreased blood glucose, evidence of edema or hepatotoxicity	[131–133]	D/C *
simvastatin	diltiazem	*CYP3A5*3/*3*	increased risk of myopathy	[99]	D
atorvastatin **lovastatin** **simvastatin**	amlodipine diltiazem verapamil	*CYP3A4*	increase the serum concentration of simvastatin acute kidney injury, hyperkalemia	[99]	D
saxagliptin	diltiazem	*CYP3A4*	may increase the serum concentration of saxagliptin	[67]	C
sitagliptin	simvastatin	*CYP3A4*	increased risk of myopathy	[162–166]	C
atorvastatin, **fluvastatin** **lovastatin** **pitavastatin** **pravastatin** **rosuvastatin** **simvastatin**	fenofibrate	Uncertain (possible additive effect)	increased risk of myopathy	[61]	C

X, avoid combination; A, no known interaction; B, no action needed; C, monitor therapy; D, consider therapy modification. The * for rosiglitazone means rosiglitazone was withdrawn from the market.

With lipid-lowering drugs, ADRs such as SAMSs, with the use of PGx testing, are preventable. In the MetS population, the concomitant use of statins and calcium channel blockers is frequent. Simvastatin and amlodipine share the same metabolic pathway through the enzyme CYP3A4. The product label advises against using them together if the dose of simvastatin exceeds 20 mg per day due to the risk of adverse effects. Similar caution should be applied to co-therapy involving amlodipine or losartan with atorvastatin and lovastatin, as both medications are also metabolized by CYP3A4 in the liver [157]. Despite existing statin clinical PGs practice guidelines recommendations, are focused primarily on polymorphisms of the SLCO1B1, ABCG2, and CYP2C9 genes. We have opted to include information on CYP3A4 polymorphisms in this text. This decision is based on the understanding that, while individual CYP3A4 variant effects may be modest, their cumulative impact or interactions with other factors (genetic, environmental, or drug-related) could hold clinical relevance.

Also, regarding statin-related toxicity, ABCG2 polymorphism should be taken into consideration when prescribing co-therapies. Potential interactions can arise between substrates (atorvastatin) and ABCG2 inhibitors (such as amlodipine, lacidipine and lercanidipine). For attending physicians, it is advisable to opt for drugs that do not inhibit the ABCG2 gene [41].

ABCG2 plays a crucial role in regulating the absorption of its substrates in the gut and facilitating their excretion into bile and urine, thereby decreasing the bioavailability of drugs that interact with it. There is a relatively common frequency of *ABCG2* polymorphisms in the population, with the genotype frequency for variants such as *ABCG2* c.421 C A reaching 10–15% among Caucasians [37]. Given the mentioned substrates, as well as inhibitors of ABCG2, there is a need for further research on the potential association of ABCG2 polymorphisms to avoid possible therapeutic difficulties.

Clinically relevant drug substrates of ABCG2 other than lipid-lowering drugs (rosuvastatin, atorvastatin, fluvastatin, ezetimibe, fibrates) are PPIs and anticoagulants (apixaban, rivaroxaban) [25–30]. Given that patients with metabolic syndrome are predisposed to cardiovascular disease (CVD), the potential DDGI is paramount, especially in prescribed anticoagulant drugs. This consideration underscores the importance of comprehensive medication management and genetic profiling in optimizing treatment efficacy and minimizing serious ADRs in this patient population.

For clinical practice, an important example of potential drug–drug interactions (DDIs) involving CYP2C9 genotypes could be the combined treatment of fluvastatin with medications commonly prescribed for comorbidities in patients with hyperlipidemia, such as losartan or valsartan (for hypertension) or glimepiride (for diabetes). While fluvastatin is a known CYP2C9 substrate, the co-administration of fluvastatin with other medications that interact with CYP2C9, such as losartan, valsartan, or glimepiride (whether as weak or moderate inhibitors or inducers), could potentially alter fluvastatin exposure. In the case of CYP2C9 inhibitors, this could lead to increased fluvastatin levels, particularly in individuals with CYP2C9 poor metabolizer genotypes, due to their inherently reduced CYP2C9 enzyme activity. This heightened exposure might increase the risk of dose-related adverse events such as myopathy. Conversely, if a co-administered medication induces CYP2C9 activity it could decrease fluvastatin levels, potentially leading to subtherapeutic concentrations.

Fibrates are dominantly favorable in the management of hypertriglyceridemia. Gemfibrozil, if given concomitantly with statin therapy, also has the potential to induce SAMSs [168–170]. On the other hand, gemfibrozil can interfere with pioglitazone. *CYP2C8*3* allele influences the variability of PK during the interaction between gemfibrozil, a CYP2C8 inhibitor, and pioglitazone, a CYP2C8 substrate. In a randomized, two-phase crossover study involving 30 healthy Caucasian participants, the findings revealed that the presence of the *CYP2C8*3* allele led to decreased plasma exposure of pioglitazone in vivo and significantly impacted the extent of the DDI between gemfibrozil and pioglitazone [139]. Furthermore, the observed effect of the genotype was consistent with findings from previous clinical studies, indicating approximately 25% to 30% lower plasma exposure of pioglitazone in carriers of the *CYP2C8*3* allele compared to individuals with the wild-type genotype [140].

Within our review, we searched for existing clinical recommendations and found that, although the PGs information of some drugs has been evaluated by CPIC and DPWG, no dosing recommendations have been made for routine clinical practice in certain cases. Examples include carvedilol (CYP2D6), glimepiride (CYP2C9), and gliclazide, glimepiride, or glipizide (G6PD genotype) [7,8]. For instance, while the impact of CYP2D6 variations on carvedilol PK may not currently necessitate dose adjustments, ongoing research could reveal subtle differences in efficacy or safety profiles among different metabolizer phenotypes. Similarly, further investigation into the effects of CYP2C9 and G6PD genotypes on the metabolism and response to antidiabetic medications like glimepiride and glipizide could potentially identify subgroups of patients who may benefit from personalized dosing strategies. Therefore, the absence of current recommendations should not be interpreted as a lack of potential clinical relevance for PGs in these cases. Rather, it highlights the need for continued research and the importance of staying abreast of emerging evidence in this rapidly evolving field.

While the interactions between one drug and a polymorphic enzyme or transporter genes is documented in some cases, our knowledge about the role of PGx in polypharmacy is still insufficient. As can be seen from Table 1, many drugs used in the treatment of MetS often share the same metabolic and transport pathways. The presence of polymorphic low- or high-activity variants of relevant genes along with drug interactions represent a significant risk for the development of ADRs and/or ineffectiveness. These are important challenges for future research on the role of PGx in the treatment of MetS.

Pharmacogenetic testing has the potential to identify patients at risk, but its widespread adoption in clinical practice faces challenges such as center availability of genetic testing, patient selection, result interpretation, and incorporation into treatment decisions. Pre-emptive pharmacogenetic analysis, coupled with assessing DDGIs, could enhance personalized drug and dose selection, reducing the incidence of ADRs.

We advocate for the integration of pharmacogenetic testing into routine clinical practice to optimize medication management in complex patient populations. By elucidating how genetic variations influence drug responses and interactions, pharmacogenomic testing offers a promising avenue for personalized treatment approaches, optimizing treatment outcomes and enhancing patient safety in the face of complex medication regimens. Further larger studies are needed and would enable us to come closer to implementing personalized treatment for patients with MetS.

Author Contributions: Conceptualization, A.B., J.M.-P. and D.V.; investigation, S.K., F.F.-A., T.B. and A.B.; data curation, S.K., F.F.-A., T.B. and A.B.; writing—original draft preparation, S.K., F.F.-A., T.B. and A.B.; writing—review and editing, all authors; supervision, A.B., T.B., J.M.-P. and D.V.; project administration, S.K. and A.B. All authors have read and agreed to the published version of the manuscript.

Funding: This research received no external funding.

Institutional Review Board Statement: Not applicable.

Informed Consent Statement: Not applicable.

Data Availability Statement: No new data were created or analyzed in this study. Data sharing is not applicable to this article.

Conflicts of Interest: The authors declare no conflicts of interest.

References

1. A Fahed, G.; Aoun, L.; BouZerdan, M.; Allam, S.; Bouferraa, Y.; Assi, H.I. Metabolic Syndrome: Updates on Pathophysiology and Management in 2021. *Int. J. Mol. Sci.* **2022**, *23*, 786. [CrossRef] [PubMed]
2. Tannenbaum, C.; Sheehan, N.L. Understanding and preventing drug-drug and drug-gene interactions. *Expert Rev. Clin. Pharmacol.* **2014**, *7*, 533–544. [CrossRef] [PubMed]

3. Malki, M.A.; Pearson, E.R. Drug–drug–gene interactions and adverse drug reactions. *Pharmacogenom. J.* **2020**, *20*, 355–366. [CrossRef]
4. UpToDate Lexidrug [Internet]. Available online: https://online.lexi.com/lco/action/login (accessed on 10 May 2024).
5. Fohner, A.E.; Brackman, D.J.; Giacomini, K.M.; Altman, R.B.; Klein, T.E. PharmGKB summary: Very important pharmacogene information for ABCG2. *Pharmacogenet. Genom.* **2017**, *27*, 420–427. [CrossRef]
6. Knox, C.; Wilson, M.; Klinger, C.M.; Franklin, M.; Oler, E.; Wilson, A.; Pon, A.; Cox, J.; Chin, N.E.; Strawbridge, S.A.; et al. DrugBank 6.0: The DrugBank Knowledgebase for 2024. *Nucleic Acids Res.* **2024**, *52*, D1265–D1275. [CrossRef] [PubMed]
7. CPIC: Clinical Pharmacogenetics Implementation Consortium of the Pharmacogenomics Research Network [Internet]. 2024. Available online: https://cpicpgx.org/ (accessed on 23 April 2024).
8. Bank, P.C.D.; Caudle, K.E.; Swen, J.J.; Gammal, R.S.; Whirl-Carrillo, M.; Klein, T.E.; Relling, M.; Guchelaar, H. Comparison of the Guidelines of the Clinical Pharmacogenetics Implementation Consortium and the Dutch Pharmacogenetics Working Group. *Clin. Pharmacol. Ther.* **2018**, *103*, 599–618. [CrossRef]
9. Pappan, N.; Rehman, A. *Dyslipidemia. StatPearls [Internet]*; StatPearls Publishing: Treasure Island, FL, USA, 2024. Available online: http://www.ncbi.nlm.nih.gov/books/NBK560891/ (accessed on 25 April 2024).
10. Abera, A.; Worede, A.; Hirigo, A.T.; Alemayehu, R.; Ambachew, S. Dyslipidemia and associated factors among adult cardiac patients: A hospital-based comparative cross-sectional study. *Eur. J. Med. Res.* **2024**, *29*, 237. [CrossRef]
11. Mach, F.; Baigent, C.; Catapano, A.L.; Koskinas, K.C.; Casula, M.; Badimon, L.; Chapman, M.J.; De Backer, G.G.; Delgado, V.; Ference, B.A.; et al. 2019 ESC/EAS Guidelines for the management of dyslipidaemias: Lipid modification to reduce cardiovascular risk: The Task Force for the management of dyslipidaemias of the European Society of Cardiology (ESC) and European Atherosclerosis Society (EAS). *Eur. Heart J.* **2020**, *41*, 111–188. [CrossRef]
12. Cooper-DeHoff, R.M.; Niemi, M.; Ramsey, L.B.; Luzum, J.A.; Tarkiainen, E.K.; Straka, R.J.; Gong, L.; Tuteja, S.; Wilke, R.A.; Wadelius, M.; et al. The Clinical Pharmacogenetics Implementation Consortium Guideline for SLCO1B1, ABCG2, and CYP2C9 genotypes and Statin-Associated Musculoskeletal Symptoms. *Clin. Pharmacol. Ther.* **2022**, *111*, 1007–1021. [CrossRef]
13. Turner, R.M.; Pirmohamed, M. Statin-Related Myotoxicity: A Comprehensive Review of Pharmacokinetic, Pharmacogenomic and Muscle Components. *J. Clin. Med.* **2019**, *9*, 22. [CrossRef]
14. Voora, D.; Baye, J.; McDermaid, A.; Narayana, S.; Wilke, R.A.; Myrmoe, A.N.; Hajek, C.; Larson, E.A. SLCO1B1*5 Allele Is Associated with Atorvastatin Discontinuation and Adverse Muscle Symptoms in the Context of Routine Care. *Clin. Pharmacol. Ther.* **2022**, *111*, 1075–1083. [CrossRef] [PubMed]
15. Turner, R.M.; Fontana, V.; Zhang, J.E.; Carr, D.; Yin, P.; FitzGerald, R.; Morris, A.P.; Pirmohamed, M. A Genome-wide Association Study of Circulating Levels of Atorvastatin and Its Major Metabolites. *Clin. Pharmacol. Ther.* **2020**, *108*, 287–297. [CrossRef] [PubMed]
16. Pasanen, M.K.; Fredrikson, H.; Neuvonen, P.J.; Niemi, M. Different effects of SLCO1B1 polymorphism on the pharmacokinetics of atorvastatin and rosuvastatin. *Clin. Pharmacol. Ther.* **2007**, *82*, 726–733. [CrossRef]
17. Mykkänen, A.J.; Tarkiainen, E.K.; Taskinen, S.; Neuvonen, M.; Paile-Hyvärinen, M.; Lilius, T.O.; Tapaninen, T.; Klein, K.; Schwab, M.; Backman, J.T.; et al. Genome-Wide Association Study of Atorvastatin Pharmacokinetics: Associations with SLCO1B1, UGT1A3, and LPP. *Clin. Pharmacol. Ther.* **2024**, *115*, 1428–1440. [CrossRef] [PubMed]
18. Božina, T.; Ganoci, L.; Karačić, E.; Šimičević, L.; Vrkić-Kirhmajer, M.; Klarica-Domjanović, I.; Križ, T.; Sertić, Z.; Božina, N. ABCG2 and SLCO1B1 gene polymorphisms in the Croatian population. *Ann. Hum. Biol.* **2022**, *49*, 323–331. [CrossRef]
19. Kalliokoski, A.; Niemi, M. Impact of OATP transporters on pharmacokinetics. *Br. J. Pharmacol.* **2009**, *158*, 693–705. [CrossRef]
20. Klaassen, C.D.; Aleksunes, L.M. Xenobiotic, bile acid, piand cholesterol transporters: Function and regulation. *Pharmacol. Rev.* **2010**, *62*, 1–96. [CrossRef]
21. International Transporter Consortium; Giacomini, K.M.; Huang, S.-M.; Tweedie, D.J.; Benet, L.Z.; Brouwer, K.L.R.; Chu, X.; Dahlin, A.; Evers, R.; Fischer, V.; et al. Membrane transporters in drug development. *Nat. Rev. Drug Discov.* **2010**, *9*, 215–236. [CrossRef]
22. Mao, Q.; Unadkat, J.D. Role of the breast cancer resistance protein (BCRP/ABCG2) in drug transport—An update. *AAPS J.* **2015**, *17*, 65–82. [CrossRef]
23. Poirier, A.; Portmann, R.; Cascais, A.-C.; Bader, U.; Walter, I.; Ullah, M.; Funk, C. The need for human breast cancer resistance protein substrate and inhibition evaluation in drug discovery and development: Why, when, and how? *Drug Metab. Dispos. Biol. Fate Chem.* **2014**, *42*, 1466–1477. [CrossRef]
24. Matsuo, H.; Takada, T.; Ichida, K.; Nakamura, T.; Nakayama, A.; Suzuki, H.; Hosoya, T.; Shinomiya, N. ABCG2/BCRP dysfunction as a major cause of gout. *Nucleosides Nucleotides Nucleic Acids* **2011**, *30*, 1117–1128. [CrossRef] [PubMed]
25. Hira, D.; Terada, T. BCRP/ABCG2 and high-alert medications: Biochemical, pharmacokinetic, pharmacogenetic, and clinical implications. *Biochem. Pharmacol.* **2018**, *147*, 201–210. [CrossRef] [PubMed]
26. Heyes, N.; Kapoor, P.; Kerr, I.D. Polymorphisms of the Multidrug Pump ABCG2: A Systematic Review of Their Effect on Protein Expression, Function, and Drug Pharmacokinetics. *Drug Metab. Dispos. Biol. Fate Chem.* **2018**, *46*, 1886–1899. [CrossRef]
27. Safar, Z.; Kis, E.; Erdo, F.; Zolnerciks, J.K.; Krajcsi, P. ABCG2/BCRP: Variants, transporter interaction profile of substrates and inhibitors. *Expert Opin. Drug Metab. Toxicol.* **2019**, *15*, 313–328. [CrossRef] [PubMed]

28. Giacomini, K.M.; Balimane, P.V.; Cho, S.K.; Eadon, M.; Edeki, T.; Hillgren, K.M.; Huang, S.-M.; Sugiyama, Y.; Weitz, D.; Wen, Y.; et al. International Transporter Consortium commentary on clinically important transporter polymorphisms. *Clin. Pharmacol. Ther.* **2013**, *94*, 23–26. [CrossRef]
29. Toyoda, Y.; Takada, T.; Suzuki, H. Inhibitors of Human ABCG2: From Technical Background to Recent Updates with Clinical Implications. *Front. Pharmacol.* **2019**, *10*, 208. [CrossRef]
30. Svedberg, A.; Jacobs, L.; Vikingsson, S.; Gréen, H. The influence of ABCG2 polymorphism on erlotinib efflux in the K562 cell line. *Pharmacol. Res. Perspect.* **2020**, *8*, e00581. [CrossRef]
31. Hofman, J.; Sorf, A.; Vagiannis, D.; Sucha, S.; Kammerer, S.; Küpper, J.-H.; Chen, S.; Guo, L.; Ceckova, M.; Staud, F. Brivanib Exhibits Potential for Pharmacokinetic Drug-Drug Interactions and the Modulation of Multidrug Resistance through the Inhibition of Human ABCG2 Drug Efflux Transporter and CYP450 Biotransformation Enzymes. *Mol. Pharm.* **2019**, *16*, 4436–4450. [CrossRef]
32. Hirota, T.; Fujita, Y.; Ieiri, I. An updated review of pharmacokinetic drug interactions and pharmacogenetics of statins. *Expert Opin. Drug Metab. Toxicol.* **2020**, *16*, 809–822. [CrossRef]
33. Klarica, D.I.; Lovrić, M.; Trkulja, V.; Petelin-Gadže, Ž.; Ganoci, L.; Čajić, I.; Božina, N. Interaction between ABCG2 421C>A polymorphism and valproate in their effects on steady-state disposition of lamotrigine in adults with epilepsy. *Br. J. Clin. Pharmacol.* **2018**, *84*, 2106–2119. [CrossRef]
34. Šušak, S.I.; Božina, N.; Klarica, D.I.; Sporiš, D.; Bašić, S.; Bašić, I.; Lovrić, M.; Ganoci, L.; Trkulja, V. Breast cancer resistance protein polymorphism ABCG2 c.421C>A (rs2231142) moderates the effect of valproate on lamotrigine trough concentrations in adults with epilepsy. *Fundam. Clin. Pharmacol.* **2024**, *38*, 351–368. [CrossRef] [PubMed]
35. Keskitalo, J.E.; Zolk, O.; Fromm, M.F.; Kurkinen, K.J.; Neuvonen, P.J.; Niemi, M. ABCG2 polymorphism markedly affects the pharmacokinetics of atorvastatin and rosuvastatin. *Clin. Pharmacol. Ther.* **2009**, *86*, 197–203. [CrossRef] [PubMed]
36. Ganoci, L.; Trkulja, V.; Živković, M.; Božina, T.; Šagud, M.; Lovrić, M.; Božina, N. ABCB1, ABCG2 and CYP2D6 polymorphism effects on disposition and response to long-acting risperidone. *Prog. Neuropsychopharmacol. Biol. Psychiatry* **2021**, *104*, 110042. [CrossRef]
37. Sakiyama, M.; Matsuo, H.; Takada, Y.; Nakamura, T.; Nakayama, A.; Takada, T.; Kitajiri, S.-I.; Wakai, K.; Suzuki, H.; Shinomiya, N. Ethnic differences in ATP-binding cassette transporter, sub-family G, member 2 (ABCG2/BCRP): Genotype combinations and estimated functions. *Drug Metab. Pharmacokinet.* **2014**, *29*, 490–492. [CrossRef] [PubMed]
38. Keskitalo, J.E.; Pasanen, M.K.; Neuvonen, P.J.; Niemi, M. Different effects of the ABCG2 c.421C>A SNP on the pharmacokinetics of fluvastatin, pravastatin and simvastatin. *Pharmacogenomics* **2009**, *10*, 1617–1624. [CrossRef]
39. Tsamandouras, N.; Guo, Y.; Wendling, T.; Hall, S.; Galetin, A.; Aarons, L. Modelling of atorvastatin pharmacokinetics and the identification of the effect of a BCRP polymorphism in the Japanese population. *Pharmacogenet. Genom.* **2017**, *27*, 27–38. [CrossRef]
40. Merćep, I.; Radman, I.; Trkulja, V.; Božina, T.; Šimičević, L.; Budimir, E.; Ganoci, L.; Božina, N. Loss of function polymorphisms in SLCO1B1 (c.521T>C, rs4149056) and ABCG2 (c.421C>A, rs2231142) genes are associated with adverse events of rosuvastatin: A case-control study. *Eur. J. Clin. Pharmacol.* **2022**, *78*, 227–236. [CrossRef]
41. Mirošević, S.N.; Macolić, S.V.; Šimić, I.; Ganoci, L.; Muačević, D.; Božina, N. ABCG2 gene polymorphisms as risk factors for atorvastatin adverse reactions: A case-control study. *Pharmacogenomics* **2015**, *16*, 803–815. [CrossRef]
42. Miroševic, S.N.; Božina, N.; Zibar, L.; Barišic, I.; Pejnovic, L.; Macolic, S.V. CYP2C9 and ABCG2 polymorphisms as risk factors for developing adverse drug reactions in renal transplant patients taking fluvastatin: A case-control study. *Pharmacogenomics* **2013**, *14*, 1419–1431. [CrossRef]
43. European Medicine Agency. Guideline on the Investigation of Drug Interactions [Internet]. 2012. Available online: https://www.ema.europa.eu/en/documents/scientific-guideline/guideline-investigation-drug-interactions-revision-1_en.pdf (accessed on 1 June 2024).
44. Draft Guidance for Industry on Drug Interaction Studies-Study Design. Data Analysis, Implications for Dosing, and Labeling Recommendations; Availability [Internet]. *Fed. Regist.* **2012**. Available online: https://www.federalregister.gov/documents/2012/02/21/2012-3958/draft-guidance-for-industry-on-drug-interaction-studies-study-design-data-analysis-implications-for (accessed on 23 April 2024).
45. Malfará, B.N.; Benzi, J.R.; Oliveira, G.C.; Zanelli, C.F.; Duarte, G.; Cavalli, R.d.C.; de Moraes, N.V. ABCG2 c.421C>A polymorphism alters nifedipine transport to breast milk in hypertensive breastfeeding women. *Reprod. Toxicol.* **2019**, *85*, 1–5. [CrossRef]
46. Ganoci, L.; Božina, T.; Mirošević, N.; Lovrić, M.; Mas, P.; Božina, N. Genetic polymorphisms of cytochrome P450 enzymes: CYP2C9, CYP2C19, CYP2D6, CYP3A4, and CYP3A5 in the Croatian population. *Drug Metab. Pers Ther.* **2017**, *32*, 11–21. [CrossRef]
47. Wilke, R.A.; Ramsey, L.B.; Johnson, S.G.; Maxwell, W.D.; McLeod, H.L.; Voora, D.; Krauss, R.M.; Roden, D.M.; Feng, Q.; Cooper-DeHoff, R.M.; et al. The clinical pharmacogenomics implementation consortium: CPIC guideline for SLCO1B1 and simvastatin-induced myopathy. *Clin. Pharmacol. Ther.* **2012**, *92*, 112–117. [CrossRef]
48. Ramsey, L.B.; Johnson, S.G.; Caudle, K.E.; Haidar, C.E.; Voora, D.; Wilke, R.A.; Maxwell, W.D.; McLeod, H.L.; Krauss, R.M.; Roden, D.M.; et al. The clinical pharmacogenetics implementation consortium guideline for SLCO1B1 and simvastatin-induced myopathy: 2014 update. *Clin. Pharmacol. Ther.* **2014**, *96*, 423–428. [CrossRef] [PubMed]
49. Mykkänen, A.J.; Taskinen, S.; Neuvonen, M.; Paile-Hyvärinen, M.; Tarkiainen, E.K.; Lilius, T.; Tapaninen, T.; Backman, J.T.; Tornio, A.; Niemi, M.; et al. Genomewide Association Study of Simvastatin Pharmacokinetics. *Clin. Pharmacol. Ther.* **2022**, *112*, 676–686. [CrossRef]

50. Zubiaur, P.; Benedicto, M.D.; Villapalos-García, G.; Navares-Gómez, M.; Mejía-Abril, G.; Román, M.; Martín-Vílchez, S.; Ochoa, D.; Abad-Santos, F. SLCO1B1 Phenotype and CYP3A5 Polymorphism Significantly Affect Atorvastatin Bioavailability. *J. Pers Med.* **2021**, *11*, 204. [CrossRef] [PubMed]
51. Luzum, J.A.; Theusch, E.; Taylor, K.D.; Wang, A.; Sadee, W.; Binkley, P.F.; Krauss, R.M.; Medina, M.W.; Kitzmiller, J.P. Individual and Combined Associations of Genetic Variants in CYP3A4, CYP3A5, and SLCO1B1 with Simvastatin and Simvastatin Acid Plasma Concentrations. *J. Cardiovasc. Pharmacol.* **2015**, *66*, 80–85. [CrossRef]
52. Lee, S.-J.; Goldstein, J.A. Functionally defective or altered CYP3A4 and CYP3A5 single nucleotide polymorphisms and their detection with genotyping tests. *Pharmacogenomics* **2005**, *6*, 357–371. [CrossRef]
53. Mulder, T.A.; Eerden, R.A.; With, M.; Elens, L.; Hesselink, D.A.; Matic, M.; Bins, S.; Mathijssen, R.H.J.; van Schaik, R.H.N. CYP3A4∗22 Genotyping in Clinical Practice: Ready for Implementation? *Front. Genet.* **2021**, *12*, 711943. [CrossRef] [PubMed]
54. Westlind-Johnsson, A.; Hermann, R.; Huennemeyer, A.; Hauns, B.; Lahu, G.; Nassr, N.; Zech, K.; Ingelmansundberg, M.; Vonrichter, O. Identification and characterization of CYP3A4*20, a novel rare CYP3A4 allele without functional activity. *Clin. Pharmacol. Ther.* **2006**, *79*, 339–349. [CrossRef] [PubMed]
55. Elens, L.; Capron, A.; Schaik, R.H.; Meyer, M.; Pauw, L.; Eddour, D.C.; Latinne, D.; Wallemacq, P.; Mourad, M.; Haufroid, V. Impact of CYP3A4*22 allele on tacrolimus pharmacokinetics in early period after renal transplantation: Toward updated genotype-based dosage guidelines. *Ther. Drug Monit.* **2013**, *35*, 608–616. [CrossRef]
56. Wang, D.; Guo, Y.; Wrighton, S.A.; Cooke, G.E.; Sadee, W. Intronic polymorphism in CYP3A4 affects hepatic expression and response to statin drugs. *Pharmacogenom. J.* **2011**, *11*, 274–286. [CrossRef]
57. Theile, D.; Hohmann, N.; Kiemel, D.; Gattuso, G.; Barreca, D.; Mikus, G.; Haefeli, W.E.; Schwenger, V.; Weiss, J. Clementine juice has the potential for drug interactions—In vitro comparison with grapefruit and mandarin juice. *Eur. J. Pharm. Sci. Off J Eur. Fed. Pharm. Sci.* **2017**, *97*, 247–256. [CrossRef] [PubMed]
58. Riedmaier, S.; Klein, K.; Hofmann, U.; Keskitalo, J.E.; Neuvonen, P.J.; Schwab, M.; Niemi, M.; Zanger, U.M. UDP-glucuronosyltransferase (UGT) polymorphisms affect atorvastatin lactonization in vitro and in vivo. *Clin. Pharmacol. Ther.* **2010**, *87*, 65–73. [CrossRef] [PubMed]
59. Keskitalo, J.E.; Kurkinen, K.J.; Neuvoneni, P.J.; Niemi, M. ABCB1 haplotypes differentially affect the pharmacokinetics of the acid and lactone forms of simvastatin and atorvastatin. *Clin. Pharmacol. Ther.* **2008**, *84*, 457–461. [CrossRef] [PubMed]
60. Birmingham, B.K.; Bujac, S.R.; Elsby, R.; Azumaya, C.T.; Wei, C.; Chen, Y.; Mosqueda-Garcia, R.; Ambrose, H.J. Impact of ABCG2 and SLCO1B1 polymorphisms on pharmacokinetics of rosuvastatin, atorvastatin and simvastatin acid in Caucasian and Asian subjects: A class effect? *Eur. J. Clin. Pharmacol.* **2015**, *71*, 341–355. [CrossRef]
61. Thompson, P.D.; Clarkson, P.; Karas, R.H. Statin-associated myopathy. *JAMA* **2003**, *289*, 1681–1690. [CrossRef]
62. Shah, M.B. Inhibition of CYP2C8 by Acyl Glucuronides of Gemfibrozil and Clopidogrel: Pharmacological Significance, Progress and Challenges. *Biomolecules* **2022**, *12*, 1218. [CrossRef]
63. Türk, D.; Hanke, N.; Wolf, S.; Frechen, S.; Eissing, T.; Wendl, T.; Schwab, M.; Lehr, T. Physiologically Based Pharmacokinetic Models for Prediction of Complex CYP2C8 and OATP1B1 (SLCO1B1) Drug-Drug-Gene Interactions: A Modeling Network of Gemfibrozil, Repaglinide, Pioglitazone, Rifampicin, Clarithromycin and Itraconazole. *Clin. Pharmacokinet.* **2019**, *58*, 1595–1607. [CrossRef]
64. Kosoglou, T.; Statkevich, P.; Johnson-Levonas, A.O.; Paolini, J.F.; Bergman, A.J.; Alton, K.B. Ezetimibe: A review of its metabolism, pharmacokinetics and drug interactions. *Clin. Pharmacokinet.* **2005**, *44*, 467–494. [CrossRef]
65. Oswald, S.; Haenisch, S.; Fricke, C.; Sudhop, T.; Remmler, C.; Giessmann, T.; Jedlitschky, G.; Adam, U.; Dazert, E.; Warzok, R. Intestinal expression of P-glycoprotein (ABCB1), multidrug resistance associated protein 2 (ABCC2), and uridine diphosphate-glucuronosyltransferase 1A1 predicts the disposition and modulates the effects of the cholesterol absorption inhibitor ezetimibe in humans. *Clin. Pharmacol. Ther.* **2006**, *79*, 206–217. [CrossRef]
66. Waart, D.R.; Vlaming, M.L.; Kunne, C.; Schinkel, A.H.; Oude, E. Complex pharmacokinetic behavior of ezetimibe depends on abcc2, abcc3, and abcg2. *Drug Metab. Dispos. Biol. Fate Chem.* **2009**, *37*, 1698–1702. [CrossRef] [PubMed]
67. Oswald, S.; König, J.; Lütjohann, D.; Giessmann, T.; Kroemer, H.K.; Rimmbach, C.; Rosskopf, D.; Fromm, M.F.; Siegmund, W. Disposition of ezetimibe is influenced by polymorphisms of the hepatic uptake carrier OATP1B1. *Pharmacogenet. Genom.* **2008**, *18*, 559–568. [CrossRef]
68. Bozina, N.; Simicevic, L.; Pecin, I. The pharmacogenomics of hypolipemics: ABCG2 as a potential predictor of hepatotoxicity. *Biochem. Med. Zagreb.* **2018**, *8*, 28.
69. Hajar, R. PCSK 9 Inhibitors: A Short History and a New Era of Lipid-Lowering Therapy. *Heart Views* **2019**, *20*, 74. [CrossRef]
70. Hindi, N.N.; Alenbawi, J.; Nemer, G. Pharmacogenomics Variability of Lipid-Lowering Therapies in Familial Hypercholesterolemia. *J. Pers. Med.* **2021**, *11*, 877. [CrossRef]
71. Zhang, Y.; Chen, H.; Liu, H.; Wang, H.; Li, B.; Zhang, M.; Li, J.; Yang, L.; Fan, L. Inclisiran: A New Generation of Lipid-Lowering SiRNA Therapeutic. *Front. Pharmacol.* **2023**, *14*. [CrossRef] [PubMed]
72. Blood Pressure Lowering Treatment Trialists' Collaboration. Blood pressure-lowering treatment based on cardiovascular risk: A meta-analysis of individual patient data. *Lancet* **2014**, *384*, 591–598. [CrossRef]
73. Franklin, S.S. Hypertension in the metabolic syndrome. *Metab. Syndr. Relat. Disord.* **2006**, *4*, 287–298. [CrossRef] [PubMed]
74. Höcht, C.; Bertera, F.M.; Mayer, M.A.; Taira, C.A. Issues in drug metabolism of major antihypertensive drugs: Beta-blockers, calcium channel antagonists and angiotensin receptor blockers. *Expert Opin. Drug Metab. Toxicol.* **2010**, *6*, 199–211. [CrossRef]

75. Collins, K.S.; Pratt, V.M.; Stansberry, W.M.; Medeiros, E.B.; Kannegolla, K.; Swart, M.; Skaar, T.C.; Chapman, A.B.; Decker, B.S.; Moorthi, R.N.; et al. Analytical validity of a genotyping assay for use with personalized antihypertensive and chronic kidney disease therapy. *Pharmacogenet. Genom.* **2019**, *29*, 18–22. [CrossRef]
76. Eadon, M.T.; Maddatu, J.; Moe, S.M.; Sinha, A.D.; Ferreira, R.M.; Miller, B.W.; Sher, S.J.; Su, J.; Pratt, V.M.; Chapman, A.B.; et al. Pharmacogenomics of Hypertension in CKD: The CKD-PGX Study. *Kidney360* **2022**, *3*, 307–316. [CrossRef] [PubMed]
77. Tanner, R.M.; Calhoun, D.A.; Bell, E.K.; Bowling, C.B.; Gutiérrez, O.M.; Irvin, M.R.; Lackland, D.T.; Oparil, S.; Warnock, D.; Muntner, P. Prevalence of apparent treatment-resistant hypertension among individuals with CKD. *Clin. J. Am. Soc. Nephrol. CJASN* **2013**, *8*, 1583–1590. [CrossRef] [PubMed]
78. US Food and Drug Administration: BiDil (Isosorbide Dinitrate and Hydralazine Hydrochloride) Prescribing Information [Package Insert]. [Internet]. Available online: https://www.accessdata.fda.gov/drugsatfda_docs/label/2019/020727s010lbl.pdf (accessed on 1 June 2024).
79. US Food and Drug Administration: Cozaar (Losartan) Prescribing Information [Package Insert] [Internet]. Available online: https://www.accessdata.fda.gov/drugsatfda_docs/label/2018/020386s062lbl.pdf (accessed on 1 June 2024).
80. US Food and Drug Administration: Lopressor (Metoprolol) Prescribing Information [Package INSERT]. [Internet]. Available online: https://www.accessdata.fda.gov/drugsatfda_docs/label/2012/018704s025lbl.pdf (accessed on 1 June 2024).
81. Annotation of DPWG Guideline for Metoprolol and CYP2D6 [Internet]. Available online: https://www.pharmgkb.org/guidelineAnnotation/PA166104995 (accessed on 1 June 2024).
82. Swen, J.J.; Nijenhuis, M.; Boer, A.; Grandia, L.; Maitland-van, A.H.; Mulder, H.; Rongen, G.A.P.J.M.; Van Schaik, R.H.N.; Schalekamp, T.; Touw, D.J.; et al. Pharmacogenetics: From bench to byte—An update of guidelines. *Clin. Pharmacol. Ther.* **2011**, *89*, 662–673. [CrossRef]
83. Zhou, Y.; Nevosadová, L.; Eliasson, E.; Lauschke, V.M. Global distribution of functionally important CYP2C9 alleles and their inferred metabolic consequences. *Hum. Genom.* **2023**, *17*, 15. [CrossRef] [PubMed]
84. Johnson, J.A.; Liggett, S.B. Cardiovascular pharmacogenomics of adrenergic receptor signaling: Clinical implications and future directions. *Clin. Pharmacol. Ther.* **2011**, *89*, 366–378. [CrossRef] [PubMed]
85. Meloche, M.; Khazaka, M.; Kassem, I.; Barhdadi, A.; Dubé, M.-P.; Denus, S. CYP2D6 polymorphism and its impact on the clinical response to metoprolol: A systematic review and meta-analysis. *Br. J. Clin. Pharmacol.* **2020**, *86*, 1015–1033. [CrossRef]
86. Dean, L. Metoprolol Therapy and CYP2D6 Genotype. In *Med Genet Summ [Internet]*; Pratt, V.M., Scott, S.A., Pirmohamed, M., Esquivel, B., Kattman, B.L., Malheiro, A.J., Eds.; National Center for Biotechnology Information (US): Bethesda, MD, USA, 2012. Available online: http://www.ncbi.nlm.nih.gov/books/NBK425389/ (accessed on 24 April 2024).
87. Collett, S.; Massmann, A.; Petry, N.J.; Heukelom, J.; Schultz, A.; Hellwig, T.; Baye, J.F. Metoprolol and CYP2D6: A Retrospective Cohort Study Evaluating Genotype-Based Outcomes. *J. Pers. Med.* **2023**, *13*, 416. [CrossRef]
88. Viviani, R.; Berres, J.; Stingl, J.C. Phenotypic Models of Drug-Drug-Gene Interactions Mediated by Cytochrome Drug-Metabolizing Enzymes. *Clin. Pharmacol. Ther.* **2024**, *116*, 592–601. [CrossRef]
89. Duricova, J.; Perinova, I.; Jurckova, N.; Kacirova, I.; Grundmann, M. Clinically important interaction between metoprolol and propafenone. *Can. Fam. Physician Med. Fam. Can.* **2013**, *59*, 373–375.
90. Luzum, J.A.; Sweet, K.M.; Binkley, P.F.; Schmidlen, T.J.; Jarvis, J.P.; Christman, M.F.; Sadee, W.; Kitzmiller, J.P. CYP2D6 Genetic Variation and Beta-Blocker Maintenance Dose in Patients with Heart Failure. *Pharm. Res.* **2017**, *34*, 1615–1625. [CrossRef]
91. Lefebvre, J.; Poirier, L.; Poirier, P.; Turgeon, J.; Lacourciere, Y. The influence of CYP2D6 phenotype on the clinical response of nebivolol in patients with essential hypertension. *Br. J. Clin. Pharmacol.* **2007**, *63*, 575–582. [CrossRef] [PubMed]
92. Whirl-Carrillo, M.; Huddart, R.; Gong, L.; Sangkuhl, K.; Thorn, C.F.; Whaley, R.; Klein, T.E. An Evidence-Based Framework for Evaluating Pharmacogenomics Knowledge for Personalized Medicine. *Clin. Pharmacol Ther.* **2021**, *110*, 563–572. [CrossRef] [PubMed]
93. Kirch, W.; Görg, K.G. Clinical pharmacokinetics of atenolol—A review. *Eur. J. Drug Metab. Pharmacokinet.* **1982**, *7*, 81–91. [CrossRef] [PubMed]
94. Bailey, D.G. Fruit juice inhibition of uptake transport: A new type of food-drug interaction. *Br. J. Clin. Pharmacol.* **2010**, *70*, 645–655. [CrossRef]
95. Jeon, H.; Jang, I.-J.; Lee, S.; Ohashi, K.; Kotegawa, T.; Ieiri, I.; Cho, J.; Yoon, S.H.; Shin, S.; Yu, K.; et al. Apple juice greatly reduces systemic exposure to atenolol. *Br. J. Clin. Pharmacol.* **2013**, *75*, 172–179. [CrossRef]
96. Tocci, G.; Battistoni, A.; Passerini, J.; Musumeci, M.B.; Francia, P.; Ferrucci, A.; Volpe, M. Calcium channel blockers and hypertension. *J. Cardiovasc. Pharmacol. Ther.* **2015**, *20*, 121–130. [CrossRef]
97. Huang, Y.; Wen, G.; Lu, Y.; Wen, J.; Ji, Y.; Xing, X.; Li, Y.; Wen, J.; Yuan, H. CYP3A4*1G and CYP3A5*3 genetic polymorphisms alter the antihypertensive efficacy of amlodipine in patients with hypertension following renal transplantation. *Int. J. Clin. Pharmacol Ther.* **2017**, *55*, 109–118. [CrossRef]
98. Zhang, Y.-P.; Zuo, X.-C.; Huang, Z.-J.; Cai, J.-J.; Wen, J.; Duan, D.D.; Yuan, H. CYP3A5 polymorphism, amlodipine and hypertension. *J. Hum. Hypertens.* **2014**, *28*, 145–149. [CrossRef]
99. Bhatnagar, V.; Garcia, E.P.; O'Connor, D.T.; Brophy, V.H.; Alcaraz, J.; Richard, E.; Bakris, G.L.; Middleton, J.P.; Norris, K.C.; Wright, J.; et al. CYP3A4 and CYP3A5 polymorphisms and blood pressure response to amlodipine among African-American men and women with early hypertensive renal disease. *Am. J. Nephrol.* **2010**, *31*, 95–103. [CrossRef]

100. Kim, K.-A.; Park, P.-W.; Lee, O.-J.; Choi, S.-H.; Min, B.H.; Shin, K.-H.; Chun, B.G.; Shin, J.G.; Park, J.Y. Effect of CYP3A5*3 genotype on the pharmacokinetics and pharmacodynamics of amlodipine in healthy Korean subjects. *Clin. Pharmacol. Ther.* **2006**, *80*, 646–656. [CrossRef]
101. Liang, H.; Zhang, X.; Ma, Z.; Sun, Y.; Shu, C.; Zhu, Y.; Zhang, Y.; Hu, S.; Fu, X.; Liu, L. Association of CYP3A5 Gene Polymorphisms and Amlodipine-Induced Peripheral Edema in Chinese Han Patients with Essential Hypertension. *Pharmacogenom. Pers. Med.* **2021**, *14*, 189–197. [CrossRef]
102. Wang, Y.-C.; Hsieh, T.-C.; Chou, C.-L.; Wu, J.-L.; Fang, T.-C. Risks of Adverse Events Following Coprescription of Statins and Calcium Channel Blockers: A Nationwide Population-Based Study. *Medicine* **2016**, *95*, e2487. [CrossRef] [PubMed]
103. Cutrell, S.; Alhomoud, I.S.; Mehta, A.; Talasaz, A.H.; Tassell, B.; Dixon, D.L. ACE-Inhibitors in Hypertension: A Historical Perspective and Current Insights. *Curr. Hypertens. Rep.* **2023**, *25*, 243–250. [CrossRef] [PubMed]
104. Sica, D.A.; Gehr, T.W.; Ghosh, S. Clinical pharmacokinetics of losartan. *Clin. Pharmacokinet.* **2005**, *44*, 797–814. [CrossRef]
105. Yasar, U.; Forslund-Bergengren, C.; Tybring, G.; Dorado, P.; Llerena, A.; Sjöqvist, F.; Eliasson, E.; Dahl, M. Pharmacokinetics of losartan and its metabolite E-3174 in relation to the CYP2C9 genotype. *Clin. Pharmacol. Ther.* **2002**, *71*, 89–98. [CrossRef] [PubMed]
106. Babaoglu, M.O.; Yasar, U.; Sandberg, M.; Eliasson, E.; Dahl, M.-L.; Kayaalp, S.O.; Bozkurt, A. CYP2C9 genetic variants and losartan oxidation in a Turkish population. *Eur. J. Clin. Pharmacol.* **2004**, *60*, 337–342. [CrossRef]
107. Sekino, K.; Kubota, T.; Okada, Y.; Yamada, Y.; Yamamoto, K.; Horiuchi, R.; Kimura, K.; Iga, T. Effect of the single CYP2C9*3 allele on pharmacokinetics and pharmacodynamics of losartan in healthy Japanese subjects. *Eur. J. Clin. Pharmacol.* **2003**, *59*, 589–592. [CrossRef]
108. Kaukonen, K.M.; Olkkola, K.T.; Neuvonen, P.J. Fluconazole but not itraconazole decreases the metabolism of losartan to E-3174. *Eur. J. Clin. Pharmacol.* **1998**, *53*, 445–449. [CrossRef]
109. Spinasse, L.B.; Santos, A.R.; Suffys, P.N.; Muxfeldt, E.S.; Salles, G.F. Different phenotypes of the NAT2 gene influences hydralazine antihypertensive response in patients with resistant hypertension. *Pharmacogenomics* **2014**, *15*, 169–178. [CrossRef]
110. Han, L.W.; Ryu, R.J.; Cusumano, M.; Easterling, T.R.; Phillips, B.R.; Risler, L.J.; Shen, D.D.; Hebert, M.F. Effect of N-Acetyltransferase 2 Genotype on the Pharmacokinetics of Hydralazine During Pregnancy. *J. Clin. Pharmacol.* **2019**, *59*, 1678–1689. [CrossRef]
111. Mazari, L.; Ouarzane, M.; Zouali, M. Subversion of B lymphocyte tolerance by hydralazine, a potential mechanism for drug-induced lupus. *Proc. Natl. Acad. Sci. USA* **2007**, *104*, 6317–6322. [CrossRef] [PubMed]
112. Schoonen, W.M.; Thomas, S.L.; Somers, E.C.; Smeeth, L.; Kim, J.; Evans, S.; Hall, A.J. Do selected drugs increase the risk of lupus? A matched case-control study. *Br. J. Clin. Pharmacol.* **2010**, *70*, 588–596. [CrossRef]
113. American Diabetes Association Professional Practice Committee. 2. Diagnosis and Classification of Diabetes: Standards of Care in Diabetes—2024. *Diabetes Care* **2023**, *47*, S20–S42. [CrossRef]
114. American Diabetes Association Professional Practice Committee. 9. Pharmacologic Approaches to Glycemic Treatment: Standards of Care in Diabetes—2024. *Diabetes Care* **2023**, *47*, S158–S178. [CrossRef]
115. Davies, M.J.; Aroda, V.R.; Collins, B.S.; Gabbay, R.A.; Green, J.; Maruthur, N.M.; Rosas, S.E.; Del Prato, S.; Mathieu, C.; Mingrone, G.; et al. Management of hyperglycaemia in type 2 diabetes, 2022. A consensus report by the American Diabetes Association (ADA) and the European Association for the Study of Diabetes (EASD). *Diabetologia* **2022**, *65*, 1925–1966. [CrossRef]
116. Imamovic, K.S.; Kulo, A.; Dujic, T. Pharmacogenetics of new classes of antidiabetic drugs. *Bosn. J. Basic Med. Sci.* **2021**, *21*, 659–671. [CrossRef]
117. Hardie, D.G. AMP-activated protein kinase as a drug target. *Annu. Rev. Pharmacol. Toxicol.* **2007**, *47*, 185–210. [CrossRef]
118. Zeng, Z.; Huang, S.-Y.; Sun, T. Pharmacogenomic Studies of Current Antidiabetic Agents and Potential New Drug Targets for Precision Medicine of Diabetes. *Diabetes Ther.* **2020**, *11*, 2521–2538. [CrossRef]
119. Pearson, E.R. New Insights Into the Genetics of Glycemic Response to Metformin. *Diabetes Care* **2024**, *47*, 193–195. [CrossRef]
120. Nasykhova, Y.A.; Tonyan, Z.N.; Mikhailova, A.A.; Danilova, M.M.; Glotov, A.S. Pharmacogenetics of Type 2 Diabetes—Progress and Prospects. *Int. J. Mol. Sci.* **2020**, *21*, 6842. [CrossRef]
121. Baye, A.M.; Fanta, T.G.; Siddiqui, M.K.; Dawed, A.Y. The Genetics of Adverse Drug Outcomes in Type 2 Diabetes: A Systematic Review. *Front. Genet.* **2021**, *12*, 675053. [CrossRef] [PubMed]
122. Rena, G.; Hardie, D.G.; Pearson, E.R. The mechanisms of action of metformin. *Diabetologia* **2017**, *60*, 1577–1585. [CrossRef] [PubMed]
123. Takane, H.; Shikata, E.; Otsubo, K.; Higuchi, S.; Ieiri, I. Polymorphism in human organic cation transporters and metformin action. *Pharmacogenomics* **2008**, *9*, 415–422. [CrossRef]
124. Florez, J.C. The pharmacogenetics of metformin. *Diabetologia* **2017**, *60*, 1648–1655. [CrossRef]
125. Peng, A.; Gong, C.; Xu, Y.; Liang, X.; Chen, X.; Hong, W.; Yan, J. Association between organic cation transporter genetic polymorphisms and metformin response and intolerance in T2DM individuals: A systematic review and meta-analysis. *Front. Public Health* **2023**, *11*, 1183879. [CrossRef]
126. Zhou, K.; Donnelly, L.A.; Kimber, C.H.; Donnan, P.T.; Doney, A.S.; Leese, G.; Hattersley, A.T.; McCarthy, M.I.; Morris, A.D.; Palmer, C.N.; et al. Reduced-function SLC22A1 polymorphisms encoding organic cation transporter 1 and glycemic response to metformin: A GoDARTS study. *Diabetes* **2009**, *58*, 1434–1439. [CrossRef] [PubMed]

127. Rotroff, D.M.; Yee, S.W.; Zhou, K.; Marvel, S.W.; Shah, H.S.; Jack, J.R.; Havener, T.M.; Hedderson, M.M.; Kubo, M.; Herman, M.A.; et al. Genetic Variants in CPA6 and PRPF31 Are Associated with Variation in Response to Metformin in Individuals with Type 2 Diabetes. *Diabetes* **2018**, *67*, 1428–1440. [CrossRef] [PubMed]
128. Zhou, K.; Yee, S.W.; Seiser, E.L.; Leeuwen, N.; Tavendale, R.; Bennett, A.J.; Groves, C.J.; Coleman, R.L.; van der Heijden, A.; Beulens, J.W.; et al. Variation in the glucose transporter gene SLC2A2 is associated with glycemic response to metformin. *Nat. Genet.* **2016**, *48*, 1055–1059. [CrossRef]
129. Gong, L.; Goswami, S.; Giacomini, K.M.; Altman, R.B.; Klein, T.E. Metformin pathways: Pharmacokinetics and pharmacodynamics. *Pharmacogenet. Genom.* **2012**, *22*, 820–827. [CrossRef]
130. Nies, A.T.; Hofmann, U.; Resch, C.; Schaeffeler, E.; Rius, M.; Schwab, M. Proton pump inhibitors inhibit metformin uptake by organic cation transporters (OCTs). *PLoS ONE* **2011**, *6*, e22163. [CrossRef]
131. Minematsu, T.; Giacomini, K.M. Interactions of tyrosine kinase inhibitors with organic cation transporters and multidrug and toxic compound extrusion proteins. *Mol. Cancer Ther.* **2011**, *10*, 531–539. [CrossRef]
132. Pellegrinotti, M.; Fimognari, F.L.; Franco, A.; Repetto, L.; Pastorelli, R. Erlotinib-induced hepatitis complicated by fatal lactic acidosis in an elderly man with lung cancer. *Ann. Pharmacother.* **2009**, *43*, 542–545. [CrossRef] [PubMed]
133. European Medicines Agency. Pioglitazone-Summary of Product Characteristics [Internet]. Available online: https://www.ema.europa.eu/en/documents/product-information/pioglitazone-actavis-epar-product-information_en.pdf (accessed on 4 April 2024).
134. European Medicine Agency. Actos: EPAR—Scientific Discussion [Internet]. 2004. Available online: https://www.ema.europa.eu/en/documents/scientific-discussion/actos-epar-scientific-discussion_en.pdf (accessed on 7 March 2024).
135. Jaakkola, T.; Laitila, J.; Neuvonen, P.J.; Backman, J.T. Pioglitazone is metabolised by CYP2C8 and CYP3A4 in vitro: Potential for interactions with CYP2C8 inhibitors. *Basic Clin. Pharmacol. Toxicol.* **2006**, *99*, 44–51. [CrossRef]
136. Pfützner, A.; Weber, M.M.; Forst, T. Pioglitazone: Update on an oral antidiabetic drug with antiatherosclerotic effects. *Expert Opin. Pharmacother.* **2007**, *8*, 1985–1998. [CrossRef] [PubMed]
137. Aquilante, C.L.; Wempe, M.F.; Spencer, S.H.; Kosmiski, L.A.; Predhomme, J.A.; Sidhom, M.S. Influence of CYP2C8*2 on the pharmacokinetics of pioglitazone in healthy African-American volunteers. *Pharmacotherapy* **2013**, *33*, 1000–1007. [CrossRef]
138. Yin, S.-J.; Qi, H.-M.; Wang, X.; Zhang, P.; Lu, Y.; Wei, M.-J.; Li, P.; Qi, G.-Z.; Lou, Y.-Q.; Lu, C.; et al. Effects of functional CYP2C8, CYP2C9, CYP3A5 and ABCB1 genetic variants on the pharmacokinetics of insulin sensitizer pioglitazone in Chinese Han individuals. *Pharmacogenet. Genom.* **2017**, *27*, 125–134. [CrossRef] [PubMed]
139. Aquilante, C.L.; Kosmiski, L.A.; Bourne, D.W.; Bushman, L.R.; Daily, E.B.; Hammond, K.P.; Hopley, C.W.; Kadam, R.S.; Kanack, A.T.; Kompella, U.B.; et al. Impact of the CYP2C8 *3 polymorphism on the drug-drug interaction between gemfibrozil and pioglitazone. *Br. J. Clin. Pharmacol.* **2013**, *75*, 217–226. [CrossRef]
140. Tornio, A.; Niemi, M.; Neuvonen, P.J.; Backman, J.T. Trimethoprim and the CYP2C8*3 allele have opposite effects on the pharmacokinetics of pioglitazone. *Drug Metab. Dispos. Biol. Fate Chem.* **2008**, *36*, 73–80. [CrossRef]
141. Yang, H.; Ye, E.; Si, G.; Chen, L.; Cai, L.; Ye, C.; Zhang, C.; Lu, X. Adiponectin gene polymorphism rs2241766 T/G is associated with response to pioglitazone treatment in type 2 diabetic patients from southern China. *PLoS ONE* **2014**, *9*, e112480. [CrossRef]
142. Dawed, A.Y.; Donnelly, L.; Tavendale, R.; Carr, F.; Leese, G.; Palmer, C.N.; Pearson, E.R.; Zhou, K. CYP2C8 and SLCO1B1 Variants and Therapeutic Response to Thiazolidinediones in Patients with Type 2 Diabetes. *Diabetes Care* **2016**, *39*, 1902–1908. [CrossRef]
143. Zhang, Y.; Si, D.; Chen, X.; Lin, N.; Guo, Y.; Zhou, H.; Zhong, D. Influence of CYP2C9 and CYP2C19 genetic polymorphisms on pharmacokinetics of gliclazide MR in Chinese subjects. *Br. J. Clin Pharmacol.* **2007**, *64*, 67–74. [CrossRef]
144. Al-Omary, F.A. Gliclazide. *Profiles Drug Subst. Excip. Relat. Methodol.* **2017**, *42*, 125–192. [CrossRef] [PubMed]
145. Klen, J.; Dolžan, V.; Janež, A. CYP2C9, KCNJ11 and ABCC8 polymorphisms and the response to sulphonylurea treatment in type 2 diabetes patients. *Eur. J. Clin. Pharmacol.* **2014**, *70*, 421–428. [CrossRef]
146. Zhou, K.; Donnelly, L.; Burch, L.; Tavendale, R.; Doney, A.S.; Leese, G.; Hattersley, A.T.; I McCarthy, M.; Morris, A.D.; Lang, C.C.; et al. Loss-of-function CYP2C9 variants improve therapeutic response to sulfonylureas in type 2 diabetes: A Go-DARTS study. *Clin. Pharmacol. Ther.* **2010**, *87*, 52–56. [CrossRef]
147. Kirchheiner, J.; Brockmöller, J.; Meineke, I.; Bauer, S.; Rohde, W.; Meisel, C.; Roots, I. Impact of CYP2C9 amino acid polymorphisms on glyburide kinetics and on the insulin and glucose response in healthy volunteers. *Clin. Pharmacol. Ther.* **2002**, *71*, 286–296. [CrossRef]
148. Niemi, M.; Cascorbi, I.; Timm, R.; Kroemer, H.K.; Neuvonen, P.J.; Kivistö, K.T. Glyburide and glimepiride pharmacokinetics in subjects with different CYP2C9 genotypes. *Clin. Pharmacol. Ther.* **2002**, *72*, 326–332. [CrossRef]
149. Wright, E.M.; Loo, D.D.; Hirayama, B.A. Biology of human sodium glucose transporters. *Physiol. Rev.* **2011**, *91*, 733–794. [CrossRef] [PubMed]
150. Francke, S.; Mamidi, R.N.; Solanki, B.; Scheers, E.; Jadwin, A.; Favis, R.; Devineni, D. In vitro metabolism of canagliflozin in human liver, kidney, intestine microsomes, and recombinant uridine diphosphate glucuronosyltransferases (UGT) and the effect of genetic variability of UGT enzymes on the pharmacokinetics of canagliflozin in humans. *J. Clin. Pharmacol.* **2015**, *55*, 1061–1072. [CrossRef]
151. Hoeben, E.; Winter, W.; Neyens, M.; Devineni, D.; Vermeulen, A.; Dunne, A. Population Pharmacokinetic Modeling of Canagliflozin in Healthy Volunteers and Patients with Type 2 Diabetes Mellitus. *Clin Pharmacokinet.* **2016**, *55*, 209–223. [CrossRef] [PubMed]

152. Marshall, J.; Liang, Y.; Sahasrabudhe, V.; Tensfeldt, T.; Fediuk, D.J.; Zhou, S.; Krishna, R.; Dawra, V.K.; Wood, L.S.; Sweeney, K. Meta-Analysis of Noncompartmental Pharmacokinetic Parameters of Ertugliflozin to Evaluate Dose Proportionality and UGT1A9 Polymorphism Effect on Exposure. *J. Clin. Pharmacol.* **2021**, *61*, 1220–1231. [CrossRef]
153. European Medicine Agency. Byetta-Summary of Product Characteristics [Internet]. Available online: https://www.ema.europa.eu/en/documents/product-information/byetta-epar-product-information_en.pdf (accessed on 3 April 2024).
154. European Medicine Agency. Ozempic-Summary of Product Characteristics [Internet]. Available online: https://www.ema.europa.eu/en/documents/product-information/ozempic-epar-product-information_en.pdf (accessed on 3 April 2024).
155. European Medicine Agency. Saxenda-Summary of Product Characteristics [Internet]. Available online: https://www.ema.europa.eu/en/documents/product-information/saxenda-epar-product-information_en.pdf (accessed on 3 April 2024).
156. European Medicine Agency. Mounjaro-Summary of product characteristics [Internet]. Available online: https://www.ema.europa.eu/en/documents/product-information/mounjaro-epar-product-information_en.pdf (accessed on 3 April 2024).
157. Heo, C.; Choi, C.-I. Current Progress in Pharmacogenetics of Second-Line Antidiabetic Medications: Towards Precision Medicine for Type 2 Diabetes. *J. Clin. Med.* **2019**, *8*, 393. [CrossRef]
158. Pathak, R.; Bridgeman, M.B. Dipeptidyl Peptidase-4 (DPP-4) Inhibitors in the Management of Diabetes. *P & T Peer-Rev. J. Formul. Manag.* **2010**, *35*, 509–513.
159. Scheen, A.J. Dipeptidylpeptitase-4 Inhibitors (Gliptins). *Clin. Pharmacokinet.* **2010**, *49*, 573–588. [CrossRef] [PubMed]
160. Herman, G.; Stevens, C.; Vandyck, K.; Bergman, A.; Yi, B.; Desmet, M.; Snyder, K.; Hilliard, D.; Tanen, M.; Tanaka, W. Pharmacokinetics and Pharmacodynamics of Sitagliptin, an Inhibitor of Dipeptidyl Peptidase IV, in Healthy Subjects: Results from Two Randomized, Double-Blind, Placebo-Controlled Studies with Single Oral Doses. *Clin. Pharmacol. Ther.* **2005**, *78*, 675–688. [CrossRef] [PubMed]
161. Prescribing Pearls: A Guide to DPP-4 Inhibitors (Gliptins)—DiabetesontheNet. Available online: https://diabetesonthenet.com/diabetes-primary-care/prescribing-pearls-dpp4is/ (accessed on 1 June 2024).
162. Khan, M.W.; Kurian, S.; Bishnoi, R. Acute-Onset Rhabdomyolysis Secondary to Sitagliptin and Atorvastatin Interaction. *Int. J. Gen. Med.* **2016**, *9*, 103–106. [CrossRef]
163. Bhome, R.; Penn, H. Rhabdomyolysis Precipitated by a Sitagliptin-Atorvastatin Drug Interaction. *Diabet. Med.* **2012**, *29*, 693–694. [CrossRef]
164. DiGregorio, R.V.; Pasikhova, Y. Rhabdomyolysis Caused by a Potential Sitagliptin-Lovastatin Interaction. *Pharmacotherapy* **2009**, *29*, 352–356. [CrossRef]
165. Kao, D.P.; Kohrt, H.E.; Kugler, J. Renal Failure and Rhabdomyolysis Associated with Sitagliptin and Simvastatin Use. *Diabet. Med.* **2008**, *25*, 1229–1230. [CrossRef]
166. Cerra. The Effects of Simvastatin on the Pharmacokinectics of Sitagliptin. *J. Popul. Ther. Clin. Pharmacol.* **2015**, *19*, e356–e360.
167. Tahrani, A.A.; Piya, M.K.; Barnett, A.H. Saxagliptin: A New DPP-4 Inhibitor for the Treatment of Type 2 Diabetes Mellitus. *Adv. Ther.* **2009**, *26*, 249–262. [CrossRef]
168. Egan, A.; Colman, E. Weighing the benefits of high-dose simvastatin against the risk of myopathy. *N. Engl. J. Med.* **2011**, *365*, 285–287. [CrossRef] [PubMed]
169. Backman, J.T.; Kyrklund, C.; Kivistö, K.T.; Wang, J.S.; Neuvonen, P.J. Plasma concentrations of active simvastatin acid are increased by gemfibrozil. *Clin. Pharmacol. Ther.* **2000**, *68*, 122–129. [CrossRef] [PubMed]
170. Schneck, D.W.; Birmingham, B.K.; Zalikowski, J.A.; Mitchell, P.D.; Wang, Y.; Martin, P.D.; Lasseter, K.C.; Brown, C.D.A.; Windass, A.S.; Raza, A. The effect of gemfibrozil on the pharmacokinetics of rosuvastatin. *Clin. Pharmacol. Ther.* **2004**, *75*, 455–463. [CrossRef] [PubMed]

diabetology

MDPI

Review

A Review of the Literature Relationship between Psychological Eating Patterns and the Risk of Type 2 Diabetes Mellitus and Metabolic Syndrome

Filip Mustač [1,*], Martina Matovinović [2,*], Tin Galijašević [3], Maja Škarić [4], Eva Podolski [5], Toma Perko [5] and Darko Marčinko [1,5]

1 Department of Psychiatry and Psychological Medicine, University Hospital Centre Zagreb, Kišpatićeva 12, 10000 Zagreb, Croatia; niarveda@gmail.com
2 Department of Internal Medicine, Division of Endocrinology, University Hospital Centre Zagreb, Croatian Referral Center for Obesity Treatment, Kišpatićeva 12, 10000 Zagreb, Croatia
3 General Hospital Varaždin, 42000 Varaždin, Croatia; kopaka@oems.hr or tin.galijasevic@gmail.com
4 Neuropsychiatric Hospital "Dr. Ivan Barbot", 44317 Popovača, Croatia; skaric.maja@gmail.com
5 School of Medicine, University of Zagreb, 10000 Zagreb, Croatia; evapodolski3@gmail.com (E.P.); toma.perko@gmail.com (T.P.)
* Correspondence: filip.mustac@gmail.com (F.M.); martina_10000@yahoo.com (M.M.)

Abstract: Mental health today includes much more than the treatment of psychiatric disorders. More and more interventions aim to bring mental health support closer to people and psychotherapeutic interventions to people with somatic conditions. Since the treatment of people with metabolic syndrome and diabetes mellitus type 2 also requires a change in lifestyle, mental health has a prominent role. This overview paper wants to offer a solution after recognizing the given patterns where psychotherapy certainly has a significant and irreplaceable role. Precisely because of this phenomenon, psychological eating patterns associated with diabetes mellitus and hence metabolic syndrome should be studied, and attempts should be made to uncover patterns in occurrence. The aim of this study is to review the literature and consider the connection among diabetes mellitus, metabolic syndrome, and psychological eating patterns such as emotional and compulsive eating, as well as through the lens of food addiction. Furthermore, we have attempted to uncover the role of psychiatry and psychotherapy in the treatment of diabetes mellitus and metabolic syndrome and delve into the complexity of recognizing these patterns and emphasize the importance of a multidisciplinary approach in the treatment of diabetes mellitus and metabolic syndrome.

Keywords: diabetes mellitus; metabolic syndrome; obesity; eating patterns; binge eating; emotional eating

1. Introduction

Nearly 80% of psychological eating patterns go undetected which is why it is crucial to better understand them as they can be connected to various other serious medical conditions, such are diabetes mellitus (DM), obesity, and metabolic syndrome (MetS) [1,2]. What is even more problematic is that often people are unaware of the psychological eating patterns, or they are unwilling to accept it, which results in poorer treatment outcomes. Instant solutions rarely lead to good treatment outcomes. Embracing balanced nutrition, considering both physical and mental well-being, is essential. Seeking guidance from healthcare professionals ensures a respectful approach to nutrition, just like how taking control over blood glucose in diabetes can certainly improve treatment outcomes in people with DM and MetS [3–5]. Therefore, knowledge about psychological eating patterns could be very helpful for both doctors and patients. One of the first warning signs would be food preoccupation which can offer insights into individuals' complex relationships with food, hinting at pathological psychological eating patterns. Since obesity is one of the most prevalent risk factors for type 2 diabetes mellitus and serious cardiovascular diseases, it remains one of the biggest public healthcare concerns of our time. Today, we recognize that obesity is but one hallmark of a more complex clinical entity—metabolic syndrome (MetS). MetS is defined as a cluster of abdominal obesity, high blood pressure, high blood sugar, high serum triglycerides, and low serum HDL. Thus, while it is clear that obesity itself represents a significant risk to an individual's health, the psychological factors that might contribute to it or be significant in these conditions remain less known, recognizable, and universal [6–8]. Exploring the psychological mechanisms that induce eating disorders like compulsive overeating or why some patients prefer unhealthy dietary choices while in heightened emotional states might present a new perspective and possibly lead to novel treatment pathways in these patients. In this review, we will examine the current literature on different eating patterns and how these might impact individuals with metabolic syndrome as well as psychiatric patients and ways that psychotherapists may approach treatment in these patients.

2. Materials and Methods

This narrative review aims to examine eating patterns and their association with metabolic syndrome, which is a significant health issue today. To this goal, five authors (F.M., T.G., M.Š., E.P., T.P.) independently identified articles they deemed relevant in this field, which were then collectively reviewed and categorized into thematic units outlined in this article, aiming for a more relevant and contemporary approach to the subtitle's theme. The analyzed articles were in English, dominantly from the Pubmed/Medline and Google Scholar databases in the period from 2015 onwards, except for papers that were even older, but represent a significant turning point in the profession, as well as capital papers that were still some of the main ones in the field of psychotherapy. The keywords we used were as follows: *eating patterns, emotional eating, dietary patterns, binge-eating, metabolic syndrome, diabetes mellitus type 2, obesity,* and *psychotherapy.* Following consultations, primarily via telephone, we extracted and structured the results of studies we considered pivotal into a narrative review format to present them in a more readable and understandable manner.

3. The Risk of Type 2 Diabetes Mellitus, Metabolic Syndrome, and Psychological Eating Patterns

3.1. The Connection between Risk and Drive—Sleep and Diet

This interconnection still represents a great challenge, but several types of eating patterns, behaviors, and trends have been researched and looked into to discern common links between them and the development of DM and MetS. Chronically high levels of insulin and insulin resistance, which is more prevalent in obese individuals [9], can impair insulin's ability to suppress motivational pathways, resulting in higher levels of stress. Individuals in negative affective states have been shown to favor the consumption of hedonically rewarding foods high in sugar and/or fat, whereas intake during happy states favors less palatable dried fruits" [10,11]. Sleep deprivation may contribute to higher levels of stress which puts people at a higher risk of developing metabolic conditions, a bigger abdominal circumference, insulin resistance, and higher blood pressure, which are all closely related to cardiovascular conditions and type II diabetes mellitus [12,13].

Certain diets are associated with a higher risk of developing MetS, including dietary patterns that include meals which are low in fiber but high in calories, cholesterol, saturated fats, sodium, and simple carbohydrates [7,8]. There are studies that observed the effects of skipping meals on the development of certain risk factors associated with the development of MetS [14]. The studies which some authors cite found that the modern lifestyle leads to people skipping meals more often [15,16], the meal most often skipped being breakfast, followed by lunch and dinner [17]. Skipping breakfast is particularly linked to a higher body weight and a higher insulin resistance [18,19]. There are parallels between skipping breakfast and a higher BMI and waist circumference, which are all risk factors associated with MetS [20,21]. The studies also concluded that people who eat multiple meals a day had a lower obesity rate than people who ate fewer than three meals a day. Some authors stated that some studies established a correlation between eating more than six or less than three meals a day and fasting plasma glucose levels [3], but another study found that there is no correlation [4], so this remains unclear. Erratic eating patterns like eating over a longer period per day and eating more than just three meals a day are widespread [5,22–27] and are associated with obesity, T2DM, MetS, and CVD [28–31]. Some studies also found that misalignment between daily rhythms of food consumption and the circadian timing system can contribute to circadian rhythm disruption which results in abnormal metabolic regulation, the disruption of metabolic homeostasis, and increased cardio-metabolic risks [32–36]. These studies presumed that time-restrictive eating (TRE) would help patients with metabolic disorders restore the normality of their circadian rhythms which would positively affect the regulation of their metabolism. The studies they cite concluded that metabolism operates at a higher and more efficient rate in the morning rather than later in the day [33,35,37,38] and that favoring higher energy intakes in the morning and keeping them low in the evening might help with losing weight and keeping glucose and lipid levels in check [39,40]. Although some review articles indicated that TRE strategies might be helpful in addressing cardio-metabolic disorders [28,33,37,41–45], a lot of the cited studies were not conducted on patients with MetS, and some conclusions cannot be made. There is a study that was conducted on animals [10,46,47] and humans [48–50] which bore no correlation between stress and the amount of food consumed, because some subjects became hypophagic, while others became hyperphagic. They suspected that this was due to different types of stressors and the duration of the stressful period. Another study suspected that lower amounts of stress induced hyperphagia, while bigger stressors induced hypophagia [51]. They also stated that under stressful situations, animals prefer foods that are high in saturated fats and rich in sugars [52–54], while humans prefer hyperpalatable, calorie-rich foods [55–57] even though there was no metabolic need for higher energy intake [58]. This effect might be more pronounced in obese individuals [50,59]. Repeated, uncontrolled, and prolonged stress can dysregulate the hypothalamic–pituitary–adrenal (HPA) axis, which is responsible for secreting glucocorticoids such as cortisol, thus influencing energy homeostasis and eating behavior.

3.2. Hormonal Basis of Relationship between Diet and Reward in MetS and Obesity

The chronic activation of the HPA axis has an effect on glucose metabolism, promoting insulin resistance and altering some appetite-related hormones [9]. The prolonged secretion of glucocorticoids promotes fat accumulation in the abdominal region which is one of the risk factors for MetS. Those under chronic stress eat hyperpalatable, energy-dense, high-fat foods more often during acute stress episodes [60]. HPA activation is linked with the activation of the reward system. A diet rich in high-fat foods sensitizes the reward system which can promote cravings and a higher intake of said foods [61]. The continued stimulation of these reward pathways progressively promotes more compulsive behavior [62]. Obese individuals have shown a stronger activation of the reward system when exposed to food while under stress compared to lean individuals [59]. Animal models demonstrated that obesity often has an effect on adipose receptors [63] which are important for the negative feedback loop and the cessation of eating. People with higher BMI scores have an increased probability of weight gain while under chronic stress compared to individuals under the same amount of stress but who have lower BMI scores [50]. Yoshida et al. [21] found that there is a significant correlation between both individuals who eat snacks after dinner and those who eat dinner before bed and a higher BMI score, higher LDL cholesterol, and abdominal circumference, while those who exhibit both behaviors have an even higher chance of presenting with the same afflictions. In some patients with MetS, we find comorbid binge eating disorder, where a person has the urge to consume enormous amounts of food at once just to satisfy an unbearable need rooted in the experience of stress and anxiety that overwhelms the person. After such binge eating episodes, patients feel temporary relief and a reduction in stress, which over time may become a compulsive pattern of behavior. This form of release represents a kind of acting out, after which an aggressive impulse is discharged, which shows that personality traits like impulsivity can also play a significant role in pathological eating patterns. Considering a person's circadian rhythm and the tendency of individuals prone to anxiety and depressive moods to be more overwhelmed with negative thoughts and feelings towards the end of the day, just before usual bedtime, it is not surprising that this phenomenon is often found in a modified form known as night eating syndrome [64]. These eating patterns play a significant role in the lives of these individuals, contributing to weight gain and obesity. Furthermore, Yoshida et al. [21] studied night eating habits and found that they are associated with dyslipidemia in both men and women. Therefore, besides addressing internal medical conditions, mental health plays an extremely important role and should be central to health. In accordance with this, treatment interventions should focus on improving the mental health of individuals with metabolic syndrome, especially those linked with compulsive overeating, as this is currently undervalued in the treatment of these patients. Thus, treatment should encompass complex psychopharmacological and non-pharmacological/psychotherapeutic interventions. Some possible pharmacological approaches include antidepressants, particularly selective serotonin reuptake inhibitors, and newer psychopharmaceuticals like Lisdexamphetamine [64].

4. Adopting Healthier Psychological Eating Patterns as Part of Treatment of Diabetes Mellitus and Metabolic Syndrome

4.1. Better Mental Health and a Healthier Lifestyle as the Root Cause of Changes in MetS and DM Type 2

The definition of MetS includes a cluster of factors such as abdominal obesity, insulin resistance, dyslipidemia, and elevated blood pressure [65]. Considering MetS a complication of obesity, losing body weight is crucial in reducing the risk of obesity-related diseases [66]. According to one study, obesity is seen as a multi-factorial disease where lifestyle traits are the most important pathogenic factors, as well as a combination of genetic, epigenetic, biological, and psychological factors that cause weight gain and disable the reduction in and retention of a healthy body weight [67]. First of all, when thinking in terms of psychiatric medications, the clinical use of psychopharmacological agents necessitates the recognition, monitoring, and management of potential adverse metabolic impacts. Switching to medications with a reduced risk of weight gain and associated metabolic issues is recommended [68]. An elevated incidence of MetS has been noticed in some groups of psychiatric patients. As de Almeida et al. [69] stressed, patients with bipolar disorder have higher rates of MetS. Other than the adverse effects of psychotropic drugs, unhealthy lifestyle choices, shared neuroendocrine and immunoinflammatory disorders, and genetic predispositions are also contributing factors. A significant neuroendocrine anomaly, the hyperactivity of the hypothalamic–pituitary–adrenal axis, predominantly associated with major depression, is implicated in the neurobiological mechanisms governing the switch processes in bipolar disorder. Moreira et al. [70] found that subjects with depression and anhedonia exhibit elevated levels of glucose, triglycerides, total cholesterol, and LDL cholesterol, alongside reductions in HDL cholesterol levels, which indicates a higher prevalence of MetS among those individuals. As suggested by Räikkönen et al. [71], psychosocial factors are predictive of the risk for developing MetS across various definitions, suggesting a potential causal role in the etiological pathway leading to MetS. Women experiencing high levels of depressive symptoms coupled with significant stressful life events at the outset of a longitudinal study demonstrated an elevated risk for developing MetS over an average follow-up period of 15 years. According to Pigsborg et al. [72], the success of weight loss interventions is influenced not only by genetics and biological processes but also by psychological and behavioral constructs. Factors related to eating behavior, societal norms, and personal psychological aspects like motivation, self-efficacy, locus of control, and self-concept play significant roles, as well as major life events [72–74].

Curis et al. [74] emphasized that the ingestion of food not only fulfills the basic need for nutrient and energy intake but also serves as a source of pleasure. Emotional instability is frequently linked to unhealthy behaviors and irrational cognitions regarding eating habits often resulting in a cascade which leads to obesity [67,74]. According to Conti et al., alexithymia, a personality trait with difficulties in recognizing and processing emotions, may also contribute to the development of MetS through binge eating and psychological distress [67,75]. Conti et al. [75] found that individuals with MetS are older, have a higher body mass index, have had obesity for a longer duration, and scored higher on scales measuring alexithymia like TAS-20, suggesting that binge eating might play a mediating role between alexithymia and metabolic syndrome.

4.2. Emotional Regulation and Psychotherapy as Significant Aids in Treatment

In our previous research, we investigated the association between alexithymia, obesity, and diabetes mellitus type 2. The paper demonstrated that recognizing and raising awareness of alexithymia, along with psychotherapy, particularly of a psychodynamic nature, could have a significant impact on improving the quality of an individual's relationships and insight into their own personality. Consequently, this may have repercussions for better diabetes mellitus control. Similarly, in the case of metabolic syndrome, it is expected that better insight and recognition of certain intrapsychic phenomena will positively affect cooperation in the treatment process [76]. Camacho-Barcia et al. [77] suggested that the excessive consumption of energy-dense foods is driven by heightened food reward sensitivity, problems with self-control, or emotional states. Implementing individual-specific psychological strategies is crucial for ensuring and sustaining weight loss. High reward sensitivity, preference for unhealthy foods, and overeating in patients with binge eating disorder and obesity underscore the need for interventions that strengthen self-control and conscientiousness, as well as developing emotion regulation skills. Furthermore, non-invasive deep magnetic brain stimulation has shown promise in reducing impulse-related behaviors linked to obesity. Mindfulness-based interventions have demonstrated positive outcomes in treating obesity by altering eating behaviors leading to mindful eating [77,78]. According to many studies, cognitive behavioral weight management treatment leads to improvements in measures of self-regulation, self-efficacy, and mood with the development of abilities to redirect attention and the management of the physiological consequences of emotions [77,79–82]. As Slabá et al. [80] mentioned, the most common character traits of obese patients predominantly include neuroticism, which manifests as anxiety, depression, impulsiveness, anger, and hostility. Marčinko et al. stressed the significant role of the spectrum of the "master emotion" of shame, as well as the importance of psychodynamic psychotherapy in the management of obesity [80,83]. Other studies recommend different psychotherapeutic approaches, such as existential therapy [80] and acceptance and commitment therapy which was found to be effective in improving weight loss in terms of BMI, psychological flexibility, and weight-related stigma [84]. In summary, the interplay of psychological, emotional, and lifestyle factors plays a significant role in the etiology and management of obesity and MetS, emphasizing the need for integrated and multifaceted therapeutic approaches [85].

Emotionally, shifts in body weight exacerbate self-esteem and body image concerns. Distorted body image perceptions, societal pressures, and underlying emotional issues drive the desire for rapid weight changes. Such fluctuations can lead to nutritional deficiencies, weakened immunity, and cardiovascular problems with rapid weight loss, while weight gain may result in metabolic issues and chronic illnesses. Achieving lasting recovery entails addressing body image and self-esteem issues alongside physical healing. Cultivating self-acceptance and self-love is crucial in this journey, supported by empathy and understanding. It is a holistic approach that fosters enduring healing by acknowledging and confronting the root causes of negative body image. The pursuit of control, which usually manifests as a constant preoccupation with food, weight, and appearance, serves as a coping mechanism in times of stress and anxiety, intertwining self-esteem with body image. Another thing to consider is the fact that studies have shown that about 50% of preadolescent girls and 30% of preadolescent boys dislike their body which shows the severity of this issue [86,87]. These behaviors disrupt daily life, elevating stress levels and affecting decision-making. This focus can strain social interactions and contribute to feelings of isolation. Other warning signs include frequent body checking, comparison with others, seeking affirmation, clothing insecurity, avoidance of social situations, and negative self-talk. Effective treatment requires a multidimensional approach, including therapy and support groups, to address underlying emotional and psychological factors. These interventions foster healthier relationships with food, body image, and self-esteem. Another important aspect to consider is the individuals' relationship with exercising. Balancing a healthy fitness routine with potential obsession is challenging. A growth-positive routine involves regular exercise for physical and mental well-being, with flexibility and joy in activities. Recognizing this balance requires understanding emotional and psychological factors. Guiding towards a balanced approach, incorporating rest and diverse activities, and nurturing positive body image are crucial for a healthy fitness routine as well as the regular control of blood glucose in the case of DM.

5. The Limitations of the Current Literature and Future Considerations

This review of the literature is predominantly narrative, although the authors have tried to select studies that they consider relevant in the field. However, this literature review was not conducted in a systematic way. Therefore, some future reviews in this area that would look at variables in a systematic way, as well as a meta-analysis of these variables, would certainly be welcome. On the other hand, psychotherapeutic phenomena are more difficult to quantify and measure than some other variables, but this does not mean that psychotherapeutic support and psychotherapeutic techniques do not have an important role in clinical work with patients. The way in which this can be examined is by providing psychotherapeutic support and comparing patients who had psychotherapeutic support with those patients who did not have it, that is, who were treated with treatment as usual, which is still dominantly present due to the stigma against psychological interventions, but today, however, it is less present than before.

6. Conclusions

It is necessary to examine the complexity of the disorder itself and with an understanding of psychological eating patterns and to be aware of these phenomena in people with DM and MetS. The complex dynamic among control of blood sugar, psychological eating patterns, pathologic behaviors, and the development of DM and MetS highlights the critical need for a holistic approach to managing this condition. While the consumption of food high in calories, cholesterol, saturated fats, and carbohydrates has been linked to a higher risk of DM and MetS, this is exacerbated by meal skipping, contributing to higher body weight and insulin resistance. We highlight the interplay of food intake with circadian rhythms and the potential benefits of time-restricted eating in metabolic regulation. The interplay between psychological well-being and metabolic health is particularly significant. Chronic stress and poor mental health can lead to maladaptive eating behaviors, further compounding the risk of DM and MetS. Effective treatment strategies must therefore include robust mental health support in addition to lifestyle interventions. Addressing emotional issues and implementing psychotherapeutic approaches are essential for the holistic care of MetS. Furthermore, recognizing and addressing unhealthy eating patterns early on are crucial. Warning signs such as extreme dietary restrictions, compulsive exercise, and rapid weight fluctuations should be recognized, and timely interventions should be implemented. Understanding eating patterns enables more effective treatment, addressing root causes and preventing escalation. Awareness helps dismantle the stigma surrounding eating disorders and obesity, encouraging open conversations and improving understanding. Creating a safe environment for individuals to express their struggles fosters empathy and promotes well-being, both mentally and emotionally, extending beyond physical health.

In this aspect, psychiatrists and psychotherapists step in as indispensable components in treating patients with DM and MetS, especially in cases where there is suspicion or confirmation of disordered eating patterns. Ultimately, reducing the prevalence and impact of DM and MetS requires a multifaceted approach that integrates medical, psychological, and lifestyle interventions. By prioritizing both physical and mental health, we can better support individuals in achieving sustainable improvements in their overall well-being. Further research is essential to refine these strategies and ensure they are effective for diverse populations, paving the way for a healthier future.

Author Contributions: Conceptualization and design of article: F.M.; literature search, writing—original draft preparation: F.M., T.G., M.Š., E.P. and T.P.; supervision: M.M. and D.M.; writing—review and editing: all authors. All authors have read and agreed to the published version of the manuscript.

Funding: This research received no external funding.

Institutional Review Board Statement: Not applicable.

Informed Consent Statement: Not applicable.

Conflicts of Interest: The authors declare no conflicts of interest.

References

1. Flament, M.F.; Henderson, K.; Buchholz, A.; Obeid, N.; Nguyen, H.N.T.; Birmingham, M.; Goldfield, G. Weight Status and DSM-5 Diagnoses of Eating Disorders in Adolescents from the Community. *J. Am. Acad. Child. Adolesc. Psychiatry* **2015**, *54*, 403–411.e2. [CrossRef] [PubMed]
2. Levinson, C.A.; Hunt, R.A.; Christian, C.; Williams, B.M.; Keshishian, A.C.; Vanzhula, I.A.; Ralph-Nearman, C. Longitudinal Group and Individual Networks of Eating Disorder Symptoms in Individuals Diagnosed with an Eating Disorder. *J. Psychopathol. Clin. Sci.* **2022**, *131*, 58–72. [CrossRef] [PubMed]
3. Carlson, O.; Martin, B.; Stote, K.S.; Golden, E.; Maudsley, S.; Najjar, S.S.; Ferrucci, L.; Ingram, D.K.; Longo, D.L.; Rumpler, W.V.; et al. Impact of Reduced Meal Frequency without Caloric Restriction on Glucose Regulation in Healthy, Normal-Weight Middle-Aged Men and Women. *Metabolism* **2007**, *56*, 1729–1734. [CrossRef] [PubMed]
4. Stote, K.S.; Baer, D.J.; Spears, K.; Paul, D.R.; Harris, G.K.; Rumpler, W.V.; Strycula, P.; Najjar, S.S.; Ferrucci, L.; Ingram, D.K.; et al. A Controlled Trial of Reduced Meal Frequency without Caloric Restriction in Healthy, Normal-Weight, Middle-Aged Adults. *Am. J. Clin. Nutr.* **2007**, *85*, 981–988. [CrossRef]
5. Suliga, E.; Kozieł, D.; Cieśla, E.; Rębak, D.; Głuszek, S. Dietary Patterns in Relation to Metabolic Syndrome among Adults in Poland: A Cross-Sectional Study. *Nutrients* **2017**, *9*, 1366. [CrossRef]
6. Chevinsky, J.D.; Wadden, T.A.; Chao, A.M. Binge Eating Disorder in Patients with Type 2 Diabetes: Diagnostic and Management Challenges. *Diabetes Metab. Syndr. Obes.* **2020**, *13*, 1117–1131. [CrossRef]
7. Pacifico, L.; Anania, C.; Martino, F.; Poggiogalle, E.; Chiarelli, F.; Arca, M.; Chiesa, C. Management of Metabolic Syndrome in Children and Adolescents. *Nutr. Metab. Cardiovasc. Dis.* **2011**, *21*, 455–466. [CrossRef]
8. Wang, H.H.; Lee, D.K.; Liu, M.; Portincasa, P.; Wang, D.Q.-H. Novel Insights into the Pathogenesis and Management of the Metabolic Syndrome. *Pediatr. Gastroenterol. Hepatol. Nutr.* **2020**, *23*, 189–230. [CrossRef]
9. Adam, T.C.; Epel, E.S. Stress, Eating and the Reward System. *Physiol. Behav.* **2007**, *91*, 449–458. [CrossRef]
10. Yau, Y.H.C.; Potenza, M.N. Stress and Eating Behaviors. *Minerva Endocrinol.* **2013**, *38*, 255–267.
11. Garg, N.; Wansink, B.; Inman, J.J. The Influence of Incidental Affect on Consumers' Food Intake. *J. Mark.* **2007**, *71*, 194–206. [CrossRef]
12. Knutson, K.L.; Van Cauter, E. Associations between Sleep Loss and Increased Risk of Obesity and Diabetes. *Ann. N. Y. Acad. Sci.* **2008**, *1129*, 287–304. [CrossRef] [PubMed]
13. Eckel, R.H.; Grundy, S.M.; Zimmet, P.Z. The Metabolic Syndrome. *Lancet* **2005**, *365*, 1415–1428. [CrossRef]
14. Alkhulaifi, F.; Darkoh, C. Meal Timing, Meal Frequency and Metabolic Syndrome. *Nutrients* **2022**, *14*, 1719. [CrossRef] [PubMed]
15. The Modern American Lunchbreak: 2 in 3 Millennials Claim to Skip Lunch in Order to "Get Ahead" at Work According to New Survey from California Walnuts. Available online: https://www.prnewswire.com/news-releases/the-modern-american-lunchbreak-2-in-3-millennials-claim-to-skip-lunch-in-order-to-get-ahead-at-work-according-to-new-survey-from-california-walnuts-300863022.html/ (accessed on 14 May 2024).
16. 31 Million Americans Skip Breakfast Each Day. Available online: https://www.huffpost.com/entry/31-million-americans-skip_n_1005076 (accessed on 14 May 2024).
17. Pendergast, F.J.; Livingstone, K.M.; Worsley, A.; McNaughton, S.A. Correlates of Meal Skipping in Young Adults: A Systematic Review. *Int. J. Behav. Nutr. Phys. Act.* **2016**, *13*, 125. [CrossRef] [PubMed]
18. McCrory, M.A.; Campbell, W.W. Effects of Eating Frequency, Snacking, and Breakfast Skipping on Energy Regulation: Symposium Overview. *J. Nutr.* **2011**, *141*, 144–147. [CrossRef]

19. Sierra-Johnson, J.; Undén, A.-L.; Linestrand, M.; Rosell, M.; Sjogren, P.; Kolak, M.; De Faire, U.; Fisher, R.M.; Hellénius, M.-L. Eating Meals Irregularly: A Novel Environmental Risk Factor for the Metabolic Syndrome. *Obesity* **2008**, *16*, 1302–1307. [CrossRef]
20. Watanabe, Y.; Saito, I.; Henmi, I.; Yoshimura, K.; Maruyama, K.; Yamauchi, K.; Matsuo, T.; Kato, T.; Tanigawa, T.; Kishida, T.; et al. Skipping Breakfast Is Correlated with Obesity. *J. Rural. Med.* **2014**, *9*, 51–58. [CrossRef]
21. Yoshida, J.; Eguchi, E.; Nagaoka, K.; Ito, T.; Ogino, K. Association of Night Eating Habits with Metabolic Syndrome and Its Components: A Longitudinal Study. *BMC Public Health* **2018**, *18*, 1366. [CrossRef]
22. Świątkiewicz, I.; Woźniak, A.; Taub, P.R. Time-Restricted Eating and Metabolic Syndrome: Current Status and Future Perspectives. *Nutrients* **2021**, *13*, 221. [CrossRef]
23. Kant, A.K.; Graubard, B.I. 40-Year Trends in Meal and Snack Eating Behaviors of American Adults. *J. Acad. Nutr. Diet.* **2015**, *115*, 50–63. [CrossRef] [PubMed]
24. Riou, J.; Lefèvre, T.; Parizot, I.; Lhuissier, A.; Chauvin, P. Is There Still a French Eating Model? A Taxonomy of Eating Behaviors in Adults Living in the Paris Metropolitan Area in 2010. *PLoS ONE* **2015**, *10*, e0119161. [CrossRef]
25. Gupta, N.J.; Kumar, V.; Panda, S. A Camera-Phone Based Study Reveals Erratic Eating Pattern and Disrupted Daily Eating-Fasting Cycle among Adults in India. *PLoS ONE* **2017**, *12*, e0172852. [CrossRef] [PubMed]
26. Gill, S.; Panda, S. A Smartphone App Reveals Erratic Diurnal Eating Patterns in Humans That Can Be Modulated for Health Benefits. *Cell Metab.* **2015**, *22*, 789–798. [CrossRef]
27. Time-Restricted Eating Effects on Body Composition and Metabolic Measures in Humans Who Are Overweight: A Feasibility Study—Chow—2020—Obesity—Wiley Online Library. Available online: https://onlinelibrary.wiley.com/doi/full/10.1002/oby.22756 (accessed on 14 May 2024).
28. Zarrinpar, A.; Chaix, A.; Panda, S. Daily Eating Patterns and Their Impact on Health and Disease. *Trends Endocrinol. Metab.* **2016**, *27*, 69–83. [CrossRef]
29. Cahill, L.E.; Chiuve, S.E.; Mekary, R.A.; Jensen, M.K.; Flint, A.J.; Hu, F.B.; Rimm, E.B. Prospective Study of Breakfast Eating and Incident Coronary Heart Disease in a Cohort of Male US Health Professionals. *Circulation* **2013**, *128*, 337–343. [CrossRef] [PubMed]
30. Pot, G.K.; Almoosawi, S.; Stephen, A.M. Meal Irregularity and Cardiometabolic Consequences: Results from Observational and Intervention Studies. *Proc. Nutr. Soc.* **2016**, *75*, 475–486. [CrossRef]
31. Ha, K.; Song, Y. Associations of Meal Timing and Frequency with Obesity and Metabolic Syndrome among Korean Adults. *Nutrients* **2019**, *11*, 2437. [CrossRef]
32. Xie, Y.; Tang, Q.; Chen, G.; Xie, M.; Yu, S.; Zhao, J.; Chen, L. New Insights into the Circadian Rhythm and Its Related Diseases. *Front. Physiol.* **2019**, *10*, 682. [CrossRef]
33. Chaix, A.; Manoogian, E.N.C.; Melkani, G.C.; Panda, S. Time-Restricted Eating to Prevent and Manage Chronic Metabolic Diseases. *Annu. Rev. Nutr.* **2019**, *39*, 291–315. [CrossRef]
34. Mason, I.C.; Qian, J.; Adler, G.K.; Scheer, F.A.J.L. Impact of Circadian Disruption on Glucose Metabolism: Implications for Type 2 Diabetes. *Diabetologia* **2020**, *63*, 462–472. [CrossRef]
35. Stenvers, D.J.; Scheer, F.A.J.L.; Schrauwen, P.; la Fleur, S.E.; Kalsbeek, A. Circadian Clocks and Insulin Resistance. *Nat. Rev. Endocrinol.* **2019**, *15*, 75–89. [CrossRef]
36. Chellappa, S.L.; Vujovic, N.; Williams, J.S.; Scheer, F.A.J.L. Impact of Circadian Disruption on Cardiovascular Function and Disease. *Trends Endocrinol. Metab.* **2019**, *30*, 767–779. [CrossRef] [PubMed]
37. Regmi, P.; Heilbronn, L.K. Time-Restricted Eating: Benefits, Mechanisms, and Challenges in Translation. *iScience* **2020**, *23*, 101161. [CrossRef]
38. Qian, J.; Scheer, F.A.J.L. Circadian System and Glucose Metabolism: Implications for Physiology and Disease. *Trends Endocrinol. Metab.* **2016**, *27*, 282–293. [CrossRef] [PubMed]
39. Mattson, M.P.; Allison, D.B.; Fontana, L.; Harvie, M.; Longo, V.D.; Malaisse, W.J.; Mosley, M.; Notterpek, L.; Ravussin, E.; Scheer, F.A.J.L.; et al. Meal Frequency and Timing in Health and Disease. *Proc. Natl. Acad. Sci. USA* **2014**, *111*, 16647–16653. [CrossRef]
40. Garaulet, M.; Gómez-Abellán, P.; Alburquerque-Béjar, J.J.; Lee, Y.-C.; Ordovás, J.M.; Scheer, F.A. Timing of Food Intake Predicts Weight Loss Effectiveness. *Int. J. Obes.* **2013**, *37*, 604–611. [CrossRef] [PubMed]
41. Sulli, G.; Manoogian, E.N.C.; Taub, P.R.; Panda, S. Training the Circadian Clock, Clocking the Drugs, and Drugging the Clock to Prevent, Manage, and Treat Chronic Diseases. *Trends Pharmacol. Sci.* **2018**, *39*, 812–827. [CrossRef]
42. de Cabo, R.; Mattson, M.P. Effects of Intermittent Fasting on Health, Aging, and Disease. *N. Engl. J. Med.* **2019**, *381*, 2541–2551. [CrossRef]
43. Panda, S. Circadian Physiology of Metabolism. *Science* **2016**, *354*, 1008–1015. [CrossRef]
44. Queiroz, J.d.N.; Macedo, R.C.O.; Tinsley, G.M.; Reischak-Oliveira, A. Time-Restricted Eating and Circadian Rhythms: The Biological Clock Is Ticking. *Crit. Rev. Food Sci. Nutr.* **2021**, *61*, 2863–2875. [CrossRef] [PubMed]
45. Asher, G.; Sassone-Corsi, P. Time for Food: The Intimate Interplay between Nutrition, Metabolism, and the Circadian Clock. *Cell* **2015**, *161*, 84–92. [CrossRef] [PubMed]
46. Levine, A.S.; Morley, J.E. Stress-Induced Eating in Rats. *Am. J. Physiol.* **1981**, *241*, R72–R76. [CrossRef] [PubMed]
47. Morley, J.E.; Levine, A.S.; Rowland, N.E. Minireview. Stress Induced Eating. *Life Sci.* **1983**, *32*, 2169–2182. [CrossRef]
48. Torres, S.J.; Nowson, C.A. Relationship between Stress, Eating Behavior, and Obesity. *Nutrition* **2007**, *23*, 887–894. [CrossRef]

49. Pasquali, R. The Hypothalamic-Pituitary-Adrenal Axis and Sex Hormones in Chronic Stress and Obesity: Pathophysiological and Clinical Aspects. *Ann. N. Y. Acad. Sci.* **2012**, *1264*, 20–35. [CrossRef]
50. Block, J.P.; He, Y.; Zaslavsky, A.M.; Ding, L.; Ayanian, J.Z. Psychosocial Stress and Change in Weight among US Adults. *Am. J. Epidemiol.* **2009**, *170*, 181–192. [CrossRef]
51. Robbins, T.W.; Fray, P.J. Stress-Induced Eating: Fact, Fiction or Misunderstanding? *Appetite* **1980**, *1*, 103–133. [CrossRef]
52. Pecoraro, N.; Reyes, F.; Gomez, F.; Bhargava, A.; Dallman, M.F. Chronic Stress Promotes Palatable Feeding, Which Reduces Signs of Stress: Feedforward and Feedback Effects of Chronic Stress. *Endocrinology* **2004**, *145*, 3754–3762. [CrossRef]
53. Dallman, M.F.; Pecoraro, N.; Akana, S.F.; La Fleur, S.E.; Gomez, F.; Houshyar, H.; Bell, M.E.; Bhatnagar, S.; Laugero, K.D.; Manalo, S. Chronic Stress and Obesity: A New View of "Comfort Food". *Proc. Natl. Acad. Sci. USA* **2003**, *100*, 11696–11701. [CrossRef]
54. la Fleur, S.E.; Houshyar, H.; Roy, M.; Dallman, M.F. Choice of Lard, but Not Total Lard Calories, Damps Adrenocorticotropin Responses to Restraint. *Endocrinology* **2005**, *146*, 2193–2199. [CrossRef] [PubMed]
55. Zellner, D.A.; Loaiza, S.; Gonzalez, Z.; Pita, J.; Morales, J.; Pecora, D.; Wolf, A. Food Selection Changes under Stress. *Physiol. Behav.* **2006**, *87*, 789–793. [CrossRef] [PubMed]
56. Epel, E.; Lapidus, R.; McEwen, B.; Brownell, K. Stress May Add Bite to Appetite in Women: A Laboratory Study of Stress-Induced Cortisol and Eating Behavior. *Psychoneuroendocrinology* **2001**, *26*, 37–49. [CrossRef] [PubMed]
57. Oliver, G.; Wardle, J.; Gibson, E.L. Stress and Food Choice: A Laboratory Study. *Psychosom. Med.* **2000**, *62*, 853–865. [CrossRef]
58. Rutters, F.; Nieuwenhuizen, A.G.; Lemmens, S.G.T.; Born, J.M.; Westerterp-Plantenga, M.S. Acute Stress-Related Changes in Eating in the Absence of Hunger. *Obesity* **2009**, *17*, 72–77. [CrossRef]
59. Jastreboff, A.M.; Sinha, R.; Lacadie, C.; Small, D.M.; Sherwin, R.S.; Potenza, M.N. Neural Correlates of Stress- and Food Cue-Induced Food Craving in Obesity: Association with Insulin Levels. *Diabetes Care* **2013**, *36*, 394–402. [CrossRef]
60. Gibson, E.L. Emotional Influences on Food Choice: Sensory, Physiological and Psychological Pathways. *Physiol. Behav.* **2006**, *89*, 53–61. [CrossRef]
61. Sinha, R. Chronic Stress, Drug Use, and Vulnerability to Addiction. *Ann. N. Y. Acad. Sci.* **2008**, *1141*, 105–130. [CrossRef]
62. Everitt, B.J.; Belin, D.; Economidou, D.; Pelloux, Y.; Dalley, J.W.; Robbins, T.W. Review. Neural Mechanisms Underlying the Vulnerability to Develop Compulsive Drug-Seeking Habits and Addiction. *Philos. Trans. R. Soc. Lond. B Biol. Sci.* **2008**, *363*, 3125–3135. [CrossRef]
63. Ikeda, H.; West, D.B.; Pustek, J.J.; Figlewicz, D.P.; Greenwood, M.R.; Porte, D.; Woods, S.C. Intraventricular Insulin Reduces Food Intake and Body Weight of Lean but Not Obese Zucker Rats. *Appetite* **1986**, *7*, 381–386. [CrossRef]
64. McCuen-Wurst, C.; Ruggieri, M.; Allison, K.C. Disordered Eating and Obesity: Associations between Binge Eating-Disorder, Night-Eating Syndrome, and Weight-Related Co-Morbidities. *Ann. N. Y. Acad. Sci.* **2018**, *1411*, 96–105. [CrossRef] [PubMed]
65. Cornier, M.-A.; Dabelea, D.; Hernandez, T.L.; Lindstrom, R.C.; Steig, A.J.; Stob, N.R.; Van Pelt, R.E.; Wang, H.; Eckel, R.H. The Metabolic Syndrome. *Endocr. Rev.* **2008**, *29*, 777–822. [CrossRef]
66. Kim, K.-K.; Haam, J.-H.; Kim, B.T.; Kim, E.M.; Park, J.H.; Rhee, S.Y.; Jeon, E.; Kang, E.; Nam, G.E.; Koo, H.Y.; et al. Evaluation and Treatment of Obesity and Its Comorbidities: 2022 Update of Clinical Practice Guidelines for Obesity by the Korean Society for the Study of Obesity. *J. Obes. Metab. Syndr.* **2023**, *32*, 1–24. [CrossRef]
67. Berkovskaya, M.A.; Tarasenko, A.A.; Fadeev, V.V.; Gurova, O.Y. [Alexithymia and its relation with eating disorders and obesity]. *Probl. Endokrinol.* **2020**, *66*, 42–48. [CrossRef] [PubMed]
68. Bhuvaneswar, C.G.; Baldessarini, R.J.; Harsh, V.L.; Alpert, J.E. Adverse Endocrine and Metabolic Effects of Psychotropic Drugs: Selective Clinical Review. *CNS Drugs* **2009**, *23*, 1003–1021. [CrossRef]
69. de Almeida, K.M.; Moreira, C.L.R.L.; Lafer, B. Metabolic Syndrome and Bipolar Disorder: What Should Psychiatrists Know? *CNS Neurosci. Ther.* **2012**, *18*, 160–166. [CrossRef]
70. Moreira, F.P.; Jansen, K.; Cardoso, T.d.A.; Mondin, T.C.; Vieira, I.S.; Magalhães, P.V. da S.; Kapczinski, F.; Souza, L.D. de M.; da Silva, R.A.; Oses, J.P.; et al. Metabolic Syndrome, Depression and Anhedonia among Young Adults. *Psychiatry Res.* **2019**, *271*, 306–310. [CrossRef]
71. Räikkönen, K.; Matthews, K.A.; Kuller, L.H. Depressive Symptoms and Stressful Life Events Predict Metabolic Syndrome among Middle-Aged Women: A Comparison of World Health Organization, Adult Treatment Panel III, and International Diabetes Foundation Definitions. *Diabetes Care* **2007**, *30*, 872–877. [CrossRef] [PubMed]
72. Pigsborg, K.; Kalea, A.Z.; De Dominicis, S.; Magkos, F. Behavioral and Psychological Factors Affecting Weight Loss Success. *Curr. Obes. Rep.* **2023**, *12*, 223–230. [CrossRef]
73. Breen, C.; O'Connell, J.; Geoghegan, J.; O'Shea, D.; Birney, S.; Tully, L.; Gaynor, K.; O'Kelly, M.; O'Malley, G.; O'Donovan, C.; et al. Obesity in Adults: A 2022 Adapted Clinical Practice Guideline for Ireland. *Obes Facts* **2022**, *15*, 736–752. [CrossRef]
74. Curis, C.; Moroianu, M.; Moroianu, L.-A.; Pintilei, D.R.; Ardeleanu, V.; Bobirca, A.; Mahler, B.; Stoian, A.P. Intuitive Nutrition Co-Factor of Emotional Equilibrium for Maintaining Nutritional Balance: A Prospective Study. *Mediterr. J. Clin. Psychol.* **2023**, *11*. [CrossRef]
75. Conti, C.; Di Francesco, G.; Severo, M.; Lanzara, R.; Richards, K.; Guagnano, M.T.; Porcelli, P. Alexithymia and Metabolic Syndrome: The Mediating Role of Binge Eating. *Eat. Weight. Disord.* **2021**, *26*, 1813–1823. [CrossRef] [PubMed]
76. Mustač, F.; Galijašević, T.; Podolski, E.; Belančić, A.; Matovinović, M.; Marčinko, D. Recent Advances in Psychotherapeutic Treatment and Understanding of Alexithymia in Patients with Obesity and Diabetes Mellitus Type 2. *Diabetology* **2023**, *4*, 481–489. [CrossRef]

77. Camacho-Barcia, L.; Lucas, I.; Miranda-Olivos, R.; Jiménez-Murcia, S.; Fernández-Aranda, F. Applying Psycho-Behavioural Phenotyping in Obesity Characterization. *Rev. Endocr. Metab. Disord.* **2023**, *24*, 871–883. [CrossRef]
78. Morillo-Sarto, H.; López-Del-Hoyo, Y.; Pérez-Aranda, A.; Modrego-Alarcón, M.; Barceló-Soler, A.; Borao, L.; Puebla-Guedea, M.; Demarzo, M.; García-Campayo, J.; Montero-Marin, J. "Mindful Eating" for Reducing Emotional Eating in Patients with Overweight or Obesity in Primary Care Settings: A Randomized Controlled Trial. *Eur. Eat. Disord. Rev.* **2023**, *31*, 303–319. [CrossRef]
79. Annesi, J.J. Coaction of Exercise and Eating Improvements Within a Behavioral Obesity Treatment: Directionality and Psychological Mechanisms. *Res. Q. Exerc. Sport.* **2023**, *94*, 826–838. [CrossRef] [PubMed]
80. Slabá, Š.; Málková, I.; Wagenknecht, M.; Riegel, K.D.; Junek, L.; Lorencová, J.; Herlesová, J.; Ondrová, V.K.; Jep, P.S.P.S.Č.O.S.Č. Psychological Aspects of Obesity. *Cas. Lek. Cesk* **2020**, *159*, 118–124.
81. Sagar, R.; Gupta, T. Psychological Aspects of Obesity in Children and Adolescents. *Indian. J. Pediatr.* **2018**, *85*, 554–559. [CrossRef] [PubMed]
82. Baygi, F.; Djalalinia, S.; Qorbani, M.; Larrabee Sonderlund, A.; Kousgaard Andersen, M.K.; Thilsing, T.; Heitmann, B.L.; Nielsen, J.B. The Effect of Psychological Interventions Targeting Overweight and Obesity in School-Aged Children: A Systematic Review and Meta-Analysis. *BMC Public Health* **2023**, *23*, 1478. [CrossRef]
83. Marčinko, D.; Bilić, V.; Jakšić, N.; Medved, S.; Levaj, S.; Mustač, F. Psychodynamics of Obesity. *Medix*, 2024, *preprint*. [CrossRef]
84. Chew, H.S.J.; Chng, S.; Rajasegaran, N.N.; Choy, K.H.; Chong, Y.Y. Effectiveness of Acceptance and Commitment Therapy on Weight, Eating Behaviours and Psychological Outcomes: A Systematic Review and Meta-Analysis. *Eat. Weight. Disord.* **2023**, *28*, 6. [CrossRef]
85. Jebeile, H.; Cardel, M.I.; Kyle, T.K.; Jastreboff, A.M. Addressing Psychosocial Health in the Treatment and Care of Adolescents with Obesity. *Obesity* **2021**, *29*, 1413–1422. [CrossRef] [PubMed]
86. Freimuth, M.; Moniz, S.; Kim, S.R. Clarifying Exercise Addiction: Differential Diagnosis, Co-Occurring Disorders, and Phases of Addiction. *Int. J. Environ. Res. Public Health* **2011**, *8*, 4069–4081. [CrossRef] [PubMed]
87. Alleva, J.M.; Sheeran, P.; Webb, T.L.; Martijn, C.; Miles, E. A Meta-Analytic Review of Stand-Alone Interventions to Improve Body Image. *PLoS ONE* **2015**, *10*, e0139177. [CrossRef] [PubMed]

diabetology

MDPI

Review

Metabolic Syndrome and Pharmacological Interventions in Clinical Development

Eugen Javor [1,*], David Šarčević [2] and Arnes Rešić [3,4]

1 Solmed Clinic, 10000 Zagreb, Croatia
2 Pharmacy Department, General Hospital Zadar, 23000 Zadar, Croatia; david.sarcevic2202@gmail.com
3 Department of Pediatric Clinical Pharmacology and Toxicology, Children's Hospital Zagreb, 10000 Zagreb, Croatia; aresic@yahoo.com
4 University Department of Health Studies, University of Split, 21000 Split, Croatia
* Correspondence: eugen.javor@gmail.com

Abstract: Metabolic syndrome prevalence is between 24 and 27% and poses a significant risk for the development of atherosclerotic cardiovascular disease (ASCVD), type 2 diabetes (T2D), or other comorbidities. Currently, no drugs are approved for metabolic syndrome treatment itself, so the risk factors are treated with therapies approved for cardiac and metabolic conditions. These are approved drugs for dyslipidemia treatment such as statins and proprotein convertase subtilisin/kexin type 9 (PCSK9) inhibitors, cornerstone antihypertensive drugs, or novel class glucagon-like peptide 1 (GLP-1) receptor agonists (GLP-1 RA) for T2D and overweight or obesity treatment. We have also evaluated new pharmacological interventions in clinical development that have reached Phase 2 and/or Phase 3 randomized clinical trials (RCTs) for the management of the risk factors of metabolic syndrome. In the pipeline are glucose-dependent insulinotropic polypeptide (GIP), GLP-1, glucagon receptor (GCGR), amylin agonists, and a combination of the latter for T2D and overweight or obesity treatment. Non-entero-pancreatic hormone-based therapies such as ketohexokinase (KHK) inhibitor, growth differentiation factor 15 (GDF15) agonists, monoclonal antibodies (mAbs) as activin type II receptors (ActRII) inhibitors, and a combination of anti-α-myostatin (GFD8) and anti-Activin-A (Act-A) mAbs have also reached Phase 2 or 3 RCTs in the same indications. Rilparencel (Renal Autologous Cell Therapy) is being evaluated in patients with T2D and chronic kidney disease (CKD) in a Phase 3 trial. For dyslipidemia treatment, novel PCSK9 inhibitors (oral and subcutaneous) and cholesteryl ester transfer protein (CETP) inhibitors are in the final stages of clinical development. There is also a surge of a new generation of an antisense oligonucleotide (ASO) and small interfering RNA (siRNA)-targeting lipoprotein(a) [Lp(a)] synthesis pathway that could possibly contribute to a further step forward in the treatment of dyslipidemia. For resistant and uncontrolled hypertension, aldosterone synthase inhibitors and siRNAs targeting angiotensinogen (AGT) messenger RNA (mRNA) are promising new therapeutic options. It would be interesting if a few drugs in clinical development for metabolic syndrome such as 6-bromotryptophan (6-BT), vericiguat, and INV-202 as a peripherally-acting CB1 receptor (CB1r) blocker would succeed in finally gaining the first drug approval for metabolic syndrome itself.

Keywords: metabolic syndrome; pharmacological interventions; research

1. Introduction

Metabolic syndrome encompasses several inter-related risk factors for the development of atherosclerotic cardiovascular disease (ASCVD), type 2 diabetes (T2D), and other various comorbidities (i.e., risk of cancer, cognitive impairment, non-alcoholic fatty liver disease (NAFLD)) [1,2]. Metabolic risk factors consist of atherogenic dyslipidemia (i.e., increased low-density lipoprotein cholesterol [LDL-C], decreased high-density lipoprotein cholesterol [HDL-C], increased levels of triglycerides), arterial hypertension, hyperglycemia, a prothrombotic state, and a proinflammatory state. Central obesity (particularly visceral adiposity) and insulin resistance represent underlying risk factors, while sedentary lifestyle, aging, hormonal imbalance, and genetic or ethnic predisposition represent other associated conditions [1]. The International Diabetes Federation (IDF) and the American Heart Association/National Heart, Lung, and Blood Institute (AHA/NHLBI) constitute the diagnosis of metabolic syndrome as the presence of any three out of five individual risk factors: elevated waist circumference, dyslipidemia (i.e., elevated triglycerides and decreased HDL-C), elevated blood pressure, and elevated fasting glucose (Table 1) [3].

Table 1. Definition of metabolic syndrome [3].

Measure	Categorical Cut Points
Elevated waist circumference *	Population- and country-specific definitions
Elevated triglycerides (drug treatment for elevated triglycerides is an alternate indicator **)	≥150 mg/dL (1.7 mmol/L)
Reduced HDL-C (drug treatment for reduced HDL-C is an alternate indicator **)	<40 mg/dL (1.0 mmol/L) in males; <50 mg/dL (1.3 mmol/L) in females
Elevated blood pressure (antihypertensive drug treatment in a patient with a history of hypertension is an alternate indicator)	Systolic ≥ 130 and/or diastolic ≥ 85 mm Hg
Elevated fasting glucose *** (drug treatment of elevated glucose is an alternate indicator)	≥100 mg/dL

HDL-C (high-density lipoprotein cholesterol). * It is recommended that the IDF cut-points be used for non-Europeans and either the IDF or AHA/NHLBI cut-points used for people of European origin until more data are available. ** The most commonly used drugs for elevated triglycerides and reduced HDL-C are fibrates and nicotinic acid. A patient taking 1 of these drugs can be presumed to have high triglycerides and low HDL-C. High dose of ω-3 fatty acids presumes high triglycerides. *** Most patients with type 2 diabetes mellitus will have metabolic syndrome by the proposed criteria.

The prevalence of metabolic syndrome in the general population is between 24 and 27% [4,5]. The MetS-Greece study reported that among individuals with metabolic syndrome, abdominal obesity (72%) was the most common abnormality. The prevalence of arterial hypertension (66%), elevated glucose (including patients with diabetes mellitus) (53%), elevated triglyceride levels (62%), and low HDL-C levels (54%) was ineligibly lower [5].

The goal of metabolic syndrome management is to reduce the risk of ASCVD and T2D development. If ASCVD or T2D are present components of metabolic syndrome, they contribute to further disease progression and risk. First-line interventions for lowering long-term and short-term risk consist of non-pharmacological interventions through lifestyle modifications (i.e., diet, exercise, weight loss, tobacco cessation) [1]. Surgical treatment strategies such as bariatric surgery can also be an option for weight loss management [6]. In individuals with a higher 10-year risk assessment of cardiovascular disease (CVD) risk on the Framingham scoring [7], pharmacological management for particular metabolic risk factors must be considered. Since metabolic syndrome lacks a single etiological factor or central pathophysiological abnormality, multiple specific pathways are targeted with several drug classes [1]. The choice of therapeutic approach depends on the individual risk factors of a patient. Currently, no drugs are approved for metabolic syndrome indication itself. Instead, metabolic syndrome risk factors are treated with therapies approved for cardiac and metabolic conditions. These treatments affect several different pathways associated with metabolic syndrome. There are several pharmacological approaches and drug classes for the management of each of the risk factors of metabolic syndrome.

1.1. *Atherogenic Dyslipidemia*

Atherogenic dyslipidemia can be modulated with statin or non-statin therapy. The primary goal for that treatment is an elevated LDL-C level, but in a case of very high (≥500 mg/dL) triglycerides, they should be the first priority. Statins, 3-hydroxy-3-methyl-glutaryl-coenzyme A (HMG-CoA) reductase inhibitors, are the cornerstone for dyslipidemia management. There are seven different statins approved by the Food and Drug Administration (FDA). They are atorvastatin, fluvastatin, lovastatin, pitavastatin, pravastatin, rosuvastatin, and simvastatin. They are additionally subdivided to low, moderate, and high intensity LDL-C, lowering the therapy depending on the type and the dose of a particular statin [8]. Non-statin therapies that may be useful in combination with statin therapy include ezetimibe (inhibits cholesterol absorption at the brush border of the small intestine mediated by the sterol transporter Niemann-Pick C1-Like-1 (NPC1L1)), bile acid sequestrants (colesevelam, colestipol, and cholestyramine), and proprotein convertase subtilisin/kexin type 9 (PCSK9) inhibitors (alirocumab, evolocumab, and inclisiran). Alirocumab and evolocumab are PCSK9 inhibitor monoclonal antibodies (mAbs), while inclisiran is a small interfering RNA (siRNA) targeting PCSK9 messenger RNA (mRNA) [9,10]. Triglyceride-lowering drugs, nicotinic acid, and fibrates (fenofibrate, fenofibric acid, gemfibrozil) may be useful in some patients with severe hypertriglyceridemia [2]. Cholesteryl ester transfer protein (CETP) inhibitors (torcetrapib, dalcetrapib, evacetrapib, anacetrapib, TA-8995) have been tested in several randomized clinical trials (RCTs) but still without proven clinical benefit or off-target effects [11,12]. Bempedoic acid, an ATP citrate lyase inhibitor, demonstrated a lower risk of major adverse cardiovascular events (MACE) among statin-intolerant patients [13].

1.2. Arterial Hypertension

For elevated blood pressure, five major drug classes are available as a first-line antihypertensive treatment. A thiazide/thiazide-like diuretic, calcium channel blocker (CCB), angiotensin-converting enzyme inhibitor (ACEi), angiotensin receptor blocker (ARB), or beta-blocker (BB) can be used depending on the individual patient risk profile. Blockers of the renin–angiotensin system (RAS) (ACEi or ARB) are considered as a common component of the general combination treatment strategy, while BBs are restricted to special clinical conditions or situations. Compelling or possible contraindications for the selection of drug classes should be evaluated when prescribing first-line antihypertensive treatment. Other antihypertensive drugs (alpha-blockers, centrally acting agents and mineralocorticoid-receptor antagonists (MRAs)) can be prescribed in some specific cases, or when blood pressure cannot be controlled by various combinations of the major drug classes [14].

1.3. Management of Hyperglycemia

There are eight classes of antihyperglycemic drugs; bigvanides (metformin), sulfonylurea (second generation particularly), thiazolidinediones (pioglitazone), dipeptidyl peptidase-4 (DPP-4) inhibitors (i.e., alogliptin, vildagliptin, sitagliptin, linagliptin, saxagliptin), insulins, sodium/glucose co-transporter 2 (SGLT-2) inhibitors (i.e., canagliflozin, dapagliflozin, empagliflozin), glucagon-like peptide 1 (GLP-1) receptor agonists (GLP-1 RAs) (i.e., dulaglutide, liraglutide, semaglutide), dual glucose-dependent insulinotropic polypeptide (GIP), and GLP-1 RA (tirzepatide), which are commonly used for hyperglycemia management in T2D. α-Glucosidase inhibitors are less commonly used, while other glucose-lowering medications (i.e., meglitinides, colesevelam, quick-release bromocriptine, and pramlintide) are rarely used [15]. Metformin is a pharmacological option in particular individuals with prediabetes, those with BMI ≥ 35 kg/m^2, those aged < 60 years, and women with prior gestational diabetes mellitus [16].

1.4. Weight Management

It is estimated that 40% of Americans suffer from obesity and 20% are overweight [17]. There are six different drug classes approved by the FDA for the treatment of obesity: orlistat, phentermine/topiramate extended release (ER), naltrexone/bupropion ER, liraglutide 3 mg, semaglutide 2.4 mg, and tirzepatide [18,19]. Incretin drugs, particularly GLP-1 RA, have revolutionized the treatment of obesity. They can help patients suffering from obesity to lose ~20 to 25% of their body weight [17].

In addition to approved drug classes that can be used in metabolic syndrome management, other targets have come up formerly in research: the so-called master metabolic regulators. They included the pathways activated by the insulin receptors, adenosine monophosphate (AMP) kinase, inflammatory cascades, endocannabinoid receptors, nuclear receptors, glucocorticoids, and mitochondrial oxidative pathways [20]. From a drug development perspective, it is problematic to conduct a clinical trial solely for metabolic syndrome [21]. As mentioned before, the metabolic syndrome risk factors are treated with therapies approved for cardiac and metabolic conditions. The questions arises as to what a comparator would be and if it is ethical to use placebo. What particular drug target could provide the highest benefit? What clinical endpoint should be used, MACE or a surrogate endpoint? Despite challenges, the metabolic syndrome risk factors are successfully treated with available pharmacological approaches.

In order to evaluate what is in the pipeline and what can be promising as potential new therapies for metabolic syndrome risk factors management, we have researched the most relevant clinical trials database.

2. Material and Methods

We have decided to research the ClinicalTrials.gov database as the most comprehensive RCTs database. ClinicalTrials.gov lists over 300,000 research studies, while the second biggest EU Clinical Trials Register lists over 34,000 clinical trials [22]. Further on, relevant RCTs that evaluate new substances that can potentially be a new standard of care are mostly multicenter and are evaluated in USA, Europe, and other parts of the world. Therefore, ClinicalTrials.gov should capture all RCTs of interest. On 13 May 2024, we have researched ClinicalTrials.gov for the records that fulfill several criteria: Phase 2 and Phase 3 RCTs, interventional RCTs, RCTs that are in recruiting, active-non recruiting, and completed phases, RCTs conducted only in adult population (>18), and with study start from 5 May 2021 to 5 May 2024. The search terms were "Metabolic syndrome", "Prediabetes", "Insulin resistance", "Obesity/Overweight", "Type 2 diabetes", "Hyperlipidemia", "Dyslipidemia", "Lipoprotein Disorder", and "Hypertension".

We have not included Phase 1 trials in our research since only 13.8% of Phase 1 trials reach drug approval [23]. Therefore, we have decided to go for Phase 2 and Phase 3 trials. Sponsors usually conducts interim analysis of RCTs that are active (in progress), and based on the given results they decide on proceeding or stopping the drug development program. Therefore, we have agreed that a three-year timeframe is long enough to catch all drugs in development that may be potential candidates to obtain drug approval. Some RCTs are conducted in parallel in more than one phase (i.e., Phase 1 and Phase 2a). In that case, we have included these studies into our research if they fulfill at least one "phase" inclusion criteria. We have excluded RCTs evaluating already known herbal remedies (i.e., herbal medicine used in traditional medicine but evaluated in RCTs in a new indication). Herbal medicines are mostly less potent and less selective than drugs themselves, and there are very small chances that an already known herbal medicine would become a new therapeutic option in metabolic syndrome treatment. We have also excluded RCTs evaluating already approved drugs used in a risk-factor treatment (e.g., inclisiran, semaglutide, tirezpatide, etc.) and RCTs in other indications/comorbidities that are not closely related to keywords of interest for metabolic syndrome (i.e., pulmonary arterial hypertension, ocular hypertension, non-alcoholic fatty liver disease (NAFLD)). The flowchart diagram of the research is present in Figure 1. Data have been extracted into the predesigned Microsoft Excel (ver. 2311, Microsoft, Redmond, WA, USA) spreadsheet.

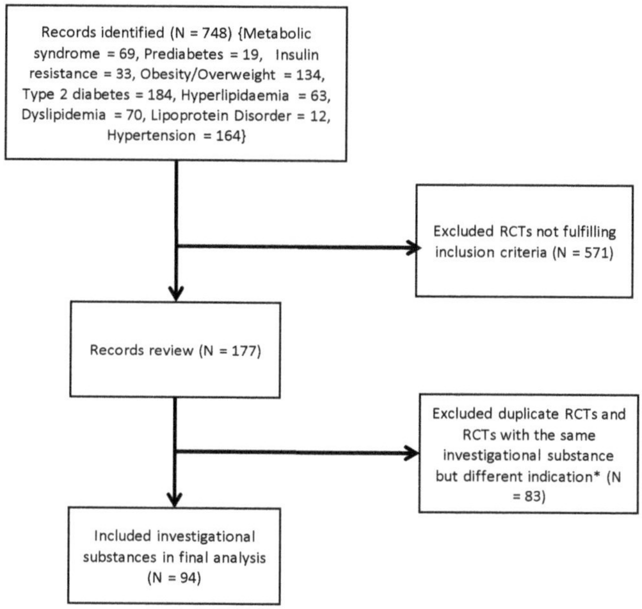

Figure 1. Flow chart diagram. * RCTs that are evaluating the same investigational substance in different indications are summarized into one record, which documented all indications for which it is in research.

3. Results

We have identified 748 records in our research. The majority of the records are for T2D and hypertension, while metabolic syndrome has 69 records (Figure 1). After selection, we have detected 94 new investigational drugs that are in the pipeline for metabolic syndrome risk factors' management (Table 2).

Half (51%) of investigational drugs have reached Phase 3 RCTs, and the other half (49%) are in a Phase 2 RCT. We have identified that the most investigational drugs are evaluated in RCTs which main clinical trials sites are located in United States of America (USA) and/or Europe (60%), less in China or South Korea (37%), and a negligible number in Brazil (1%). RCTs with main clinical trials located in USA and/or Europe and in China are represented with 2%. We could not find any information on the mechanism of action for 17 (18%) investigational drugs, of which 15 (88%) were tested in China or South Korea, 1 (6%) in Brazil, and 1 (6%) in USA and/or Europe. From all investigational drugs evaluated in the main trial sites located in China or South Korea, for 43% of them we could not find mechanism of action of investigational drugs.

Most investigational drugs are evaluated in T2D (41%), obesity and/or overweight (31%), dyslipidemia and/or hyperlipidemia and/or lipoprotein disorder (29%), and hypertension (19%) indications (Table 2).

Table 2. Pharmacological interventions in clinical development.

N	Investigational Drug	Mechanism of Action	Indication	Main Site Location	Phase	NCT
1	6-bromotryptophan (6-BT)	Endogenous plasma microbiome-derived tryptophan metabolite	Metabolic Syndrome	USA and/or Europe	Phase 1 Phase 2	NCT05971524
2	AD-209	N/A	Essential Hypertension	South Korea	Phase 2	NCT05631990
3	AD-218	N/A	Dyslipidemia	South Korea	Phase 3	NCT05631990
4	AD-221 and AD-221A	N/A	Primary Hypercholesterolemia	China	Phase 3	NCT05131997
5	AD-223	N/A	Essential Hypertension	South Korea	Phase 3	NCT06052748
6	ALN-KHK	RNAi targeting ketohexokinase	Type 2 Diabetes Mellitus with Obesity	USA and/or Europe	Phase 1 Phase 2	NCT05761301
7	ALT-801 (SP-1373)	Dual GCGR and GLP-1 receptor agonist	Obesity	USA and/or Europe	Phase 2	NCT05295875
8	AP-325	Binds and modulates the GABAA receptor (an ionotropic receptor and ligand-gated ion channel)	Type 2 Diabetes Mellitus	USA and/or Europe	Phase 2	NCT05160272
9	APHD-012	Distal jejunal-release dextrose	Obesity	USA and/or Europe	Phase 2	NCT05385978
10	ATB-1011 and ATB-1012	N/A	Essential Hypertension and Type 2 Diabetes Mellitus	China	Phase 3	NCT05573477
11	AZD0780	Oral PCSK9 Inhibitor	Dyslipidemia	USA and/or Europe	Phase 2	NCT06173570
12	AZD8233	ASO targeting PCSK9	Hyperlipidaemia	USA and/or Europe	Phase 2	NCT04964557, NCT06173570
13	AZD9550	Dual GCGR and GLP-1 receptor agonist	Type 2 Diabetes Mellitus with Overweight or Obesity	USA and/or Europe	Phase 1 Phase 2	NCT06151964
14	Baxdrostat (CIN-107)	Aldosterone synthase inhibitors	Uncontrolled Hypertension and Resistant Hypertension; Uncontrolled Hypertension and Chronic Kidney Disease	USA and/or Europe	Phase 2 Phase 3	NCT06344104, NCT05432167
15	BC Lispro (THDB0206)	Insulin	Type 2 Diabetes Mellitus	China	Phase 3	NCT05834868
16	Berlim 25/2	N/A	Type 2 Diabetes Mellitus and Dyslipidemia	Brazil	Phase 3	NCT04602754

Table 2. *Cont.*

N	Investigational Drug	Mechanism of Action	Indication	Main Site Location	Phase	NCT
17	Bimagrumab	mAb inhibitor of ActRII	Overweight or Obesity	USA and/or Europe	Phase 2	NCT05616013
18	BMF-219	Oral irreversible covalent inhibitor of menin	Type 2 Diabetes Mellitus	USA and/or Europe	Phase 1 Phase 2	NCT05731544
19	BR1017A and BR1017B	N/A	Essential Hypertension and Primary Hypercholesterolemia	South Korea	Phase 3	NCT05930028
20	BR1018B and BR1018C	N/A	Essential Hypertension and Primary Hypercholesterolemia	South Korea	Phase 3	NCT06165250
21	Cagrilintide	Amylin receptor agonist	Type 2 Diabetes Mellitus; Overweight or Obesity	USA and/or Europe	Phase 2 Phase 3	NCT05813925, NCT04982575
22	CKD-391 and CKD-331	N/A	Primary Hypercholesterolemia	China, South Korea	Phase 3	NCT05657574
23	CPL207280	GPR40 (also known as FFA receptor 1) agonist	Type 2 Diabetes Mellitus	USA and/or Europe	Phase 2	NCT05248776
24	D064 and D702	N/A	Essential Hypertension	South Korea	Phase 3	NCT06121518
25	D150, D745 and D759	N/A	Type 2 Diabetes Mellitus	South Korea	Phase 3	NCT05566028
26	Dapiglutide	Dual GLP-1R/GLP-2R agonist	Obesity	USA and/or Europe	Phase 2	NCT05788601
27	Denatonium Acetate (ARD-101)	Oral potential TAS2R agonist	Obesity	USA and/or Europe	Phase 2	NCT05121441
28	DW1125 and DW1125A	N/A	Primary Hypercholesterolemia or Dyslipidemia	South Korea	Phase 3	NCT05970679
29	DWP16001	SGLT2 inhibitor	Type 2 Diabetes Mellitus	China, South Korea	Phase 3	NCT05376930, NCT05505994
30	Ecnoglutide (XW003)	Long-acting cAMP Signaling Biased GLP-1 Analog	Obesity; Type 2 Diabetes Mellitus	USA and/or Europe, China	Phase 2 Phase 3	NCT05111912, NCT05813795, NCT05680155, NCT05680129
31	Efsitora Alfa (BIF, LY3209590, or insulin efsitora alfa)	Basal Insulin Fc	Type 2 Diabetes Mellitus	USA and/or Europe	Phase 3	NCT05462756

Table 2. *Cont.*

N	Investigational Drug	Mechanism of Action	Indication	Main Site Location	Phase	NCT
32	GLY-200	Mucin-complexing polymer	Obesity; Type 2 Diabetes Mellitus	USA and/or Europe	Phase 2	NCT06259981, NCT05478525
33	GSBR-1290	Oral GLP-1 receptor agonist	Type 2 Diabetes Mellitus, and Overweight or Obesity	USA and/or Europe	Phase 1 Phase 2	NCT05762471
34	GZR18	GLP-1 receptor agonist	Type 2 Diabetes Mellitus; Overweight or Obesity	China	Phase 1 Phase 2	NCT06256523, NCT06256536, NCT06256562
35	GZR4	INSR agonist	Type 2 Diabetes Mellitus	China	Phase 2	NCT06202079
36	HCP1803	N/A	Essential Hypertension	South Korea	Phase 3	NCT05362110
37	HCP1904-3	N/A	Essential Hypertension	South Korea	Phase 3	NCT05199129
38	HCP2102	N/A	Essential Hypertension	South Korea	Phase 3	NCT05450601
39	HD-6277	Selective GPR40 agonist	Type 2 Diabetes Mellitus	South Korea	Phase 2	NCT05666128
40	HEC88473	Dual FGF21 receptor and GLP-1 receptor agonist	Type 2 Diabetes Mellitus	China	Phase 2	NCT06148649
41	HRS9531	Dual GIP and GLP-1 receptor agonist	Obesity; Type 2 Diabetes Mellitus	China	Phase 2	NCT05881837, NCT05966272
42	HS-20094	Dual GIP and GLP-1 receptor agonist	Type 2 Diabetes Mellitus; Overweight or Obesity	China	Phase 2	NCT06118008, NCT06118021
43	HSG4112	Analog of glabridin	Overweight or Obesity	South Korea	Phase 2	NCT05197556
44	iGlarLixi vs. IDegAsp	Insulins	Type 2 Diabetes Mellitus	China	Phase 3	NCT05413369
45	INS068	Long-acting insulin analog	Type 2 Diabetes Mellitus	South Korea	Phase 3	NCT05702073, NCT05699408
46	Insulin Efsitora Alfa (LY3209590)	Basal Insulin Fc (BIF)	Type 2 Diabetes Mellitus	USA and/or Europe	Phase 3	NCT05662332, NCT05275400
47	INV-202	CB1R inverse agonist	Obesity and Metabolic Syndrome; Type 2 Diabetes Mellitus	USA and/or Europe	Phase 2	NCT05891834, NCT05514548

Table 2. *Cont.*

N	Investigational Drug	Mechanism of Action	Indication	Main Site Location	Phase	NCT
48	ION904 (IONIS-AGT-LRx)	Hepatocyte-directed ASO targeting AGT mRNA	Uncontrolled Hypertension	USA and/or Europe	Phase 2	NCT05314439
49	JS002	Humanized anti-PCSK9 mAb	Hyperlipidaemia	China	Phase 3	NCT05532800
50	JW0101+C2101	Livalo (pitavastatin)	Dyslipidemia and Hypertension	South Korea	Phase 3	NCT05331014
51	JW0201	N/A	Type 2 Diabetes Mellitus	South Korea	Phase 3	NCT05814393
52	Lepodisiran (LY3819469)	siRNA (binds to the hepatic asialoglycoprotein receptor) targeting Lp(a)	Elevated Lipoprotein(a)	USA and/or Europe	Phase 2 Phase 3	NCT05565742, NCT06292013
53	Lerodalcibep (LIB003)	PCSK9 Inhibitor	Hyperlipidaemia and High risk Cardiovascular Disease (CVD)	USA and/or Europe	Phase 3	NCT05004675, NCT05234775
54	Lorundrostat (MLS-101)	Aldosterone synthase inhibitor	Resistant Hypertension; Uncontrolled Hypertension	USA and/or Europe	Phase 2 Phase 3	NCT06153693, NCT05968430, NCT05001945
55	Eloralintide (LY3841136)	Amylin receptor agonist	Overweight or Obesity	USA and/or Europe	Phase 2	NCT06230523
56	MAR001	Maresin 1 (MaR1) specialised pro-resolving lipid mediator	Metabolic dysfunction at screening (triglyceride levels > 2.8 mmol/L)	USA and/or Europe	Phase 1 Phase 2	NCT05896254
57	Maridebart cafraglutide (AMG 133)	Dual GIP and GLP-1 receptor agonist	Overweight or Obesity With or Without Type 2 Diabetes Mellitus	USA and/or Europe	Phase 2	NCT05669599
58	Mazdutide (IBI362, LY3305677)	Dual GCGR and GLP-1 receptor agonist	Type 2 Diabetes Mellitus with Obesity; Overweight or Obesity	USA and/or Europe, China	Phase 2 Phase 3	NCT06184568, NCT06143956, NCT04904913
59	MBL949	GDF15 agonist (agonist at the GFRAL/RET receptor)	Obesity with or without Type 2 Diabetes Mellitus	USA and/or Europe	Phase 2	NCT05199090
60	MK-0616	Oral PCSK9 inhibitor	Hyperlipidaemia	USA and/or Europe	Phase 3	NCT05952856
61	Muvalaplin (LY3473329)	Orally active inhibitor of Lp(a)	Elevated Lipoprotein(a) at High Risk for Cardiovascular Events	USA and/or Europe	Phase 2	NCT05563246
62	NNC0165-1875	NPY2R or Y2R agonist	Obesity	USA and/or Europe	Phase 2	NCT04969939
63	NNC0480-0389	N/A	Type 2 Diabetes Mellitus	USA and/or Europe	Phase 2	NCT05144984

Table 2. *Cont.*

N	Investigational Drug	Mechanism of Action	Indication	Main Site Location	Phase	NCT
64	NNC0519-0130	Dual GIP and GLP-1 receptor agonist	Overweight or Obesity, Type 2 Diabetes Mellitus	USA and/or Europe	Phase 2	NCT06326060, NCT06326047
65	NST-1024 (SEFA-1024)	CETP inhibitor	Hypertriglyceridemia	USA and/or Europe	Phase 2	NCT05889156
66	Obicetrapib (AMG-899, DEZ-001, TA-8995)	CETP inhibitor	Hyperlipidaemia; Heterozygous familial hypercholesterolemia (HeFH) and/or atherosclerotic cardiovascular disease (ASCVD) or multiple ASCVD risk factors	USA and/or Europe	Phase 2 Phase 3	NCT05421078, NCT06005597, NCT05266586
67	Ocedurenone(KBP-5074)	Third-generation non-steroidal MRA	Uncontrolled Hypertension and Moderate or Severe Chronic Kidney Disease	USA and/or Europe	Phase 3	NCT04968184
68	Olezarsen (ISIS 678354, AKCEA-APOCIII-LRx)	ASO targeting mRNA for APOC3	Hypertriglyceridemia and Atherosclerotic Cardiovascular Disease, or With Severe Hypertriglyceridemia; Severe Hypertriglyceridemia	USA and/or Europe	Phase 3	NCT05552326, NCT05079919, NCT05610280
69	Olpasiran (AMG-890, ARO-LPA)	siRNA (binds to the hepatic asialoglycoprotein receptor) targeting Lp(a)	Atherosclerotic cardiovascular disease (ASCVD) and elevated Lipoprotein(a).	USA and/or Europe	Phase 3	NCT05581303
70	Orforglipron (LY3502970)	Non-peptide GLP-1 receptor agonist	Type 2 Diabetes Mellitus with Overweight or Obesity; Type 2 Diabetes Mellitus; Overweight or Obesity and related comorbidities, Overweight or Obesity	USA and/or Europe	Phase 3	NCT05803421, NCT06010004, NCT05869903, NCT05872620, NCT05051579, NCT05048719
71	PB-201	Glucokinase activator (partial, pancreas- and liver-dual activator of glucokinase)	Type 2 Diabetes Mellitus	China	Phase 3	NCT05102149
72	Pegozafermin (BIO89-100)	FGF21 analog	Severe Hypertriglyceridemia	USA and/or Europe	Phase 3	NCT05852431

Table 2. *Cont.*

N	Investigational Drug	Mechanism of Action	Indication	Main Site Location	Phase	NCT
73	Pelacarsen (IONIS-APO(a)-LRx, AKCEA-APO(a)-LRx, or TQJ230)	Apo(a) inhibitor, hepatocyte-directed ASO targeting mRNA transcribed from the *LPA* gene	Hyperlipoproteinemia(a) and Established Cardiovascular Disease	USA and/or Europe	Phase 3	NCT05305664, NCT05900141
74	Pemafibrate (K-877, LY3473329)	Selective peroxisome proliferator-activated receptor (PPAR)-α modulator (SPPARM)	Hypercholesterolemia and statin intolerance; Elevated Lipoprotein(a)	USA and/or Europe	Phase 2 Phase 3	NCT05923281, NCT05563246
75	Plozasiran (ARO-APOC3)	siRNA targeting mRNA for APOC3	Hypertriglyceridemia; Severe Hypertriglyceridemia; Dyslipidemia	USA and/or Europe	Phase 2 Phase 3	NCT06347133, NCT06347016, NCT05413135, NCT04720534, NCT04998201
76	RAY1225	Dual GIP and GLP-1 receptor agonist	Type 2 Diabetes Mellitus; Obesity	China	Phase 2	NCT06254274, NCT06254261
77	Recaticimab (SHR-1209)	mAb against PCSK9	Hyperlipidaemia	China	Phase 3	NCT04885218
78	Rilparencel (Renal Autologous Cell Therapy-REACT®)	Renal Autologous Cell Therapy	Type 2 Diabetes Mellitus and Chronic Kidney Disease	USA and/or Europe	Phase 3	NCT05099770
79	Retatrutide (LY3437943)	Triple GIP, GLP-1 and GCGR receptor agonist	Overweight or Obesity and Chronic Kidney Disease With or Without Type 2 Diabetes Mellitus; Type 2 Diabetes Mellitus; Overweight or Obesity; Type 2 Diabetes Mellitus with Overweight or Obesity; Overweight or Obesity with Cardiovascular Disease	USA and/or Europe	Phase 2 Phase 3	NCT05936151, NCT06297603, NCT05929066, NCT05929079, NCT05882045, NCT04881760
80	RGT-075	Oral GLP-1 receptor agonist	Overweight or Obesity	USA and/or Europe	Phase 2	NCT06277934
81	Solbinsiran (LY3561774)	siRNA that targets ANGPTL3	Dyslipidemia	USA and/or Europe	Phase 2	NCT05256654
82	SPC1001	N/A	Essential Hypertension	South Korea	Phase 2	NCT06212648
83	SPH3127	Renin inhibitor (direct)	Essential Hypertension	China	Phase 3	NCT05359068

Table 2. *Cont.*

N	Investigational Drug	Mechanism of Action	Indication	Main Site Location	Phase	NCT
84	Supaglutide	GLP-1 receptor agonist	Type 2 Diabetes Mellitus	China	Phase 2 Phase 3	NCT04994288, NCT04998032
85	Survodutide (BI 456906)	Dual GCGR and GLP-1 receptor agonist	Type 2 Diabetes Mellitus with Overweight or Obesity; Obesity; Overweight or Obesity	USA and/or Europe	Phase 3	NCT06066528, NCT06176365, NCT06066515, NCT06077864
86	TLC-3595 (S-723595)	Allosteric inhibitor of acetyl-CoA carboxylase 2 (ACC2)	Insulin Resistance	USA and/or Europe	Phase 2	NCT05665751
87	Trevogrumab (REGN1033) and Garetosmab (REGN2477)	Trevogrumab is GFD8 fully humanized mAb, Garetosmab (REGN2477) Act-A mAb	Obesity	USA and/or Europe	Phase 2	NCT06299098
88	Vericiguat	Stimulator of soluble guanylate cyclase (sGC)	Metabolic Syndrome and Coronary Vascular Dysfunction	USA and/or Europe	Phase 2	NCT05711719
89	VK2735	Dual GIP and GLP-1 receptor agonist	Overweight or Obesity	USA and/or Europe	Phase 2	NCT06068946
90	XXB750	mAb, NPR1 agonist	Resistant Hypertension	USA and/or Europe	Phase 2	NCT05562934
91	Yogliptin	DPP-4 inhibitor	Type 2 Diabetes Mellitus	China	Phase 3	NCT05318326
92	Zerlasiran (SLN360)	siRNA (binds to the hepatic asialoglycoprotein receptor) targeting Lp(a)	Elevated lipoprotein(a) at high risk of atherosclerotic cardiovascular disease events	USA and/or Europe	Phase 2	NCT05537571
93	Zilebesiran (ALN-AGT)	siRNA targeting AGT mRNA	High cardiovascular risk and Uncontrolled Hypertension; Hypertension	USA and/or Europe	Phase 2	NCT06272487, NCT04936035, NCT05103332
94	Zodasiran (ARO-ANG3)	siRNA that targets ANGPTL3	Dyslipidemia	USA and/or Europe	Phase 2	NCT04832971

ACC2: acetyl-CoA carboxylase 2; Act-A: Activin-A; ActRII: activin type II receptors; AGT: angiotensinogen; ANGPTL3: angiopoietin-like protein 3; Apo(a): apolipoprotein(a); APOC3: apolipoprotein C-III; ASO: antisense oligonucleotide; CB1R: Cannabinoid receptor-1; CETP: cholesteryl ester transfer protein; FGF21: fibroblast growth factor 21; GCCR: glucagon receptor; GDF15: growth differentiation factor 15; GFD8: α-myostatin; GIP: glucose-dependent insulinotropic polypeptide; GLP-1: glucagon-like peptide 1; GPR40: class A G-protein coupled receptor (GPCR); INSR: insulin receptor; KHK: ketohexokinase; Lp(a): lipoprotein(a) gene; mAbs: monoclonal antibodies; MRA: mineralocorticoid-receptor antagonists; N/A: not applicable; NPR1: natriuretic peptide receptor 1; NPY2R: neuropeptide Y receptor type 2; PCSK9: proprotein convertase subtilisin/kexin type 9; SGLT2: Sodium-glucose cotransporter-2; siRNA: small interfering RNA; TAS2R: Bitter Taste Receptor.

3.1. Type 2 Diabetes, Obesity and/or Overweight

In T2D, obesity, and/or overweight treatment, new entero-pancreatic hormone-based pharmacotherapies are under development. Ecnoglutide (XW003) is a long-acting GLP-1 RA administered as a once-weekly injection that has demonstrated positive results in a Phase 2 trial in Chinese patients with T2D [24]. The dual glucagon receptor (GCGR) and GLP-1 receptor agonists AZD9550, mazdutide (IBI362, LY3305677) [25], maridebart cafraglutide (AMG 133), and survodutide (BI 456906) [26] are strengthening the pipeline for the incretin pathway in obesity or overweight treatment with or without T2D. In addition to the approved tirzepatide [27], other dual GIP and GLP-1 receptor agonists, HRS9531, HS-20094, and RAY1225 are being evaluated in China in patients with obesity or T2D. NNC0519-0130 is also under development in the USA and/or Europe. Retatrutide (LY-3437943) is a triple GIP, GLP-1, and GCGR agonist that is tested in several indications (overweight or obesity and chronic kidney disease with or without T2D, T2D, obesity or overweight, T2D with obesity or overweight, obesity or overweight with cardiovascular disease) (Table 2) [28]. Cagrilintide and eloralintide (LY3841136) as amylin receptor agonists are evaluated in T2D or obesity/overweight indications (Table 2). Amylin is involved in postprandial satiety regulation. Cagrilintide, as a new long-acting amylin analog, is combined with semaglutide 2.4 mg once weekly (CagriSema) in patient with obesity [29]. NNC0165-1875 is a neuropeptide Y receptor type 2 agonist (NPY2R agonist or Y2R agonist) and has finished the Phase 2 trial but with no results posted for now. Y2R inhibits food intake by acting centrally on the hypothalamus [30].

Also, the new non-entero-pancreatic hormone-based pharmacotherapy is in clinical development. Oral denatonium acetate (ARD-101) is a potential bitter taste receptor (TAS2R) agonist [31] and is being evaluated in obesity treatment in a Phase 2 trial. ALN-KHK belongs to a new treatment approach with siRNA, which is conjugated with a new class of degraders, a triantennary N-acetylgalactosamine (GalNAc). GalNAc is the ligand of the asialoglycoprotein receptor (ASGPR), a lysosomal targeting receptor specifically expressed on liver cells. Conjugation with GalNAc enables the extracellular protein targets to be successfully internalized and delivered into the lysosome for degradation in the liver [32]. ALN-KHK targets ketohexokinase (KHK). It is considered that the inhibition of KHK prevents fructose-induced metabolic dysfunction, such as insulin resistance, de novo lipogenesis (DNL), and hepatic steatosis [33]. Bimagrumab is a human mAb inhibitor of activin type II receptors (ActRII), which consequently stimulates skeletal muscle growth and causes a reduction in fat mass and weight loss [34]. The other different mechanism of action in obesity or T2D treatment is BMF-219, as an oral irreversible covalent inhibitor of menin. Pbk is a serine/threonine protein kinase, essential for high-fat diet induced beta cell proliferation. The menin inhibition disrupts the menin–JunD interaction and augments Pbk transcription [35]. CPL207280 is a GPR40 agonist (also known as an FFA receptor 1 agonist). GPR40 is a class A G-protein coupled receptor (GPCR), the activation of which after a meal ingestion induces the secretion of incretins in the gut, including GLP-1, GIP, and peptide YY (PYY), the latter controlling appetite and glucose metabolism [36]. PYY is also known as an NPY2R agonist (Y2R agonist), since PYY is rapidly cleaved by DPP-4 to its active form (PYY 3-36), which acts on a Y2R [37]. GLY-200 as a mucin-complexing polymer and MBL949 as a growth differentiation factor 15 (GDF15) agonist (agonist at the GFRAL/RET receptor) are also in clinical development. GDF15, which is a non-homeostatic regulator of food intake and body weight, is emerging as having the potential for a new mechanism in obesity treatment. GDF-15 is a stress-induced cytokine, which is expressed in multiple cell types including cardiomyocytes, adipocytes, and macrophages [38]. At the moment, the Phase 2 trial with MBL949 has been completed and we are awaiting publication of the results. Other mAbs under development are trevogrumab (REGN1033) as an α-myostatin (GFD8), fully humanized mAb and the garetosmab (REGN2477) Activin-A (Act-A) mAb. Act-A is a second "myostatin" that appears to be a more important regulator of muscle mass. The addition of garetosmab (anti-Activin A) to trevogrumab (anti-GDF8) is expected to increase thigh muscle volume and decrease fat mass [39]. In the exciting cell and gene therapy (CGT) field, we have detected the ProKidney's rilparencel (Renal Autologous Cell Therapy-REACT®) that is being evaluated in patients with T2D and chronic kidney disease (CKD) in the Regen-006 Phase 3 trial. The aim of the autologous cellular therapy is not only to slow and stabilize the progression of CKD, but in some cases possibly drive meaningful improvement in kidney function [40].

3.2. Dyslipidemia and Lipoprotein Disorder

For strengthening the already known approach of PCSK9 inhibition in dyslipidemia, AZD0780 and MK-0616 as oral and lerodalcibep (LIB003) as subcutaneous (SC) PCSK9 inhibitors, are in clinical development. AZD8233 is an antisense oligonucleotide (ASO), targeting PCSK9 as well. China is developing JS002 and recaticimab (SHR-1209) as mAbs targeting PCSK9.

In dyslipidemia and lipoprotein disorders, particularly lipoprotein(a) (Lp(a)), we are approaching a new era with two classes of nucleic acid therapeutics, ASOs and siRNAs. Elevated Lp(a) is one of the last untreatable frontiers of cardiovascular risk. Lp(a) is genetically regulated but due to extensive variability in Lp(a) levels between individuals, a potential role for non-genetic factors cannot be disregarded [41]. Lp(a) is produced from the binding of apolipoprotein(a) (apo(a)) to apolipoprotein B (apo B). Silencing the transcription of the *LPA* gene minimizes the mRNA that encodes for apo(a). ASOs and siRNAs are covalently linked with GalNAc which is rapidly cleaved in the liver, allowing the RNA interference therapy to degrade the mRNA that encodes for apo(a). Olezarsen (ISIS 678354, AKCEA-APOCIII-LRx) and pelacarsen (AKCEA-APO(a)-LRx or TQJ230) are ASOs, while lepodisiran (LY3819469), olpasiran, plozasiran (ARO-APOC3), solbinsiran (LY3561774), zerlasiran (SLN360), and zodasiran (ARO-ANG3) are siRNAs targeting the Lp(a) synthesis pathway. Plozasiran, an apolipoprotein (apo) C-III (APOC3) antagonist, is being evaluated in dyslipidemia. Plozasiran is an GalNAc-bound RNA i that targets APOC3 mRNA within the cytoplasm of hepatocytes, resulting in prolonged suppression of apo C-III. In patients with dyslipidemia, plozasiran reduced triglycerides and atherogenic lipoproteins [42,43]. Olezarsen is also an GalNAc-conjugated ASO that targets mRNA for APOC3. Olezarsen is being evaluated in severe hypertriglyceridemia in a Phase 3 trial, after a Phase 2b trial in patients with moderate hypertriglyceridemia and an elevated cardiovascular risk demonstrated encouraging results in the reduction in triglycerides, apo B, and non-HDL cholesterol [44]. Lepodisiran in a Phase 1 trial demonstrated a significant reduction in serum Lp(a) concentrations in patients with elevated Lp(a) [45]. Solbinsiran and zodasiran areangiopoietin like protein 3 (ANGPTL3) inhibitors. ANGPTL3 regulates lipoprotein metabolism by inhibiting lipoprotein and endothelial lipases. It is known that the ANGPTL3 loss-of-function carriers have decreased circulating triglycerides, LDL-C, and HDL-C. In the ARCHES-2 dose-ranging Phase 2b trial, zodisiran decreased atherogenic triglyceride-rich lipoproteins, LDL-C, and total apo B in patients with mixed hyperlipidemia [46]. In the APOLLO Phase 1 trial, zerlasiran demonstrated a reduction in Lp(a) concentrations in patients with elevated Lp(a) and established ASCVD [47]. Muvalaplin (LY3473329) is an orally administered small molecule inhibitor of Lp(a). It demonstrated positive results in a Phase 1 trial and proceeded to a Phase 2 trial in the clinical development [48].

NST-1024 (SEFA-1024) and obicetrapib (AMG-899, DEZ-001, TA-8995) are the new hope for CETP inhibitors in hypertriglyceridemia and dyslipidemia treatment, respectively (Table 2). Results from a completed Phase 2 trial with obicetrapib in patients with dyslipidemia on a high-intensity statin are encouraging [49]. Pemafibrate (K-877, LY3473329) is a selective peroxisome proliferator-activated receptor (PPAR)-α modulator (SPPARM) and offers a new approach to the treatment of hypercholesterolemia and statin intolerance or elevated Lp(a). It is approved for the treatment of hyperlipidemia in Japan due to a favorable risk–benefit ratio [50].

3.3. Hypertension

For the subgroup of patients with metabolic syndrome that have uncontrolled or resistant hypertension, there are currently several drug classes in clinical development. Baxdrostat (CIN-107) and lorundrostat (MLS-101) are aldosterone synthase inhibitors. Baxdrostat (CIN-107) is in a Phase 3 trial and recruiting. Baxdrostat demonstrated positive effect on the reduction in blood pressure in a Phase 2 trial, the BrigHTN trial, in resistant hypertension [51]. However, the HALO (efficacy and safety of baxdrostat in patients with uncontrolled hypertension) trial did not demonstrate a significant blood pressure-lowering benefit of baxdrostat compared to placebo [52]. Lorundrostat is at the moment in a Phase 3 RCT, since the Target-HTN Phase 2 trial demonstrated a significant, double-digit reduction in systolic blood pressure in an uncontrolled hypertension [53]. Ocedurenone (KBP-5074) is a third-generation non-steroidal MRA evaluated in uncontrolled or resistant hypertension and chronic kidney disease [54]. ION904 (IONIS-AGT-L_{Rx}) is an ASO conjugated with GalNAc that inhibits angiotensinogen (AGT) mRNA in hepatocytes. In a Phase 2 trial in patients with uncontrolled hypertension, it significantly reduced plasma AGT levels and reduced blood pressure when given SC monthly [55]. Zilebesiran (ALN-AGT) is also an siRNA conjugated with GalNAc and targeting AGT which has the potential for biannual dosing. Recent KARDIA-2 trial results demonstrated a significant systolic blood pressure reduction in patients with uncontrolled hypertension [56]. XXB750 is a fully humanized mAb long-acting natriuretic peptide receptor 1 (NPR1) agonist. Atrial natriuretic peptide (ANP) induces vasodilation via NPR1 in the vasculature [57]. XXB750 reduced blood pressure in a dose-dependent manner in a Phase 1 trial [58].

3.4. Metabolic Syndrome and Insulin Resistance

For metabolic syndrome treatment itself, 6-bromotryptophan (6-BT) and vericiguat are in Phase 2 trials and recruiting. 6-bromotryptophan (6-BT) is an endogenous plasma microbiome-derived tryptophan metabolite, and vericiguat is a stimulator of soluble guanylyl cyclase. Vericiguat showed favorable results on the reduction of death from any cause or hospitalization for heart failure in patients with high-risk heart failure in the VICTORIA trial [59]. It would be interesting to see its results in an ongoing trial with metabolic syndrome and coronary vascular dysfunction. INV-202 as a peripherally acting CB1 receptor (CB1r) blocker showed promising results on weight loss and biomarkers in metabolic syndrome patients in a Phase 1b trial. It is believed that INV-202 has very low central nervous system (CNS) penetration in contrast to former cannabinoid blockers such as rimonabant, which was compromised with serious neuropsychiatric adverse effects [60,61].

TLC-3595 (formerly S-723595), a small molecule, allosteric inhibitor of acetyl-CoA carboxylase 2 (ACC2), is recruiting patients with insulin resistance in a Phase 2 trial. The inhibition of ACC2 may increase fatty acid oxidation (FAO), reduce ectopic lipid accumulation, and improve insulin sensitivity in skeletal muscle and liver [62,63]. We did not find any relevant RCT for prediabetes treatment.

4. Discussion

The pharmacological treatment of the metabolic syndrome requires a comprehensive approach targeting several different pathways, depending on the individual risk factors of a patient. There is a vast number of available drug classes for cardiac and metabolic conditions treatments, but there is still a need for more efficacious, safe, and more convenient dosing pharmacological options. We have identified that the investigational drugs in our research are tested the most in T2D (41%), obesity and/or overweight (31%), dyslipidemia and/or hyperlipidemia, and/or lipoprotein disorders (29%), and more treatment options will probably emerge in these indications. For some investigational drugs, we could not find a mechanism of action, mostly for the main clinical sites located in China and/or South Korea. It is unknown if these drugs are under development with the new mechanism of action or with the same mechanism of action as approved drugs already on the market (e.g., as like drugs).

SGLT-2 inhibitors and GLP-1 RA have revolutionized T2D treatment, as well as the GLP-1 RA obesity treatment [16–18]. New combinations in entero-pancreatic hormone-based pharmacotherapies are in clinical development, mostly in Phase 3 trials. China is developing the dual GIP and GLP-1 receptor agonists HRS9531, HS-20094, and RAY1225 for obesity or T2D, while in the USA and/or Europe NNC0519-0130 is under development. The other combination includes the dual GCGR and GLP-1 receptor agonists AZD9550, AZD9550, mazdutide (IBI362, LY3305677) [25], maridebart cafraglutide (AMG 133), and survodutide (BI 456906) [26] for obesity or overweight treatment with or without T2D. In a Phase 2 trial, survodutide demonstrated a dose-dependent effect on body weight reduction, ranging from −6.2% to −14.9%, in patients suffering from obesity without T2D. Adverse effects (AEs) occurred in 91% patients on survodutide, and most were primarily gastrointestinal (GIT) (75%) [64]. The triple combination of receptor agonism is retatrutide as a triple GIP, GLP-1, and GCGR agonist for which Eli Lilly has big expectations [65]. In a Phase 2 trial in overweight patients with or obesity, retatrutide also demonstrated a dose-dependent effect (ranging from −8.7% to −24.2%) on body weight reduction, as well as dose related AEs, mostly GIT AEs with mild to moderate severity [28]. Another combination is cagrilintide as a new long-acting amylin analog, combined with GLP-1 RA semaglutide 2.4 mg once weekly (CagriSema) in patients with obesity or T2D. In the Phase 2 trial, in patients with T2D, the combination showed a more pronounced effect on body weight reduction than cagrilintide or semaglutide alone [29]. NNC0165-1875 as the Y2R agonist is a new approach that has yet to be proven in regard to efficacy and safety.

Non-entero-pancreatic hormone-based pharmacotherapy offers new therapeutic approaches as denatonium acetate a TAS2R agonist and ALN-KHK as siRNA conjugated with GalNAc targeting KHK. The GalNAc delivery system increased the surge of siRNA and ASO therapies, mostly in dyslipidemia or elevated Lp(a) treatment. Bimagrumab is a mAb inhibitor of ActRII, which demonstrated in a Phase 2 trial in patients with a T2D fat mass (FM) a reduction of −20.5%, body mass −6.5%, and lean mass (LM) gain 3.6% [34]. Other mAbs include the trevogrumab α-myostatin (GFD8) and garetosmab Act-A mAbs combination, and it would be interesting to see if they provide a similar beneficial effect on weight loss and LM gain. GDF-15 induces weight loss through a reduction in food intake through actions in the CNS [66]. MBL949 is under development as a GDF15 agonist. CGT therapy with rilparencel (Renal Autologous Cell Therapy-REACT®) in patients with T2D and moderate to severe CKD is novel and in early development. The first interim results of the REGEN-006 trial are expected in late 2024 [40]. A Phase 2 trial of rilparencel administered as bilateral percutaneous kidney injections into the kidney cortex demonstrated less decline in eGFR compared to the standard care group, while post-hoc analysis indicated a kidney function stabilization in patients with Stage 4 CKD and a severe urine albumin-to-creatinine ratio (UACR) [67,68]

For dyslipidemia treatment, novel PCSK9 inhibitors are in the pipeline: AZD0780 and MK-0616 as oral (daily administration) and AZD8233 and lerodalcibep as SC (monthly administration) PCSK9 inhibitors. In China, JS002 and recaticimab as mAbs against PCSK9 are under development. A new era of elevated Lp(a) and dyslipidemia treatment is occurring with ASO and siRNAs, covalently linked with GalNAc and targeting the mRNA that encodes apo(a). Olezarsen and pelacarsen are an ASO while lepodisiran olpasiran, plozasiran, solbinsiran, zerlasiran, and zodasiran are siRNAs, and muvalaplin is an orally administered small molecule inhibitor of Lp(a). Results in earlier phases (Phase 1 and Phase 2) in dyslipidemia and/or elevated Lp(a) with or without ASCVD with these new therapies are very encouraging and will probably be a new standard of care as an add-on therapy or monotherapy for these indications [42–48,69].

CEPT inhibitors have been evaluated in several RCTs, but without the expected benefit [11,12]. However, NST-1024 (SEFA-1024) and obicetrapib are a new hope for CETP inhibitors in hypertriglyceridemia and dyslipidemia treatment. In a Phase 2 trial, obicetrapib in combination with ezetimibe significantly lowered LDL-C (63.4%) in patients with dyslipidemia and high-intensity statin therapy [49]. Pemafibrate is a novel SPPARM that has the potential to demonstrate positive results outside Japan, where it is approved for the treatment of hyperlipidemia. Compared to other PPARα agonists, pemafibrate does not significantly increase alanine aminotransferase (ALT) or γ-glutamyltransferase (GGT), and it is also excreted via the liver [50].

Baxdrostat and lorundrostat aldosterone synthase inhibitors have proved efficacy in Phase 2 trials for resistant and uncontrolled hypertension, respectively [51,53]. ION904 as an ASO conjugated with GalNAc inhibits AGT mRNA. In a Phase 2 trial in patients with uncontrolled hypertension, ION904 significantly reduced plasma AGT levels and blood pressure [54]. Zilebesiran as an siRNA conjugated with GalNAc and targeting AGT also demonstrated a significant systolic blood pressure reduction in patients with uncontrolled hypertension [56]. XXB750, a fully humanized mAb NPR1 agonist, reduced blood pressure in a dose-dependent manner in a Phase 1 trial [58].

Metabolic syndrome has no approved drugs for itself. It would be interesting to see if 6-BT may prove beneficial as an endogenous plasma microbiome-derived tryptophan metabolite or vericiguat as a stimulator of soluble guanylyl cyclase. INV-202, as a peripherally acting CB1r blocker, has shown promising results on weight loss and biomarkers in metabolic syndrome patients in a Phase 1b trial [60]. TLC-3595 as an ACC2 inhibitor has for now no published results in patients with insulin resistance.

5. Conclusions

Metabolic syndrome prevalence is between 24 and 27% and poses a significant risk for the development of ASCVD, T2D, or other various comorbidities. Currently, no drugs are approved for metabolic syndrome treatment itself, so the risk factors are treated with therapies approved for cardiac and metabolic conditions. There are many new pharmacological approaches and drug classes that have reached Phase 2 and Phase 3 RCT for the management of each of the risk factors of metabolic syndrome. GIP, GLP-1, GCGR, and amylin agonists, as well as their combinations, are under development in T2D and overweight or obesity. Non-entero-pancreatic hormone-based therapies have created several new pathways to act as a KHK inhibitor, GDF15 agonist, and mAbs as an ActRII inhibitor and to target GFD8 and Act-A. For dyslipidemia treatment, in addition to the novel PCSK9 inhibitors (oral and SC) and CETP inhibitors, a new generation of ASO and siRNAs targeting the Lp(a) synthesis pathway is on the way. For resistant and uncontrolled hypertension, aldosterone synthase inhibitors and siRNAs targeting AGT are promising new therapeutic options. It will be interesting to see whether metabolic syndrome will finally gain the first drug approval for metabolic syndrome itself.

Author Contributions: E.J.: Conceptualization, methodology, investigation, formal analysis, visualization, writing—original draft. D.Š.: Investigation, review and editing. A.R.: Validation, writing—review and editing. All authors have read and agreed to the published version of the manuscript.

Funding: This research received no external funding.

Data Availability Statement: Data are available on request from the corresponding author.

Acknowledgments: The authors thank Darko Galić for proofreading the article.

Conflicts of Interest: The authors declare no conflicts of interest.

References

1. Grundy, S.M.; Cleeman, J.I.; Daniels, S.R.; Donato, K.A.; Eckel, R.H.; Franklin, B.A.; Gordon, D.J.; Krauss, R.M.; Savage, P.J.; Smith, S.C., Jr.; et al. Diagnosis and management of the metabolic syndrome: American Heart Association/National Heart, Lung, and Blood Institute Scientific Statement: Executive summary. *Circulation* **2005**, *112*, e285–e290. [CrossRef] [PubMed]
2. Rask Larsen, J.; Dima, L.; Correll, C.U.; Manu, P. The pharmacological management of metabolic syndrome. *Expert Rev. Clin. Pharmacol.* **2018**, *11*, 397–410. [CrossRef] [PubMed]

3. Alberti, K.G.M.M.; Eckel, R.H.; Grundy, S.M.; Zimmet, P.Z.; Cleeman, J.I.; Donato, K.A.; Fruchart, J.-C.; James, W.P.T.; Loria, C.M.; Smith, S.C., Jr.; et al. Harmonizing the metabolic syndrome: A joint interim statement of the International Diabetes Federation Task Force on Epidemiology and Prevention; National Heart, Lung, and Blood Institute; American Heart Association; World Heart Federation; International Atherosclerosis Society; and International Association for the Study of Obesity. *Circulation* **2009**, *120*, 1640–1645. [CrossRef] [PubMed]
4. Ford, E.S.; Giles, W.H.; Mokdad, A.H. Increasing prevalence of the metabolic syndrome among u.s. Adults. *Diabetes Care* **2004**, *27*, 2444–2449. [CrossRef] [PubMed]
5. Athyros, V.G.; Bouloukos, V.I.; Pehlivanidis, A.N.; Papageorgiou, A.A.; Dionysopoulou, S.G.; Symeonidis, A.N.; Petridis, D.I.; Kapousouzi, M.I.; Satsoglou, E.A.; Mikhailidis, D.P. The prevalence of the metabolic syndrome in Greece: The MetS-Greece Multicentre Study. *Diabetes Obes. Metab.* **2005**, *7*, 397–405. [CrossRef] [PubMed]
6. Batsis, J.A.; Romero-Corral, A.; Collazo-Clavell, M.L.; Sarr, M.G.; Somers, V.K.; Lopez-Jimenez, F. Effect of bariatric surgery on the metabolic syndrome: A population-based, long-term controlled study. *Mayo Clin. Proc.* **2008**, *83*, 897–906. [CrossRef] [PubMed]
7. D'Agostino, R.B.; Vasan, R.S.; Pencina, M.J.; Wolf, P.A.; Cobain, M.; Massaro, J.M.; Kannel, W.B. General cardiovascular risk profile for use in primary care: The Framingham heart study. *Circulation* **2008**, *117*, 743–753. [CrossRef] [PubMed]
8. Grundy, S.M.; Stone, N.J.; Bailey, A.L.; Beam, C.; Birtcher, K.K.; Blumenthal, R.S.; Braun, L.T.; de Ferranti, S.; Faiella-Tommasino, J.; Forman, D.E.; et al. 2018 AHA/ACC/AACVPR/AAPA/ABC/ACPM/ADA/AGS/APhA/ASPC/NLA/PCNA guideline on the management of blood cholesterol: American College of Cardiology/American Heart Association on clinical practice guidelines. *Circulation* **2019**, *139*, 25. [CrossRef] [PubMed]
9. Kaddoura, R.; Orabi, B.; Salam, A.M. PCSK9 monoclonal antibodies: An overview. *Heart Views* **2020**, *21*, 97–103. [CrossRef] [PubMed]
10. Zhang, Y.; Chen, H.; Hong, L.; Wang, H.; Li, B.; Zhang, M.; Li, J.; Yang, L.; Liu, F. Inclisiran: A new generation of lipid-lowering siRNA therapeutic. *Front. Pharmacol.* **2023**, *14*, 1260921. [CrossRef]
11. Shrestha, S.; Wu, B.J.; Guiney, L.; Barter, P.J.; Rye, K.A. Cholesteryl ester transfer protein and its inhibitors. *J. Lipid Res.* **2018**, *59*, 772–783. [CrossRef] [PubMed]
12. Fiorentino, R.; Chiarelli, F. Treatment of dyslipidaemia in children. *Biomedicines* **2021**, *9*, 1078. [CrossRef] [PubMed]
13. Nissen, S.E.; Lincoff, A.M.; Brennan, D.; Ray, K.K.; Mason, D.; Kastelein, J.J.P.; Thompson, P.D.; Libby, P.; Cho, L.; Plutzky, J.; et al. Bempedoic acid and cardiovascular outcomes in statin-intolerant patients. *N. Engl. J. Med.* **2023**, *388*, 1353–1364. [CrossRef] [PubMed]
14. Mancia, G.; Kreutz, R.; Brunström, M.; Burnier, M.; Grassi, G.; Januszewicz, A.; Muiesan, M.L.; Tsioufis, K.; Agabiti-Rosei, E.; Algharably, E.A.; et al. 2023 ESH guidelines for the management of arterial hypertension the task force for the management of arterial hypertension of European Society of Hypertension: Endorsed by the International Society of Hypertension (ISH) and the European Renal Association (ERA). *J. Hypertens.* **2023**, *41*, 1874–2071. [CrossRef] [PubMed]
15. Davies, M.J.; Aroda, V.R.; Collins, B.S.; Gabbay, R.A.; Green, J.; Maruthur, N.M.; Rosas, S.E.; Del Prato, S.; Mathieu, C.; Mingrone, G.; et al. Management of hyperglycemia in type 2 diabetes, 2022. A consensus report by the American Diabetes Association (ADA) and the European Association for the Study of Diabetes (EASD). *Diabetes Care* **2022**, *45*, 2753–2786. [CrossRef] [PubMed]
16. American Diabetes Association. 3. Prevention or delay of type 2 diabetes: Standards of medical care in diabetes—2021. *Diabetes Care* **2021**, *44*, S34–S39. [CrossRef] [PubMed]
17. Spector, R. A revolution in the treatment of obesity. *Am. J. Med.* **2024**, *22*, S0002934324003346. [CrossRef] [PubMed]
18. ElSayed, N.A.; Aleppo, G.; Aroda, V.R.; Bannuru, R.R.; Brown, F.M.; Bruemmer, D.; Collins, B.S.; Hilliard, M.E.; Isaacs, D.; Johnson, E.L.; et al. 8. Obesity and weight management for the prevention and treatment of type 2 diabetes: Standards of care in diabetes—2023. *Diabetes Care* **2023**, *46*, S128–S139. [CrossRef] [PubMed]
19. U.S. Food and Drug Administration (FDA). FDA Approves New Medication for Chronic Weight Management. 2023. Available online: https://www.fda.gov/news-events/press-announcements/fda-approves-new-medication-chronic-weight-management (accessed on 28 June 2024).
20. Grundy, S.M. Drug therapy of the metabolic syndrome: Minimizing the emerging crisis in polypharmacy. *Nat. Rev. Drug Discov.* **2006**, *5*, 295–309. [CrossRef]
21. Matfin, G. Developing therapies for the metabolic syndrome: Challenges, opportunities, and... the unknown. *Ther. Adv. Endocrinol. Metab.* **2010**, *1*, 89–94. [CrossRef] [PubMed]
22. Global Observatory on Health Research and Development. Clinical Trials. Available online: https://www.who.int/observatories/global-observatory-on-health-research-and-development/resources/databases/databases-on-processes-for-r-d/clinical-trials (accessed on 28 May 2024).
23. Wong, C.H.; Siah, K.W.; Lo, A.W. Estimation of clinical trial success rates and related parameters. *Biostatistics* **2019**, *20*, 273–286. [CrossRef] [PubMed]
24. Zhu, D.; Qin, H.H.; Zheng, Q.; Ning, J.; Zhu, Z.; Mengying, G.; Bu, Y.; Jones, C.; Fenaux, M.; Xu, S.; et al. 755-p: A phase 2 evaluation of a novel GLP-1 analog ecnoglutide (Xw003) for glycemic control in adults with type 2 diabetes. *Diabetes* **2023**, *72*, 755-P. [CrossRef]

25. Ji, L.; Jiang, H.; An, P.; Deng, H.; Liu, M.; Li, L.; Feng, L.; Song, B.; Han-Zhang, H.; Ma, Q.; et al. IBI362 (LY3305677), a weekly-dose GLP-1 and glucagon receptor dual agonist, in Chinese adults with overweight or obesity: A randomised, placebo-controlled, multiple ascending dose phase 1b study. *EClinicalMedicine* **2021**, *39*, 101088. [CrossRef] [PubMed]
26. Zimmermann, T.; Thomas, L.; Baader-Pagler, T.; Haebel, P.; Simon, E.; Reindl, W.; Bajrami, B.; Rist, W.; Uphues, I.; Drucker, D.J.; et al. BI 456906: Discovery and preclinical pharmacology of a novel GCGR/GLP-1R dual agonist with robust anti-obesity efficacy. *Mol. Metab.* **2022**, *66*, 101633. [CrossRef] [PubMed]
27. Nauck, M.A.; D'Alessio, D.A. Tirzepatide, a dual GIP/GLP-1 receptor co-agonist for the treatment of type 2 diabetes with unmatched effectiveness regrading glycaemic control and body weight reduction. *Cardiovasc. Diabetol.* **2022**, *21*, 169. [CrossRef] [PubMed]
28. Jastreboff, A.M.; Kaplan, L.M.; Frías, J.P.; Wu, Q.; Du, Y.; Gurbuz, S.; Coskun, T.; Haupt, A.; Milicevic, Z.; Hartman, M.L.; et al. Triple–hormone-receptor agonist retatrutide for obesity—A phase 2 trial. *N. Engl. J. Med.* **2023**, *389*, 514–526. [CrossRef] [PubMed]
29. Frias, J.P.; Deenadayalan, S.; Erichsen, L.; Knop, F.K.; Lingvay, I.; Macura, S.; Mathieu, C.; Pedersen, S.D.; Davies, M. Efficacy and safety of co-administered once-weekly cagrilintide 2·4 mg with once-weekly semaglutide 2·4 mg in type 2 diabetes: A multicentre, randomised, double-blind, active-controlled, phase 2 trial. *Lancet* **2023**, *402*, 720–730. [CrossRef] [PubMed]
30. Kopelman, P.G.; Grace, C. New thoughts on managing obesity. *Gut* **2004**, *53*, 1044–1053. [CrossRef] [PubMed]
31. Niethammer, A.G.; Zheng, Z.; Timmer, A.; Lee, T.L. First-in-human evaluation of oral denatonium acetate (ARD-101), a potential bitter taste receptor agonist: A randomized, double-blind, placebo-controlled phase 1 trial in healthy adults. *Clin. Pharmacol. Drug Dev.* **2022**, *11*, 997–1006. [CrossRef] [PubMed]
32. Zhou, Y.; Teng, P.; Montgomery, N.T.; Li, X.; Tang, W. Development of triantennary N-Acetylgalactosamine conjugates as degraders for extracellular proteins. *ACS Cent. Sci.* **2021**, *7*, 499–506. [CrossRef] [PubMed]
33. Gutierrez, J.A.; Liu, W.; Perez, S.; Xing, G.; Sonnenberg, G.; Kou, K.; Blatnik, M.; Allen, R.; Weng, Y.; Vera, N.B.; et al. Pharmacologic inhibition of ketohexokinase prevents fructose-induced metabolic dysfunction. *Mol. Metab.* **2021**, *48*, 101196. [CrossRef] [PubMed]
34. Heymsfield, S.B.; Coleman, L.A.; Miller, R.; Rooks, D.S.; Laurent, D.; Petricoul, O.; Praestgaard, J.; Swan, T.; Wade, T.; Perry, R.G.; et al. Effect of bimagrumab vs placebo on body fat mass among adults with type 2 diabetes and obesity: A phase 2 randomized clinical trial. *JAMA Netw. Open* **2021**, *4*, e2033457. [CrossRef] [PubMed]
35. Ma, J.; Xing, B.; Cao, Y.; He, X.; Bennett, K.E.; Tong, C.; An, C.; Hojnacki, T.; Feng, Z.; Deng, S.; et al. Menin-regulated Pbk controls high fat diet-induced compensatory beta cell proliferation. *EMBO Mol. Med.* **2021**, *13*, e13524. [CrossRef] [PubMed]
36. Guan, H.P.; Xiong, Y. Learn from failures and stay hopeful to GPR40, a GPCR target with robust efficacy, for therapy of metabolic disorders. *Front. Pharmacol.* **2022**, *13*, 1043828. [CrossRef] [PubMed]
37. Neary, N.M.; Small, C.J.; Druce, M.R.; Park, A.J.; Ellis, S.M.; Semjonous, N.M.; Dakin, C.L.; Filipsson, K.; Wang, F.; Kent, A.S.; et al. Peptide YY3-36 and glucagon-like peptide-17-36 inhibit food intake additively. *Endocrinology* **2005**, *146*, 5120–5127. [CrossRef] [PubMed]
38. Benichou, O.; Coskun, T.; Gonciarz, M.D.; Garhyan, P.; Adams, A.C.; Du, Y.; Dunbar, J.D.; Martin, J.A.; Mather, K.J.; Pickard, R.T.; et al. Discovery, development, and clinical proof of mechanism of LY3463251, a long-acting GDF15 receptor agonist. *Cell Metab.* **2023**, *35*, 274–286.e10. [CrossRef] [PubMed]
39. Nielsen, T.L.; Vissing, J.; Krag, T.O. Antimyostatin treatment in health and disease: The story of great expectations and limited success. *Cells* **2021**, *10*, 533. [CrossRef] [PubMed]
40. ProKidney Corp. (Nasdaq: PROK). ProKidney Receives Allowance from the UK Medicines and Healthcare Products Regulatory Agency (MHRA) for proact 1 (REGEN-006) and EMA Scientific Advice on Phase 3 Protocols of REACT for Diabetic Chronic Kidney Disease. 2022. Available online: https://investors.prokidney.com/news-releases/news-release-details/prokidney-receives-allowance-uk-medicines-and-healthcare (accessed on 28 June 2024).
41. Enkhmaa, B.; Berglund, L. Non-genetic influences on lipoprotein(A) concentrations. *Atherosclerosis* **2022**, *349*, 53–62. [CrossRef]
42. Vasas, S.; Azizad, M.; Clifton, P.; Gaudet, D.; Goldenberg, R.; Modesto, K.; Chang, T.; Melquist, S.; Fu, R.; San Martin, J.; et al. Abstract 17091: ARO-APOC3, an investigational RNAi therapeutic, silences APOC3 and reduces atherosclerosis-associated lipoproteins in patients with mixed dyslipidemia: MUIR study results. *Circulation* **2023**, *148*, A17091. [CrossRef]
43. Gaudet, D.; Pall, D.; Watts, G.F.; Nicholls, S.J.; Rosenson, R.S.; Modesto, K.; San Martin, J.; Hellawell, J.; Ballantyne, C.M. Plozasiran (ARO-APOC3) for severe hypertriglyceridemia: The SHASTA-2 randomized clinical trial. *JAMA Cardiol.* **2024**, *9*, 620–630. [CrossRef] [PubMed]
44. Bergmark, B.A.; Marston, N.A.; Prohaska, T.A.; Alexander, V.J.; Zimerman, A.; Moura, F.A.; Murphy, S.A.; Goodrich, E.L.; Zhang, S.; Gaudet, D.; et al. Olezarsen for hypertriglyceridemia in patients at high cardiovascular risk. *N. Engl. J. Med.* **2024**, *390*, 1770–1780. [CrossRef] [PubMed]
45. Nissen, S.E.; Linnebjerg, H.; Shen, X.; Wolski, K.; Ma, X.; Lim, S.; Michael, L.F.; Ruotolo, G.; Gribble, G.; Navar, A.M.; et al. Lepodisiran, an extended-duration short interfering RNA targeting lipoprotein(A): A randomized dose-ascending clinical trial. *JAMA* **2023**, *330*, 2075–2083. [CrossRef] [PubMed]
46. Rosenson, R.S.; Gaudet, D.; Hegele, R.A.; Ballantyne, C.M.; Nicholls, S.J.; Lucas, K.J.; San Martin, J.; Zhou, R.; Muhsin, M.A.; Chang, T.; et al. Zodasiran, an RNAi therapeutic targeting ANGPTL3, for mixed hyperlipidemia. *N. Engl. J. Med.* **2024**, NEJMoa2404147. [CrossRef] [PubMed]

47. Nissen, S.E.; Wolski, K.; Watts, G.F.; Koren, M.J.; Fok, H.; Nicholls, S.J.; Rider, D.A.; Cho, L.; Romano, S.; Melgaard, C.; et al. Single ascending and multiple-dose trial of zerlasiran, a short interfering RNA targeting lipoprotein(A): A randomized clinical trial. *JAMA* **2024**, *331*, 1534. [CrossRef] [PubMed]
48. Nicholls, S.J.; Nissen, S.E.; Fleming, C.; Urva, S.; Suico, J.; Berg, P.H.; Linnebjerg, H.; Ruotolo, G.; Turner, P.K.; Michael, L.F.; et al. Muvalaplin, an oral small molecule inhibitor of lipoprotein(A) formation: A randomized clinical trial. *JAMA* **2023**, *330*, 1042–1053. [CrossRef] [PubMed]
49. Ballantyne, C.M.; Ditmarsch, M.; Kastelein, J.J.P.; Nelson, A.J.; Kling, D.; Hsieh, A.; Curcio, D.L.; Maki, K.C.; Davidson, M.H.; Nicholls, S.J. Obicetrapib plus ezetimibe as an adjunct to high-intensity statin therapy: A randomized phase 2 trial. *J. Clin. Lipidol.* **2023**, *17*, 491–503. [CrossRef] [PubMed]
50. Yokote, K.; Yamashita, S.; Arai, H.; Araki, E.; Suganami, H.; Ishibashi, S. Long-term efficacy and safety of pemafibrate, a novel selective peroxisome proliferator-activated receptor-α modulator (SPPARMα), in dyslipidemic patients with renal impairment. *Int. J. Mol. Sci.* **2019**, *20*, 706. [CrossRef] [PubMed]
51. Freeman, M.W.; Halvorsen, Y.D.; Marshall, W.; Pater, M.; Isaacsohn, J.; Pearce, C.; Murphy, B.; Alp, N.; Srivastava, A.; Bhatt, D.L.; et al. Phase 2 trial of baxdrostat for treatment-resistant hypertension. *N. Engl. J. Med.* **2023**, *388*, 395–405. [CrossRef] [PubMed]
52. Presented by Bhatt, D.L. *Results from a Phase 2, Double-Blind, Placebo-Controlled Trial Evaluating the Efficacy and Safety of Baxdrostat in Patients with Uncontrolled Hypertension*; Session 403-08; ACC Scientific Session: New Orleans, LA, USA, 2023. [CrossRef]
53. Laffin, L.J.; Rodman, D.; Luther, J.M.; Vaidya, A.; Weir, M.R.; Rajicic, N.; Slingsby, B.T.; Nissen, S.E. Aldosterone synthase inhibition with lorundrostat for uncontrolled hypertension: The Target-HTN randomized clinical trial. *JAMA* **2023**, *330*, 1140. [CrossRef] [PubMed]
54. Morgan, E.; Duran, J.M.; Weinland, J.; Lin, T.; Mullick, A.E.; Geary, R.; Tsimikas, S. Abstract 17395: Effect ION904, an antisense inhibitor of angiotensinogen production: Results of phase 1 and phase 2 pilot studies. *Circulation* **2023**, *148*, A17395. [CrossRef]
55. Bakris, G.L.; Yang, Y.F.; McCabe, J.M.; Liu, J.R.; Tan, X.J.; Benn, V.J.; Pitt, B. Efficacy and safety of ocedurenone: Subgroup analysis of the BLOCK-CKD study. *Am. J. Hypertens.* **2023**, *36*, 612–618. [CrossRef] [PubMed]
56. Presented by Bakris, G.L. Zilebesiran in Combination with a Standard-of-Care Antihypertensive in Patients with Inadequately Controlled Hypertension—KARDIA-2. 2024. Available online: https://www.acc.org/Latest-in-Cardiology/Clinical-Trials/2024/04/05/04/26/kardia-2 (accessed on 28 May 2024).
57. Tokudome, T.; Otani, K.; Mao, Y.; Jensen, L.J.; Arai, Y.; Miyazaki, T.; Sonobe, T.; Pearson, J.T.; Osaki, T.; Minamino, N.; et al. Endothelial natriuretic peptide receptor 1 play crucial role for acute and chronic blood pressure regulation by atrial natriuretic peptide. *Hypertension* **2022**, *79*, 1409–1422. [CrossRef] [PubMed]
58. He, Y.L.; Wu, X.; Serra Roma, A.; Markiewicz, M.; Healy, E.; Yan, J.-H.; Bitsaktsis, C.; Kulmatycki, K.; Kinhikar, A.; Zhang, T.; et al. 23281: Safety and Blood Pressure Lowering Effects of a Novel and Long-Acting Natriuretic Peptide Receptor 1 Agonist in Healthy Participants: A First-in-Human Clinical Study. Late-breaking science abstracts and featured science abstracts from the American Heart Association's scientific sessions 2023 and late-breaking abstracts in resuscitation science from the resuscitation science symposium 2023. *Circulation* **2023**, *148*, 25. [CrossRef]
59. Armstrong, P.W.; Pieske, B.; Anstrom, K.J.; Ezekowitz, J.; Hernandez, A.F.; Butler, J.; Lam, C.S.P.; Ponikowski, P.; Voors, A.A.; Jia, G.; et al. Vericiguat in patients with heart failure and reduced ejection fraction. *N. Engl. J. Med.* **2020**, *382*, 1883–1893. [CrossRef] [PubMed]
60. Crater, G.D.; Lalonde, K.; Ravenelle, F.; Harvey, M.; Després, J.P. Effects of CB1R inverse agonist, INV-202, in patients with features of metabolic syndrome. A randomized, placebo-controlled, double-blind phase 1b study. *Diabetes Obes. Metab.* **2024**, *26*, 642–649. [CrossRef] [PubMed]
61. King, A. Neuropsychiatric adverse effects signal the end of the line for rimonabant. *Nat. Rev. Cardiol.* **2010**, *7*, 602. [CrossRef] [PubMed]
62. Glund, S.; Schoelch, C.; Thomas, L.; Niessen, H.G.; Stiller, D.; Roth, G.J.; Neubauer, H. Inhibition of acetyl-CoA carboxylase 2 enhances skeletal muscle fatty acid oxidation and improves whole-body glucose homeostasis in db/db mice. *Diabetologia* **2012**, *55*, 2044–2053. [CrossRef] [PubMed]
63. Vijayakumar, A.; Murakami, E.; Huss, R.S.; Sroda, N.; Shimazaki, A.; Kashiwagi, Y.; Myers, R.P.; Subramanian, M.; Shulman, G.I. 849-P: Antidiabetic effects of TLC-3595, a selective ACC2 inhibitor, in ZDF rats. *Diabetes* **2023**, *72*, 849-P. [CrossRef]
64. Le Roux, C.W.; Steen, O.; Lucas, K.J.; Startseva, E.; Unseld, A.; Hennige, A.M. Glucagon and GLP-1 receptor dual agonist survodutide for obesity: A randomised, double-blind, placebo-controlled, dose-finding phase 2 trial. *Lancet Diabetes Endocrinol.* **2024**, *12*, 162–173. [CrossRef] [PubMed]
65. Naeem, M.; Imran, L.; Banatwala, U.E.S.S. Unleashing the power of retatrutide: A possible triumph over obesity and overweight: A correspondence. *Health Sci. Rep.* **2024**, *7*, e1864. [CrossRef] [PubMed]
66. Asrih, M.; Wei, S.; Nguyen, T.T.; Yi, H.S.; Ryu, D.; Gariani, K. Overview of growth differentiation factor 15 in metabolic syndrome. *J. Cell. Mol. Med.* **2023**, *27*, 1157–1167. [CrossRef] [PubMed]
67. Stavas, J.; Silva, A.L.; Wooldridge, T.D.; Aqeel, A.; Saad, T.; Prakash, R.; Bakris, G. Rilparencel (Renal autologous cell therapy-REACT®) for chronic kidney disease and type 1 and type 2 diabetes: Phase 2 trial design evaluating bilateral kidney dosing and redosing triggers. *Am. J. Nephrol.* **2024**, *55*, 389–398. [CrossRef] [PubMed]

68. European Renal Association. 61st ERA Congress, Congress Review. 2024. Available online: https://www.era-online.org/wp-content/uploads/2024/06/ERA24-Congress-Review.pdf (accessed on 28 June 2024).
69. Bejar, N.; Tat, T.T.; Kiss, D.L. RNA therapeutics: The next generation of drugs for cardiovascular diseases. *Curr. Atheroscler. Rep.* **2022**, *24*, 307–321. [CrossRef] [PubMed]

diabetology

Systematic Review

Comparative Analysis of Cardiovascular Outcomes in Type 2 Diabetes Patients Engaging in Aerobic, Resistance, and Combined Training: A Systematic Review

Sayed Alireza Mousavi Zadeh [1], Giuseppe Caminiti [2,*], Maurizio Aracri [1], Massimo Pieri [3], Anna Paola Mitterhofer [4], Antonino De Lorenzo [5], Sergio Bernardini [3], Pasquale Farsetti [1], Maurizio Volterrani [2,6], Rosario Barone [7], Ferdinando Iellamo [1] and Marco Alfonso Perrone [1,*]

1 Department of Clinical Sciences and Translational Medicine, University of Rome Tor Vergata, 00133 Rome, Italy; alirezamosavi332@gmail.com (S.A.M.Z.); maurizio.aracri@ptvonline.it (M.A.); farsetti@med.uniroma2.it (P.F.); iellamo@uniroma2.it (F.I.)
2 Department of Human Science and Promotion of Quality of Life, San Raffaele Open University, 00163 Rome, Italy; maurizio.volterrani@uniroma5.it
3 Department of Experimental Medicine, University of Rome Tor Vergata, 00133 Rome, Italy; massimo.pieri@uniroma2.it (M.P.); bernardini@med.uniroma2.it (S.B.)
4 Department of Systems Medicine, University of Rome Tor Vergata, 00133 Rome, Italy; annapaola.mitter@uniroma2.it
5 Department of Biomedicine and Prevention, University of Rome Tor Vergata, 00133 Rome, Italy; delorenzo@uniroma2.it
6 IRCCS San Raffaele Roma, 00166 Rome, Italy
7 Department of Biomedicine, Neurosciences and Advanced Diagnostics, University of Palermo, 90127 Palermo, Italy; rosario.barone@unipa.it
* Correspondence: giuseppe.caminiti@uniroma5.it (G.C.); marco.perrone@uniroma2.it (M.A.P.)

Abstract: Background: Among individuals with type 2 diabetes (T2D), cardiovascular disease (CVD) is the leading cause of death, demanding prevention approaches. Exercise is a powerful option for non-pharmacological strategies to improve cardiovascular outcomes. This systematic review aims to evaluate the effects of aerobic, resistance, and combined training on CVD in individuals with T2D. **Methods:** From 2013 through the end of 2023, PubMed, Scopus, and Web of Science were systematically searched for articles. The studies included 15 articles lasting at least eight weeks and involving 1794 participants each. The cardiac events measured were blood pressure, lipid levels, heart rate variability (HRV), and inflammatory markers such as C-reactive protein (CRP) and interleukin-6 (IL-6). **Results:** Aerobic training reduced systolic and diastolic blood pressure by 6 mmHg and 3 mmHg, respectively, while significantly enhancing lipid profiles, evidenced by an 8% reduction in LDL cholesterol and a 5% rise in HDL cholesterol. In addition, improvements in lean muscle mass, insulin sensitivity, and slight changes in inflammatory markers support the benefits of resistance training. The most pronounced effects emerged from combined training, which resulted in a 9 mmHg decrease in systolic blood pressure, a 6 mmHg decrease in diastolic pressure, a 10% reduction in LDL cholesterol, a 15% increase in HRV, and a 10% reduction in CRP and IL-6 levels. **Conclusions:** Combined training has more favorable effects on several key CVD risk factors than aerobic or resistance training alone. It can be regarded as the most effective exercise modality for decreasing CVD risk in adults with T2D.

Keywords: type 2 diabetes; cardiovascular outcomes; aerobic exercise; resistance training; combined training; heart rate variability; inflammatory markers

1. Introduction

1.1. Global Impact of Type 2 Diabetes and Cardiovascular Disease

Type 2 Diabetes (T2D) affects over half a billion individuals worldwide and could impact over 640 million by 2030 due to aging populations, urbanization, and increasing obesity [1,2]. Beyond metabolic health consequences, T2D strongly predisposes individuals to cardiovascular disease (CVD), accounting for nearly 70% of deaths among diabetics [3]. This dual risk illustrates that interventions addressing glycemic control alone may be insufficient; interventions targeting cardiovascular complications associated with T2D will also be necessary and imperative.

1.2. Role of Exercise in Cardiovascular Health for T2D

CVD in T2D results from a complex interaction involving chronic hyperglycemia, insulin resistance, and systemic factor inflammation. These promote endothelial dysfunction, atherosclerosis, and dyslipidemia marked by elevated triglycerides (TG), low high-density lipoprotein (HDL), and small, dense low-density lipoprotein (LDL) particles [4,5]. Moreover, hypertension in about 80% of T2D patients exacerbates vascular injury, accelerating atherosclerotic plaque progression and heightening cardiovascular event risk [6].

Physical activity is solidly established as fundamental to T2D management, conferring metabolic and cardiovascular benefits beyond drugs. Regular exercise enhances insulin sensitivity, boosts glucose uptake, reduces visceral fat, and improves blood pressure and lipid profiles [6,7]. The American Diabetes Association (ADA) advocates moderate-to-vigorous aerobic activity and resistance training as integral to diabetes care [7]. However, the comparative efficacy of aerobic, resistance, and combined training modes in improving cardiovascular outcomes in T2D individuals remains an active research area.

Recent studies suggest aerobic exercise mainly benefits cardiovascular fitness and lipids, while resistance training improves muscle strength and insulin sensitivity. Combined training and blending both hold promise for synergistic effects [8–10]. Nevertheless, gaps persist in understanding the long-term comparative effectiveness of these exercise regimens regarding key cardiovascular endpoints such as blood pressure regulation, lipid metabolism, heart rate variability (HRV), and systemic inflammation markers [11,12].

While high-intensity interval training (HIIT) and flexibility-based exercises may provide cardiovascular benefits, these modalities were excluded due to insufficient long-term outcome data and a lack of consistency in cardiovascular endpoints reported across T2D populations. In contrast, aerobic, resistance, and combined training have been extensively investigated and are commonly included in international guidelines, making them more suitable for systematic comparison.

1.3. Study Objectives and Contributions

This article aims to systematically review the literature and consolidate evidence regarding the impact of aerobic, resistance, and combined training on cardiovascular health in individuals with T2D patients. By incorporating key insights from recent clinical trials with mechanistic studies, in this review, we strive to provide a clearer understanding of the physiological pathways by which the observed benefits of each exercise modality are observed. In addition, implications for clinical practice are discussed, including evidence supporting structured exercise interventions to mitigate CVD risk and sustain health in T2D individuals.

This study contributes to the growing evidence supporting exercise as a cost-effective, non-drug strategy for managing T2D. It highlights the promising capability of combined exercise training as an integrated strategy to tackle the complex issues of T2D-related cardiovascular risk. This synthesis is aimed at both clinical and policy stakeholders interested in developing evidence-based guidance on exercise prescription specific to the unique needs of patients with T2D to optimize long-term engagement with exercise and follow-up health benefits.

2. Methodology

2.1. Research Design

Taking on the systematic review method, this study examines the effects of categories in which exercise modes can be divided by looking at aerobic exercise methods, the resistance category, and aerobic and anaerobic integration exercises that affect cardiovascular results for T2D patients. It synthesizes findings from several studies to examine the impact of these exercise modalities on key markers of cardiovascular health, including blood pressure, lipid profiles, HRV, and inflammation. These outcomes were selected based on strong evidence of responsiveness to exercise interventions and direct relevance to cardiovascular health risk [13].

2.2. Rationale for the Systematic Review

This review summarizes the exercise modality of choice concerning attenuating cardiovascular risk in T2D. It also maintains transparency and reproducibility by abiding by and adhering to the Preferred Reporting Items for Systematic Reviews and Meta-Analyses (PRISMA) guidelines [14]. It provides a methodical framework for collecting and qualitatively evaluating available studies, identifying the specific form of exercise that most significantly improves cardiovascular outcomes. The lipid profiles and HRV outcomes also highlight their association with physiological processes, including increased lipid metabolism and an improved autonomic nervous system. Such mechanisms help lower systemic inflammation as well [6].

2.3. Research Questions and Hypotheses

Below are the detailed questions and hypotheses that will guide the systematic review and the analysis and interpretation of the findings.

- Main Question:

What type of exercise (i.e., aerobic, resistance, or combined training) strongly affects cardiovascular outcomes in T2D?

- Secondary Questions:
    1. How do exercise intensity, frequency, and duration impact cardiovascular risk factors?
    2. Is combined training more synergistic or superior to single-modality training?

While aerobic, resistance, and combined training have each shown individual benefits for cardiometabolic health, there is a lack of comparative synthesis assessing their distinct and overlapping impacts on cardiovascular markers in T2D. Most prior studies evaluated these modalities independently, often in small samples or with heterogeneous outcome definitions. Furthermore, the long-term effectiveness of each modality, particularly in relation to HRV and inflammatory biomarkers, remains insufficiently clarified. This review was thus designed to address these knowledge gaps directly.

- H1: Aerobic activity leads to more pronounced blood pressure drops and cholesterol profile enhancements compared to strength training [6].
- H2: Strength training improves performance, indirectly lowers inflammation, improves cardiovascular health, and increases muscle mass and glucose metabolism [10].
- H3: Individuals can achieve the greatest cardiovascular benefits by improving muscle strength and cardiorespiratory fitness through resistance and aerobic exercise. This may lead to a greater reduction in cardiovascular risks [9].

2.4. Inclusion and Exclusion Criteria

This review included studies meeting the following inclusion and exclusion criteria to ensure relevance and quality:

- Inclusion Criteria:
  1. Population: Adults 18 years and older diagnosed with T2D.
  2. Interventions: Exercise interventions must be aerobic, resistance training, or both (combined) and at least 8 weeks long. Such a period is the minimum for detecting relevant cardiovascular and metabolic effects adaptations.
  3. Outcomes: Eligible studies should report cardiovascular outcomes, including blood pressure, lipid profiles (LDL, HDL, TG), HRV, and inflammatory biomarkers (e.g., C-reactive protein (CRP) and interleukin-6 (IL-6)).
  4. Study Design: Randomized controlled trials (RCTs), cohort studies, and longitudinal designs that isolate exercise intervention effects on cardiovascular outcomes.

Note on Multi-Component Interventions:

Studies that included additional lifestyle components, such as dietary advice, were only included if the effects of exercise on cardiovascular outcomes were reported independently and could be analyzed separately from the dietary intervention.

- Exclusion Criteria:
  1. Non-T2D Populations: Studies focused on and/or only included non-T2D populations or pharmacological intervention without distinction of exercise effect [5].
  2. Pharmacological Interventions: This review will exclude any studies that combine exercise interventions with pharmacological medications (e.g., insulin or metformin) in which exercise is not examined separately, as it focuses solely on the effects of exercise on cardiovascular outcomes [6].
  3. Duration of Intervention: Interventions lasting fewer than eight weeks were excluded, as this duration is generally insufficient to produce meaningful cardiovascular or metabolic changes.
  4. Language and Publication Type: Only peer-reviewed, English-language publications were included to enhance methodological rigor and ensure consistency in quality assessment. While this approach reduces heterogeneity in study design and reporting, we acknowledge that the exclusion of non-English studies and gray literature may introduce language and publication bias.

Consideration of Medication Use

While we excluded studies where the contribution of pharmacological therapy could not be disentangled from exercise, some participants in the included trials may have been taking stable glucose-lowering agents such as SGLT2 inhibitors or GLP-1 receptor agonists. Given their established cardioprotective properties, these medications may have partly influenced the observed cardiovascular outcomes. Future research should stratify results by medication use or adjust for pharmacologic confounders to better isolate the effects of exercise.

2.5. Data Sources and Search Strategy

The systematic review included a comprehensive search of electronic databases, specifically PubMed, Scopus, and Web of Science. These databases were selected because they cover extensive medical and exercise science literature. The search was conducted for studies published between 2013 and 2023 [14].

Key search terms and Boolean operators were used to refine the search results. Examples include:

- "Type 2 Diabetes" AND "Cardiovascular Outcomes";
- "Aerobic Exercise" OR "Resistance Training" OR "Combined Training";
- "Blood Pressure" AND "Lipid Profiles" AND "Heart Rate Variability";
- "Inflammation" AND "C-reactive Protein" AND "IL-6".

Studies were included if they reported on adults diagnosed with T2D, were written in English, and adhered to ethical standards. The search identified 800 primary studies, which were systematically evaluated based on the inclusion and exclusion criteria [15].

2.6. Study Selection Process

In the study selection stage, methodological rigor and transparency were strictly followed using the PRISMA guidelines. The multi-stage screening method used involved the following [14]:

- Title and Abstract Screening: The titles and abstracts of 800 studies were initially reviewed to eliminate duplicates and irrelevant studies. Studies unrelated to cardiovascular outcomes or not involving exercise interventions were removed at this stage.
- Full-Text Review: 200 articles were reviewed in detail to assess their adherence to inclusion criteria. Only studies that met the specified intervention, population, and outcome requirements were included.
- Eligible Articles: For the final analysis, 15 studies with around 1794 subjects each were included. The above-mentioned studies included a wide range of exercise protocols and targeted several cardiovascular disease-mediated endpoints related to the management of T2D (see Figure 1).

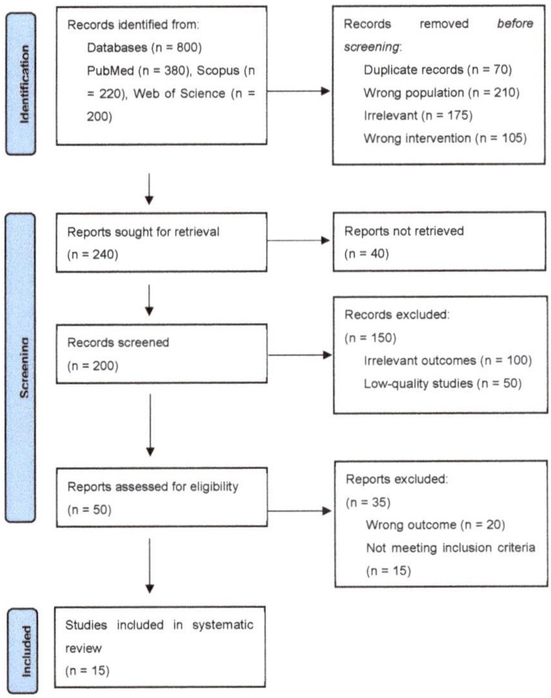

Figure 1. PRISMA 2020 flowchart showing the selection process of studies included in the systematic review. This includes identification, screening, eligibility assessment, and final inclusion, with reasons for exclusion detailed at each stage. Note: Gray literature, preprints, and non-English studies were not considered in this review.

2.7. Data Extraction and Management

Data extraction was conducted in a standardized manner, gathering all necessary information from the articles to fulfill our study's objectives.

Two independent reviewers performed data extraction using a standardized data extraction form. Data were extracted and compared, and discrepancies were resolved by consensus or, if necessary, in discussion with a third reviewer. No automation tools were employed, and the authors of the studies were not contacted; all data were extracted from the published reports.

- Study Information: The authors, year of publication, and journal information are provided as input.
- Demographic characteristics: Details regarding the age, gender, and duration of T2D among participants were extracted.
- Intervention characteristics: The type of exercise intervention, including intensity, frequency, and duration, were recorded.
- Cardiovascular Outcomes: The cardiovascular outcomes examined (e.g., blood pressure, cholesterol levels, and HRV) were recorded.

Besides the primary outcomes, study setting, participant recruitment strategies, and funding sources, when reported, were also extracted. In cases where there was missing or unclear information (e.g., incomplete intervention description on intensity or participant demographics), assumptions were made based either on the context of the study or according to best practices in exercise science. If it was not reasonable to infer values for the variable, then it was recorded as 'not reported' to avoid distortions of the data and maintain methodological transparency.

The outcome domains most frequently extracted from studies met are systolic and diastolic blood pressure, components of the lipid profile (LDL, HDL, TG), HRV, and inflammatory biomarkers (CRP, IL-6). When studies reported outcomes at multiple time points or used various measurement tools, we prioritized post-intervention outcomes and the longest follow-up period. Such a method provided comparability between studies and accounted for the sustained impact of exercise interventions on CVD outcomes in those with T2D.

It is important to note that, although some studies did not provide full baseline data, we included this information where available. Confidence intervals and effect sizes are shown when available in the original publications.

2.8. Quality Assessment

The quality of each study was assessed using the Cochrane Risk of Bias tool, which evaluates several key factors:

- Randomization: Whether participants were randomly assigned to different exercise groups [15].
- Blinding: Whether the outcome assessors were blinded to group assignments.
- Incomplete Data: How the study managed missing or incomplete data, such as participant dropouts.
- Selective Reporting: Whether the study reported all expected outcomes or only favorable results.

Two reviewers independently assessed the risk of bias for each included study, and any disagreements were resolved through discussion or consultation with a third reviewer. No automation tools were used in the risk of bias assessment process. The risk of bias due to missing results or publication bias across studies was not formally assessed, as no meta-analysis or publication bias analysis (e.g., funnel plots) was conducted.

2.9. Data Synthesis

A narrative synthesis described the findings by type of exercise intervention. Studies were classified as aerobic, resistance, or combined training. Cardiovascular outcomes, such as blood pressure, lipid profiles, HRV, and inflammatory markers, were compared qualitatively within each category. Subgroup analyses examined differences in results regarding exercise intensity and duration frequency.

Effect measures used in the synthesis included mean differences (e.g., mmHg for blood pressure, changes in VO_2max) and percentage changes (e.g., lipid profiles, HRV, CRP, IL-6), depending on the format used in each included study.

Information on individual studies and their synthesis was systematically presented in structured summary tables. Characteristics of individual studies included in qualitative synthesis are shown in Table 1, including sample size, type of intervention, duration, intensity, and measures of outcome. In addition, Table 2 summarizes the risk of bias for each included study according to the Cochrane criteria. Domains assessed include randomization, blinding, incomplete data, selective reporting, and overall risk rating.

Our data were further adapted into figures, which illustrate key trends and differences across training modalities, emphasizing the relative magnitude of effects on outcomes, such as blood pressure, lipid profile, HRV, and inflammatory markers.

A meta-analysis was not conducted due to high variability in intervention types, outcome measures, and follow-up durations across the included studies, which limited the feasibility of quantitative synthesis. A qualitative subgroup analysis based on intervention duration ($\geq$24 weeks vs. <24 weeks) was conducted to account for variability. However, due to inconsistent reporting across studies, subgroup analysis by exercise intensity was not feasible. Furthermore, time-to-event outcome data were not reported in any of the included studies, making Kaplan–Meier survival analysis inappropriate in this context [16].

Table 1. Summary of included studies evaluating aerobic, resistance, and combined training in patients with T2D. Table includes study design, sample size, intervention characteristics, and cardiovascular outcomes.

No.	Study (Author, Year)	First Author	Total Participants	Average Age	Gender Distribution	Intervention Type	Frequency (per Week)	Duration (Weeks)	Intensity	Primary Outcomes	Secondary Outcomes	Statistical Measures (Mean, SD, Significance)
1	Cassidy et al., 2019 [17]	Cassidy, Sophia—Houghton, David	22.0	60 ± 2 years	17 males	HIIT (3 sessions per week) vs. control with standard care	3	12.0	High-intensity	Glycemic Control (HbA1c): Significant improvement in the HIIT group (7.13% to 6.87%, $p = 0.03$); HRV: No significant changes; Blood Pressure Variability: Some variations but not statistically significant	Negative correlation between HbA1c and BRS	HbA1c improvement: Mean change, $p = 0.03$
2	Byrkjeland et al., 2017 [18]	Byrkjelan, Rune	137.0	63.1 ± 7.9 years	Predominantly Caucasian	Exercise Program: 12-month combined aerobic and resistance training (150 min/week); Control Group: Standard follow-up	3 (150 min total)	52.0	Moderate	Glycemic Control (HbA1c): Significant decrease in HbA1c in the exercise group, correlated with reductions in endothelial biomarkers (E-selectin, ICAM-1, VCAM-1)	Endothelial Function: No direct improvement, but reduced endothelial activation correlated with HbA1c improvements	HbA1c and endothelial markers: Correlation observed, exact values not specified
3	Karjalainen et al., 2015 [19]	Karjalainen, Jaana	1.046	Not specified	Not specified	LTPA and Home-Based Exercise Training: 2-year controlled trial including endurance and strength training	Varied (No LTPA, irregular LTPA, LTPA > 3 times weekly)	104.0	Varied (endurance and strength)	Cardiovascular Events: Minor improvement in exercise capacity (0.2 ± 0.8 MET for T2D); Blood Pressure: Reduced systolic and diastolic pressure in CAD patients with T2D; Glycemic Control (HbA1c): Slight, non-significant reduction	Composite End Points: LTPA reduced CV morbidity and mortality; controlled exercise training showed no significant effect on CV risk factors	Exercise capacity: Mean ± SD; HbA1c reduction: Not significant
4	Verma et al., 2018 [20]	Verma, Shalini	60.0	Not specified	Not specified	Low-intensity, low-volume; Low-intensity, high-volume; High-intensity, high-volume	Varied: 3–5 sessions per week	12.0	Varied: Low to High Intensity	Primary outcomes include maximal oxygen consumption (VO_2max), oxidative stress markers (SOD, CAT, GPX, NO), and cardiac autonomic function (HRR, HRV)	Secondary outcomes include body composition, lipid profiles, glycemic control (HbA1c, fasting glucose)	ANOVA (split-plot), Bonferroni post hoc, significance level set at $p < 0.05$
5	Rech et al., 2019 [21]	Rech, Anderson	39.0	68 ± 6.5 years (AC); 70.5 ± 7.4 years (RT)	Not specified	RT Group: 12-week, 3×/week resistance training with functional and traditional exercises; AC Group: Low-intensity stretching exercises once per week	RT: 3; AC: 1	12.0	RT: Resistance exercises; AC: Low-intensity stretching	Inflammatory Markers: TNF-α and IL-1β decreased significantly in both groups; No changes in CRP, IL-6, or IL-10	Endothelial Function: No significant improvements in FMD or BAD; Lipid Profile: No significant changes in triglycerides, HDL, LDL, or total cholesterol; Glycemic Control: No significant improvement in HbA1c and fasting glycemia	Inflammatory markers: Significant decrease in TNF-α and IL-1β; Lipid profile and glycemic control: No significant changes
6	Ghardashi et al., 2020 [22]	Ghardashi, Afousi	74.0	45–60 years	Not specified	HIIT: Six intervals of 4 min at 85–90% HRmax, with 3 min at 45–50% HRmax, 3×/week for 12 weeks; Control group with no intervention	3	12.0	HIIT: High-intensity (85–90% HRmax)	Carotid Intima-Media Thickness (cIMT): Significant reduction in HIIT group (from 0.83 ± 0.17 to 0.71 ± 0.14 mm); Serum Markers (Dkk-1, Sclerostin): Both decreased significantly, correlating with cIMT reduction	Cardiorespiratory Fitness (VO2 Peak): Increased by 6.2 mL/kg/min in HIIT, with inverse correlation with cIMT, Dkk-1, and sclerostin levels	cIMT, VO2 Peak, Dkk-1, Sclerostin: Mean ± SD; Correlations with cIMT noted

Table 1. *Cont.*

No.	Study (Author, Year)	First Author	Total Participants	Average Age	Gender Distribution	Intervention Type	Frequency (per Week)	Duration (Weeks)	Intensity	Primary Outcomes	Secondary Outcomes	Statistical Measures (Mean, SD, Significance)
7	Seyedizadeh et al., 2020 [23]	Seyedizadeh, Seyedeh Hoda	24.0	45–65 years	Female only	Combined Training: Resistance and aerobic exercises, 3×/week for 8 weeks; Resistance Training: 2–3 sets, 8–12 reps with progressive load; Aerobic Training: Interval running at 50–65% HRR, progressively increased in duration and intensity	3	8.0	Resistance: Progressive load; Aerobic: 50–65% HRR	Serum Kinesin-1: No significant change in either group; Aerobic Endurance: Slight decline in both groups, greater decrease in control	Lower Body Strength: Significant improvement in experimental group compared to decline in control group	Aerobic endurance and lower body strength: Relative changes observed; significance noted in strength improvements
8	Li et al., 2022 [24]	Li, Jun	37.0	32–47 years	Not specified	HIIT: 10 rounds of 1 min power cycling at 80–95% VO_2max, 1 min rest at 25–30% VO_2max, 5×/week; MICT: Continuous cycling at 50–70% VO_2max for 30 min, 5×/week; Control: Standard counseling on exercise and diet	5	12.0	HIIT: High-intensity (80–95% VO_2max); MICT: Moderate-intensity (50–70% VO_2max)	Body Composition: Weight reduction significant in MICT (−3.52 kg); BMI reduction in MICT (from 26.75 ± 4.20 to 25.45 ± 3.51 kg/m²); Cardiorespiratory Fitness: VO_2max increased in HIIT (0.53 L/min) and MICT (0.31 L/min)	Glycemic Control: FBG and HbA1c reduced in HIIT and MICT; Fasting Insulin: Reduced in HIIT (−2.39 pmol/L) and MICT (−0.99 pmol/L)	Weight, BMI, VO_2max, FBG, HbA1c, and FI: Mean ± SD, significant reductions in MICT and HIIT
9	Otten et al., 2019 [25]	Otten, Julia	22.0	30–70 years	Not specified	Both groups followed a Paleolithic diet for 12 weeks; PD-EX group engaged in 3 h of supervised exercise/week, combining aerobic and resistance training	3 h of exercise for PD-EX	12.0	Aerobic and resistance training for PD-EX	Cardiac and Metabolic Measures: MTG reduced by 45% in PD-EX; Improvements in LV mass-to-volume ratio and end-diastolic volume in PD-EX; Significant increase in VO_2max in PD-EX	Weight Loss and HbA1c: Significant reductions in both groups, with more pronounced changes in PD-EX	MTG, LV remodeling, VO_2max, weight loss, and HbA1c: Mean ± SD; significant changes noted in PD-EX group
10	Naylor et al., 2016 [26]	Naylor, Louise	13.0	13–21 years	10 female, 3 male	Exercise Protocol: Personalized gym-based sessions, 3×/week for 12 weeks; Combined aerobic (65–85% HRmax) and resistance (55–70% MVC) training; Control Group: Usual activity levels without additional training	3	12.0	Aerobic: 65–85% HRmax; Resistance: 55–70% MVC	Vascular Health: FMD increased in the exercise group (+2.2%, $p < 0.05$); Microvascular function improved in exercise group; Body Composition: Fat mass decreased by 1.10 kg in exercise group; Lean mass increased by 1.35 kg in exercise group	Strength: Total strength increased significantly in exercise group; Glycemic Control: No significant changes in insulin sensitivity	FMD, fat mass, lean mass, and strength: Mean ± SD; significance noted for FMD and strength increases
11	MacDonald et al., 2020 [27]	MacDonald, Christopher	98.0	54.4 ± 9.0 years	Not specified	U-TURN group divided into tertiles by accumulated exercise volume (12 months); Lower Tertile: 178 min/week; Intermediate Tertile: 296 min/week; Upper Tertile: 380 min/week; Standard Care: Lifestyle advice without structured exercise	Lower: 178; Intermediate: 296; Upper: 380	52.0	Varied by tertile	Medication Discontinuation: 48% (lower), 60% (intermediate), 70% (upper) discontinued meds; 16% in standard care group	Glycemic Control: HbA1c reduction in intermediate and upper tertiles; Fasting glucose and insulin improved in both tertiles; Body Composition: Reduction in body mass in intermediate and upper tertiles; VO_2max increased significantly in upper tertile only	Medication discontinuation and glycemic control measures: Percentages noted; significant reductions in body mass and increases in VO_2max

Table 1. *Cont.*

No.	Study (Author, Year)	First Author	Total Participants	Average Age	Gender Distribution	Intervention Type	Frequency (per Week)	Duration (Weeks)	Intensity	Primary Outcomes	Secondary Outcomes	Statistical Measures (Mean, SD, Significance)
12	Amaravadi et al., 2024 [28]	Amaravadi, Sampath Kumar	160.0	30–65 years	Not specified	Structured exercise regimen, including aerobic, resistance, and combined exercises, 3–5 times weekly for 12 weeks; Conducted at a diabetic clinic with ongoing monitoring and adherence checks	3–5	12.0	Aerobic and resistance exercises	Insulin Resistance (HOMA-IR): 30.06% improvement in exercise group vs. 14.9% increase in control; Fasting Insulin: 24.34% reduction in exercise group vs. 8.11% increase in control	Glycemic Control: FBS decreased by 14.24% and PPBS by 12.66% in exercise group; HbA1c reduced by 0.55 points; Quality of Life: Significant improvements in WHOQOL-BREF across all domains; Functional Capacity: 27.43% improvement in Six-Minute Walk Test in exercise group	Insulin resistance, fasting insulin, glycemic control, and quality of life measures: Mean ± SD; significance noted for improvements
13	Kluding et al., 2015 [29]	Kluding, Patricia	18.0	58.1 years (SD = 5)	13 females, 5 males	16-week supervised aerobic exercise program, 3×/week; Sessions: 30–50 min, progressing from 50% to 70% VO2R	3	16.0	50% to 70% VO2R	Adverse Events: 57 non-serious events reported, mainly in initial weeks (joint pain, hypoglycemia, hyperglycemia); Cardiovascular Fitness (VO2peak): Increased by 1.1 mL/kg/min ($p < 0.05$)	Body Composition: 1% reduction in total body fat ($p < 0.01$) and 1780 g fat mass reduction; Peripheral Blood Flow: Improved by 2.27%; Fatigue: Significant reduction in general and physical fatigue scores	VO2peak, body fat, and fatigue scores: Mean ± SD; significance noted for improvements
14	Taylor et al., 2014 [30]	Taylor, J. David	21.0	MOD: 52.2 years; HIGH: 54.4 years	Not specified	MOD Group: Resistance at 75% of 8-RM, aerobic at 30–45% HRR; HIGH Group: Resistance at 100% of 8-RM, aerobic at 50–65% HRR; Both groups trained for 3 months, resistance exercises twice weekly, aerobic three times weekly	Resistance: 2; Aerobic: 3	12.0	MOD: 75% 8-RM, 30–45% HRR; HIGH: 100% 8-RM, 50–65% HRR	Physical Fitness: Muscle strength improved in both groups, no significant difference; Exercise capacity and physical function improved in both groups without significant differences	Glycemic Control: Blood glucose decreased immediately and 1 h after exercise; MOD: 204.5 to 172.0 mg/dL; HIGH: 140.0 to 118.5 mg/dL	Muscle strength, exercise capacity, and blood glucose measures: Mean ± SD; significance noted in blood glucose reductions
15	Cassidy et al., 2016 [31]	Cassidy, Sophia—Thoma Christian	23.0	Around 60 years	Not specified	HIIT: 12-week cycling-based high-intensity interval training, 3x/week, intervals at 80–90% HRmax; Control: Standard care without structured exercise	3	12.0	80–90% heart rate max	Cardiac Function: LV Wall Mass increased in HIIT (104 ± 17 g to 116 ± 20 g); Stroke volume increased from 76 ± 16 mL to 87 ± 19 mL; Early diastolic filling rate improved in HIIT; Liver Fat: 39% relative reduction in liver fat, correlated with improvements in HbA1c	Glycemic Control: HbA1c reduced from 7.1% to 6.8% in HIIT; No improvement in control group; Other glycemic markers: No significant changes in fasting glucose or insulin sensitivity	Cardiac and liver fat measures: Mean ± SD; significance noted for LV mass and stroke volume changes

Abbreviations: HIIT = high-intensity interval training; RT = resistance training; AC = aerobic conditioning; LTPA = leisure-time physical activity; HbA1c = hemoglobin A1c; TNF-α = tumor necrosis factor-alpha; BRS = baroreflex sensitivity. BMI, HbA1c, and other baseline measures are reported when available. Statistical significance, confidence intervals, and effect sizes are included when clearly reported in the original studies.

Percentage changes presented in the summary table were derived from approximate averages across the included studies and rounded to the nearest 5–10%. These values were extracted directly from individual study outcomes and are not based on pooled statistical analysis.

2.10. Ethical Considerations

All 15 studies included in this review reported ethical approval from a recognized ethics committee and informed consent from participants. Table 3 provides a summary of these details for each study.

Table 2. Risk of bias assessment using the Cochrane tool for included studies. Domains assessed include randomization, blinding, incomplete data, and selective reporting.

Study (Author, Year)	Randomization	Blinding	Incomplete Data	Selective Reporting	Overall Risk
Cassidy et al., 2019 [17]	Low	High	Low	Low	Moderate
Byrkjeland et al., 2017 [18]	Low	High	Low	Low	Low
Karjalainen et al., 2015 [19]	Low	High	Low	Low	Moderate
Verma et al., 2018 [20]	Low	High	Low	Low	High
Rech et al., 2019 [21]	Low	High	Low	Low	Moderate
Ghardashi et al., 2020 [22]	Low	Unclear	Low	Low	Moderate
Seyedizadeh et al., 2020 [23]	Low	Unclear	Low	Low	Moderate
Li et al., 2022 [24]	Low	Unclear	Low	Low	Moderate
Otten et al., 2019 [25]	Low	Unclear	Low	Low	Low
Naylor et al., 2016 [26]	Low	High	Low	Low	Moderate
MacDonald et al., 2020 [27]	Low	High	High	Low	Low
Amaravadi et al., 2024 [28]	Low	High	Low	Low	Low
Kluding et al., 2015 [29]	Unclear	Unclear	Low	Low	Moderate
Taylor et al., 2014 [30]	Low	High	Unclear	Low	Moderate
Cassidy et al., 2016 [31]	Low	High	Low	Low	Low

Table 3. Ethical approval and informed consent status of all studies included in this systematic review.

Study (Author, Year)	Ethical Approval	Informed Consent
Cassidy et al., 2019 [17]	Yes	Yes
Byrkjeland et al., 2017 [18]	Yes	Yes
Karjalainen et al., 2015 [19]	Yes	Yes
Verma et al., 2018 [20]	Yes	Yes
Rech et al., 2019 [21]	Yes	Yes
Ghardashi et al., 2020 [22]	Yes	Yes
Seyedizadeh et al., 2020 [23]	Yes	Yes
Li et al., 2022 [24]	Yes	Yes
Otten et al., 2019 [25]	Yes	Yes
Naylor et al., 2016 [26]	Yes	Yes
MacDonald et al., 2020 [27]	Yes	Yes
Amaravadi et al., 2024 [28]	Yes	Yes
Kluding et al., 2015 [29]	Yes	Yes
Taylor et al., 2014 [30]	Yes	Yes
Cassidy et al., 2016 [31]	Yes	Yes

3. Results

3.1. Search Strategy and Study Selection

A systematic search across PubMed, Scopus, and Web of Science identified 800 articles. After screening and applying strict inclusion criteria (e.g., T2D, adult populations, interventions $\geq$8 weeks, and cardiovascular outcome metrics), 15 studies involving a combined total of approximately 1794 participants (sample sizes: 50–1046) were included for analysis [17–31].

The included studies involved aerobic training, resistance training, or a combination of aerobic and resistance training interventions. Each modality yielded distinct yet complementary insights into cardiovascular and metabolic adaptations in those with T2D (discussed below).

3.2. *Study Characteristics and Intervention Protocols*

The included studies featured structured exercise interventions with differing protocols for specific exercise modalities. The interventions lasted 8 to 104 weeks and provided short and long-term perspectives.

Aerobic Training: Most aerobic protocols involve moderate-intensity exercise (60–75% VO_2max) lasting 30–50 min per session, performed 3–5 times weekly. This modality affects cardiovascular efficiency, lipid profile, and HRV, which are critical to managing T2D [17].

- Resistance Training: Training protocols were designed to improve muscle strength and insulin sensitivity. They typically involve 2–4 sets of 8–12 repetitions performed 2–3 times weekly. Exercises target large muscle groups to enhance vascular health and glucose metabolism [20,21,23–28,31].
- Combined Training: Protocols integrate aerobic and resistance components within the same intervention. These programs vary, with some studies combining both modalities in a single session and others alternating between them. Combined training was particularly effective in simultaneously addressing multiple cardiovascular and metabolic risk factors [18,24,25,27].

The effect of such interventions was examined in terms of cardiovascular health markers such as blood pressure, lipid patterns, HRV, and inflammatory biomarkers like CRP and IL-6.

3.3. *Cardiovascular Outcomes by Exercise Modality*

3.3.1. Aerobic Training

Eight studies reported the effects of aerobic training on cardiovascular outcomes post-screening (intervention duration: 8–52 weeks).

- Blood Pressure: Aerobic exercise reduced blood pressure, with an average decrease of 6 mmHg systolic and 3 mmHg diastolic. Systolic pressure reduction ranged from 4 to 8 mmHg, while diastolic decreases ranged from 2 to 5 mmHg [19,26]. These results can be explained by improved endothelial function and reduced arterial stiffness.
- Lipid Profiles: LDL cholesterol decreased by 8%, while HDL cholesterol increased by 5%. Study sub-analyses also showed a 6% reduction in TG [30]. Aerobic exercise enhances lipid metabolism in T2D patients by increasing lipid oxidation and lipoprotein lipase activity, facilitating transport and hydrolysis of lipids.
- HRV: Aerobic training modestly improved HRV, indicating positive changes in autonomic control. Four studies showed increased time-domain HRV measures, reflecting parasympathetic dominance and better cardiovascular flexibility [17,20].
- Inflammatory Markers: CRP and IL-6 dropped 5–7%, indicating that aerobic exercises have anti-inflammatory effects. This may result from improved insulin sensitivity, reduced adiposity, and better lipid profiles, which decrease chronic low-grade inflammation tied to T2D-associated cardiovascular disease [22].

3.3.2. Resistance Training

Six studies targeted resistance training, with study durations of 8–52 weeks.

- Blood Pressure: Resistance training reduced systolic and diastolic blood pressure by 5 mmHg and 3 mmHg [21], respectively. While these reductions were slightly smaller than those achieved with aerobic training, they were clinically meaningful.
- Lipid Profiles: Resistance training increased HDL cholesterol by 6%, with minor decreases in TG levels. These changes highlight the potential of resistance exercise to improve lipid metabolism [28].

- Muscle Mass and Insulin Sensitivity: Participants showed a 2 kg rise in lean muscle mass, which improved glucose uptake by muscle tissue. The improved insulin sensitivity lowers hyperglycemia and cardiovascular risk by reducing oxidative stress and inflammation [25].
- Inflammatory Markers: An average study of resistance training found that five studies showed a 5% fall in CRP levels, with changes in IL-6 being variable. This suggests a modest anti-inflammatory effect to resistance training and raises the hope that it could reduce atherosclerosis development in T2D [21].

3.3.3. Combined Training

The five studies on combined training used interventions ranging from 8 to 104 weeks. Combined training consistently demonstrated the most substantial cardiovascular improvements.

- Blood Pressure: Combining training methods yielded the most significant reductions—9 mmHg systolic and 6 mmHg diastolic—showing the benefits of merging aerobic and resistance training exercises [18].
- Lipid Profiles: Combined training reduced LDL cholesterol by an average of 10% and increased HDL cholesterol by 8%. These changes far exceed those from aerobic or strength training alone, suggesting a synergistic effect. Combined exercise may influence lipid metabolism by altering enzymes and increasing mitochondrial function mass [24].
- HRV: Improvements (15%) surpassed those seen with aerobic or resistance training, emphasizing better autonomic function regulation [26].
- Inflammatory Markers: Combined training had the largest effect on inflammation markers: CRP and IL-6 decreased by around 10%. This result underscores the potential of combined training to mitigate chronic inflammation associated with atherosclerosis and other cardiovascular complications in T2D [27].

Overall Comparison of Modalities

A comparative overview of outcome improvements across all three training modalities is presented in Figure 2.

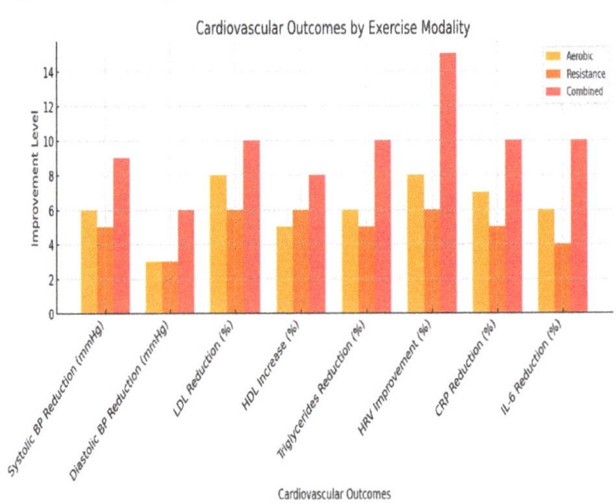

Figure 2. Comparative summary of cardiovascular outcome improvements across three exercise modalities: aerobic, resistance, and combined training. Parameters include blood pressure, lipid profile, HRV, and inflammatory markers (CRP and IL-6), averaged from the reviewed studies. Combined training yielded the most pronounced improvements across most metrics.

3.4. Short-Term vs. Long-Term Effects

Intervention duration significantly influenced outcomes. Long-term interventions (≥24 weeks) yielded more pronounced improvements compared to short-term programs (<24 weeks). The comparative changes in lipid profiles by intervention duration are presented in Figure 3.

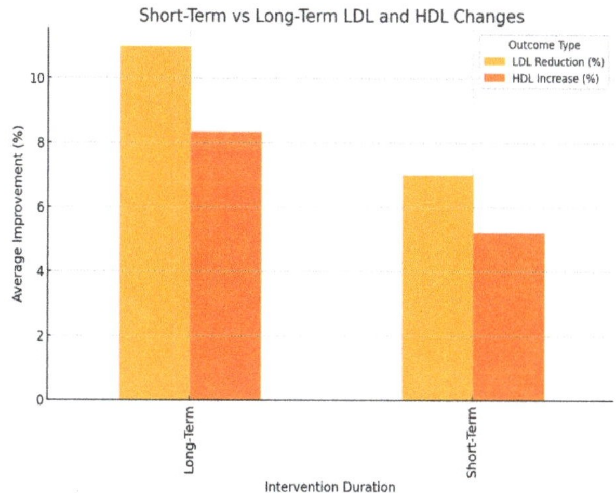

Figure 3. Comparative effects of short-term (<24 weeks) versus long-term (≥24 weeks) exercise interventions on lipid profiles in individuals with T2D. The figure illustrates average changes in LDL and HDL cholesterol. Long-term interventions showed greater improvements in both lipid parameters.

- Blood Pressure: Long-term combined training significantly reduced systolic and diastolic pressures, likely due to improved cardiovascular health remodeling [18,21].
- Lipid Profiles: Longer interventions led to greater reductions in LDL levels and higher increases in HDL cholesterol levels.
- HRV: Long-term studies have shown greater improvements, highlighting sustained exercise's importance for autonomic health [26]. These HRV improvements are illustrated in Figure 4.

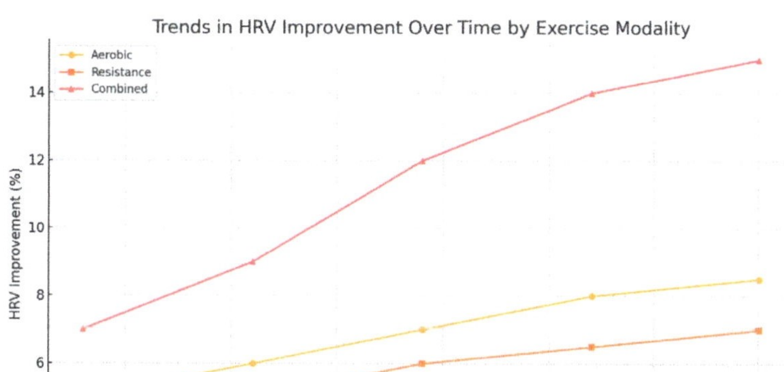

Figure 4. Effect of aerobic, resistance, and combined training on HRV in individuals with T2D. Combined training resulted in the highest increase in HRV, indicating enhanced autonomic regulation.

- Inflammatory Markers: Prolonged interventions led to larger reductions in CRP and IL-6, highlighting the benefits of sustained exercise routines [27,32].

4. Summary of Findings

Combined training provides the best cardiovascular results, with 24-week or longer interventions producing the most robust benefit. Variations in effectiveness highlight the importance of designing long-term exercise programs that combine aerobic and resistance training to reduce CVD risk in those with T2D. These programs are the cornerstone of CVD care and primary or secondary prevention for persons with T2D [18,24,28].

The overall summary of cardiovascular improvements across exercise modalities is shown in Table 4.

Table 4. Summary of cardiovascular outcome improvements across exercise modalities in patients with T2D.

Exercise Modality	Systolic BP Reduction (mmHg)	Diastolic BP Reduction (mmHg)	LDL Reduction (%)	HDL Increase (%)	TG Reduction (%)	HRV Improvement (%)	CRP Reduction (%)	IL-6 Reduction (%)
Aerobic	6	3	8	5	6	8	7	6
Resistance	5	3	6	6	5	6	5	4
Combined	9	6	10	8	10	15	10	10

Abbreviations: BP = blood pressure; mmHg = millimeters of mercury. Note: Values represent the approximate average changes observed across the included studies, rounded to the nearest 5–10% where applicable. In cases where the study-level data varied, median or typical values were used to provide a comprehensive summary. Exact values can be found in the individual study result descriptions.

5. Discussion

5.1. Overview of Finding

This systematic review presents significant results associated with structured exercise programs and cardiovascular benefits among people with T2D. Aerobic, resistance, and combination training modalities conferred unique and clinically meaningful benefits in managing cardiovascular risk factors. Combined training was the most successful approach, preventing the most unfavorable impact by comprehensively improving several cardiovascular endpoints, such as blood pressure, lipid profiles, HRV, and inflammatory markers [8].

5.2. Aerobic Training and Cardiovascular Outcomes

The aerobic exercise led to significant reductions in systolic (–6 mmHg) and diastolic (–3 mmHg) blood pressure and improved lipid profile, characterized by an 8% decrease in LDL cholesterol and a 5% increase in HDL cholesterol [33]. The benefits are likely attributable to increased nitric oxide (NO) production, leading to decreased arterial stiffness and increased vasodilation [34]. Moreover, it enhances lipid metabolism by increasing lipoprotein lipase activity, balancing lipid influx and efflux, improving the HDL-to-LDL ratio, and boosting mitochondrial density, which reduces the atherogenic risk profile and promotes vascular health. In addition, the positive impact of aerobic exercise on autonomic balance and the decrease of sympathetic nervous system activity also leads to more appropriate blood pressure regulation [35].

Although formal subgroup analysis was not conducted, studies suggest that higher-intensity aerobic training, such as HIIT, may induce larger improvements than moderate-intensity continuous training in insulin sensitivity and lipid parameters [36]. This is mainly attributed to superior mitochondrial adaptations and more stimulation of the glucose transporter (GLUT-4). However, head-to-head studies with larger T2D populations to confirm this effect remain to be demonstrated.

Aerobic exercise's anti-inflammatory effects, such as decreased CRP and IL-6, support it as a low-cost, non-pharmacological approach [37].

5.3. Resistance Training and Cardiovascular Benefits

Resistance exercise offers distinct advantages, especially in muscle mass and insulin sensitivity. Improvements in HDL cholesterol levels (6%) and a 5 mmHg decrease in systolic blood pressure have been reported [38]. Resistance training induces glucose uptake by increasing the expression of Glucose Transporter Type 4 (GLUT4) receptors and promotes lean muscle mass, thereby lowering oxidative stress and inflammation [39]. Though modest, reductions in inflammatory markers such as CRP highlight resistance training's potential to slow the progression of atherosclerosis in T2D populations [40].

5.4. Combined Training as a Superior Modality

Combined training produced the most vigorous improvements across all cardiovascular metrics. These included reductions of 9 mmHg systolic and 6 mmHg diastolic blood pressure, a 10% reduction in LDL cholesterol, and a 15% increase in HRV, demonstrating the additive effects of combining aerobic and resistance exercise [41]. The synergistic effects are likely a result of complementary mechanisms of both modalities, such as improved vascular compliance and lipid metabolism [35]. In addition, the highest decreases in inflammatory markers were observed in the combined training group. CRP and IL-6 declined by 10%, highlighting the possibility of reducing the perpetuation of low-grade chronic inflammation in T2D-related CVD [42].

Combined training produced the most vigorous improvements across all cardiovascular metrics. These comparisons are based on narrative synthesis and are not derived from pooled statistical tests. The reported values reflect commonly observed effects across the included studies.

5.5. Practical Considerations and Real-World Applicability

These findings are based on qualitative synthesis across studies; no formal statistical tests (e.g., ANOVA or meta-analysis) were performed. Based on overall trends, combined training was seen to provide the greatest benefit across most heart-related outcomes. Despite its effectiveness, combined training can be harder to apply in real life. Some people may not have enough time, equipment, or motivation. In chronic conditions like T2D, adherence to structured exercise interventions is a key determinant of long-term success. However, not all included studies reported detailed adherence or dropout data. This restricts our understanding of the practical applicability of these long-duration training regimes. Trials moving forward need to be consistent with reporting adherence metrics and include behavioral support methods (e.g., digital monitoring tools, motivational counseling, or group-based programs) to promote patient engagement and, consequently, limit attrition.

Additionally, aerobic or resistance training alone may be more practical for older adults or individuals with mobility issues, and they also help improve heart health [43]. That is why it is important to choose a training program that fits everyone's needs and daily life [44]. A future meta-analysis using more consistent and standardized data could provide stronger statistical support for our conclusions.

5.6. Clinical Implications and Recommendations

This comprehensive systematic review indicates that patients with T2D are most likely to achieve optimal cardio-metabolic health when aerobic and resistance training synergistically affect their cardiovascular and skeletal systems. Aerobic training is targeted at 150–300 min/week of moderate-intensity (60–75% VO_2max) exercise (e.g., brisk walking and swimming), which should be performed 3–5 days/week to improve lipid profiles and blood pressure management. Resistance training should be included 2 to 3 days/week, targeting large muscle groups at moderate intensity for 2 to 3 sets of 8 to 12 repetitions to improve strength and insulin sensitivity. During combined training, whether performed in distinct workouts or within the same workout, 45–60 minutes of moderate-intensity training should be prioritized to accumulate cardiovascular benefits [45]. It has been shown that these strategies need to be customized for every person to fit individual preferences and health status to achieve compliance and sustainable outcomes.

These improvements have significant clinical importance. For instance, every 10 mmHg decrease in systolic BP is associated with a roughly 20% lower relative risk of major cardiovascular events such as myocardial infarction and stroke. Likewise, a 10% lowering of LDL cholesterol and reductions in CRP and IL-6 have been associated with decreased atherosclerosis progression and improved vascular health [46]. The present results, therefore, also lend support to the widespread use of exercise prescriptions to improve glycemic control and as a cornerstone approach to cardiovascular prevention in T2D. A visual comparison of the effects across training modalities on cardiovascular parameters is presented in Figure 5.

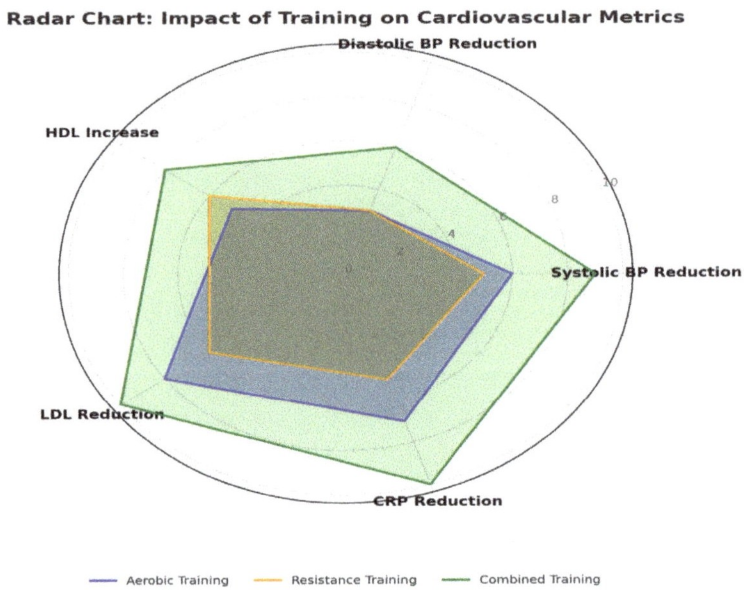

Figure 5. Radar chart comparing the effects of aerobic, resistance, and combined training on five key cardiovascular outcomes in individuals with T2D: systolic blood pressure (SBP), diastolic blood pressure (DBP), LDL, HDL, and CRP. Combined training demonstrated the most favorable overall impact across these parameters.

5.7. Behavioral Strategies and Sustainability

Behavioral interventions can improve adherence, including SMART (Specific, Measurable, Achievable, Relevant, and Time-bound) goals, digital tools such as fitness trackers, and mobile applications. Such approaches enable patients to track progress and remain inspired [47]. Social support gets you moving, whether it is a neighborhood exercise group or accountability [48]. Breaking goals into manageable and realistic steps may help prevent burnout caused by unrealistic expectations and support long-term adherence to physical activity, especially in patients with diabetes. Clinicians should reposition exercise as a long-term lifestyle strategy, highlighting the many (even in a few with diabetes) benefits it confers beyond managing the disease, including enhanced mood, energy, and mobility [49].

5.8. Future Directions

Future studies should also assess the long-term impact of combined training in different populations, focusing on innovative digital tools for remote monitoring and providing feedback. Low-cost community programs may increase access, especially for populations with less access. Such initiatives can serve as additional resources to allow all T2D patients to engage in exercise programs that are both sustainable and sufficient to address not only cardiovascular risk factors but also improve quality of life [50–52].

6. Conclusions

The results of this systematic review indicate that aerobic, resistance, and combined training provide significant cardiovascular benefits to individuals with T2D. Exercise consistently demonstrated benefits in the most important parameters and outcomes of interest, including blood pressure, lipid profile, HRV, and inflammatory markers. However, combined training showed the most significant improvements across the modes in potential cross-benefits for cardiovascular health and metabolism. Aerobic training significantly improved endothelial function and reduced inflammation, whereas resistance training distinctively increased muscle mass and improved insulin sensitivity. These findings emphasize the significant role of physical activity, particularly mode-specific training, as part of the comprehensive treatment and prevention of T2D. These effects must be sustained through long-term compliance with structured exercise programs. We recommend that prospective studies standardize exercise protocols, assess long-term outcomes, and incorporate innovative strategies to improve adherence and outcomes.

Funding: This research received no external funding.

Conflicts of Interest: All authors declare no conflicts of interest.

References

1. Cantley, J.; Ashcroft, F.M. Q&A: Insulin secretion and type 2 diabetes: Why do β-cells fail? *BMC Biol.* **2015**, *13*, 33. [CrossRef]
2. Saeedi, P.; Petersohn, I.; Salpea, P.; Malanda, B.; Karuranga, S.; Unwin, N.; Colagiuri, S.; Guariguata, L.; Motala, A.A.; Ogurtsova, K.; et al. Global and regional diabetes prevalence estimates for 2019 and projections for 2030 and 2045: Results from the International Diabetes Federation Diabetes Atlas, 9th edition. *Diabetes Res. Clin. Pract.* **2019**, *157*. [CrossRef] [PubMed]
3. Viigimaa, M.; Sachinidis, A.; Toumpourleka, M.; Koutsampasopoulos, K.; Alliksoo, S.; Titma, T. Macrovascular Complications of Type 2 Diabetes Mellitus. Available online: https://www.eurekaselect.com/article/97859 (accessed on 22 April 2025).
4. Chakraborty, S.; Verma, A.; Garg, R.; Singh, J.; Verma, H. Cardiometabolic Risk Factors Associated With Type 2 Diabetes Mellitus: A Mechanistic Insight. *Clin. Med. Insights Endocrinol. Diabetes* **2023**, *16*, 11795514231220780. [CrossRef]
5. Wu, L.; Parhofer, K.G. Diabetic dyslipidemia. *Metabolism* **2014**, *63*, 1469–1479. [CrossRef] [PubMed]
6. Colberg, S.R.; Sigal, R.J.; Fernhall, B.; Regensteiner, J.G.; Blissmer, B.J.; Rubin, R.R.; Chasan-Taber, L.; Albright, A.L.; Braun, B. Exercise and Type 2 Diabetes: The American College of Sports Medicine and the American Diabetes Association: Joint position statement. *Diabetes Care* **2010**, *33*, e147. [CrossRef]
7. Dugan, J.A. Exercise recommendations for patients with type 2 diabetes. *J. Am. Acad. Physician Assist.* **2016**, *29*, 13–18. [CrossRef]
8. Yavari, A.; Najafipoor, F.; Aliasgharzadeh, A.; Niafar, M.; Mobasseri, M. Effect of aerobic exercise, resistance training or combined training on glycaemic control and cardiovascular risk factors in patients with type 2 diabetes. *Biol. Sport* **2012**, *29*, 135–143. [CrossRef]
9. Sigal, R.J.; Kenny, G.P.; Wasserman, D.H.; Castaneda-Sceppa, C.; White, R.D. Physical Activity/Exercise and Type 2 Diabetes. *Diabetes Care* **2006**, *29*, 1433–1438. [CrossRef]
10. Church, T.S.; Blair, S.N.; Cocreham, S.; Johannsen, N.; Johnson, W.; Kramer, K.; Mikus, C.R.; Myers, V.; Nauta, M.; Rodarte, R.Q.; et al. Effects of Aerobic and Resistance Training on Hemoglobin A_{1c} Levels in Patients With Type 2 Diabetes: A Randomized Controlled Trial. *JAMA* **2010**, *304*, 2253. [CrossRef]

11. Moore, M.N.; Climie, R.E.; Otahal, P.; Schultz, M.G. Exercise blood pressure and cardiovascular disease risk: A systematic review and meta-analysis of cross-sectional studies. *J. Hypertens.* **2021**, *39*, 2395–2402. [CrossRef]
12. Zanuso, S.; Jimenez, A.; Pugliese, G.; Corigliano, G.; Balducci, S. Exercise for the management of type 2 diabetes: A review of the evidence. *Acta Diabetol.* **2010**, *47*, 15–22. [CrossRef]
13. Shoelson, S.E.; Lee, J.; Goldfine, A.B. Inflammation and insulin resistance. *J. Clin. Investig.* **2006**, *116*, 1793–1801. [CrossRef] [PubMed]
14. Moher, D.; Liberati, A.; Tetzlaff, J.; Altman, D.G.; Group, T.P. Preferred Reporting Items for Systematic Reviews and Meta-Analyses: The PRISMA Statement. *PLoS Med.* **2009**, *6*, e1000097. [CrossRef] [PubMed]
15. Higgins, J.P.T.; López-López, J.A.; Becker, B.J.; Davies, S.R.; Dawson, S.; Grimshaw, J.M.; McGuinness, L.A.; Moore, T.H.M.; Rehfuess, E.A.; Thomas, J.; et al. Synthesising quantitative evidence in systematic reviews of complex health interventions. *BMJ Glob. Health* **2019**, *4*, e000858. [CrossRef]
16. Xiao, M.-X.; Lu, C.-H.; Ta, N.; Wei, H.-C.; Haryadi, B.; Wu, H.-T. Machine learning prediction of future peripheral neuropathy in type 2 diabetics with percussion entropy and body mass indices. *Biocybern. Biomed. Eng.* **2021**, *41*, 1140–1149. [CrossRef]
17. Cassidy, S.; Houghton, D.; Zalewski, P.; Seferovic, J.P.; Hallsworth, K.; MacGowan, G.A.; Trenell, M.I.; Jakovljevic, D.G. Unsupervised high-intensity interval training improves glycaemic control but not cardiovascular autonomic function in type 2 diabetes patients: A randomised controlled trial. *Diab. Vasc. Dis. Res.* **2019**, *16*, 69–76. [CrossRef] [PubMed]
18. Byrkjeland, R.; Njerve, I.U.; Arnesen, H.; Seljeflot, I.; Solheim, S. Reduced endothelial activation after exercise is associated with improved HbA_{1c} in patients with type 2 diabetes and coronary artery disease. *Diab. Vasc. Dis. Res.* **2017**, *14*, 94–103. [CrossRef]
19. Karjalainen, J.J.; Kiviniemi, A.M.; Hautala, A.J.; Piira, O.-P.; Lepojärvi, E.S.; Perkiömäki, J.S.; Junttila, M.J.; Huikuri, H.V.; Tulppo, M.P. Effects of Physical Activity and Exercise Training on Cardiovascular Risk in Coronary Artery Disease Patients with and Without Type 2 Diabetes. *Diabetes Care* **2015**, *38*, 706–715. [CrossRef]
20. Verma, S.; Moiz, J.A.; Anwer, S.; Alghadir, A.H.; Hussain, M.E. A dose-response study of aerobic training for oxygen uptake, oxidative stress and cardiac autonomic function in type 2 diabetes mellitus: Study protocol for a randomized controlled trial. *Trials* **2018**, *19*, 289. [CrossRef]
21. Rech, A.; Botton, C.E.; Lopez, P.; Quincozes-Santos, A.; Umpierre, D.; Pinto, R.S. Effects of short-term resistance training on endothelial function and inflammation markers in elderly patients with type 2 diabetes: A randomized controlled trial. *Exp. Gerontol.* **2019**, *118*, 19–25. [CrossRef]
22. Ghardashi-Afousi, A.; Davoodi, M.; Hesamabadi, B.K.; Asvadi-Fard, M.; Bigi, M.A.B.; Izadi, M.R.; Gaeini, A.A. Improved carotid intima-media thickness-induced high-intensity interval training associated with decreased serum levels of Dkk-1 and sclerostin in type 2 diabetes. *J. Diabetes Complicat.* **2020**, *34*, 107469. [CrossRef]
23. Seyedizadeh, S.H.; Cheragh-Birjandi, S.; Hamedi Nia, M.R. The Effects of Combined Exercise Training (Resistance-Aerobic) on Serum Kinesin and Physical Function in Type 2 Diabetes Patients with Diabetic Peripheral Neuropathy (Randomized Controlled Trials). *J. Diabetes Res.* **2020**, *2020*, 6978128. [CrossRef]
24. Li, J.; Cheng, W.; Ma, H. A Comparative Study of Health Efficacy Indicators in Subjects with T2DM Applying Power Cycling to 12 Weeks of Low-Volume High-Intensity Interval Training and Moderate-Intensity Continuous Training. *J. Diabetes Res.* **2022**, *2022*, 1–13. [CrossRef] [PubMed]
25. Otten, J.; Andersson, J.; Ståhl, J.; Stomby, A.; Saleh, A.; Waling, M.; Ryberg, M.; Hauksson, J.; Svensson, M.; Johansson, B.; et al. Exercise Training Adds Cardiometabolic Benefits of a Paleolithic Diet in Type 2 Diabetes Mellitus. *J. Am. Heart Assoc.* **2019**, *8*, e010634. [CrossRef] [PubMed]
26. Naylor, L.H.; Davis, E.A.; Kalic, R.J.; Paramalingam, N.; Abraham, M.B.; Jones, T.W.; Green, D.J. Exercise training improves vascular function in adolescents with type 2 diabetes. *Physiol. Rep.* **2016**, *4*, e12713. [CrossRef]
27. MacDonald, C.S.; Johansen, M.Y.; Nielsen, S.M.; Christensen, R.; Hansen, K.B.; Langberg, H.; Vaag, A.A.; Karstoft, K.; Lieberman, D.E.; Pedersen, B.K.; et al. Dose-Response Effects of Exercise on Glucose-Lowering Medications for Type 2 Diabetes: A Secondary Analysis of a Randomized Clinical Trial. *Mayo Clin. Proc.* **2020**, *95*, 488–503. [CrossRef]
28. Amaravadi, S.K.; Maiya, G.A.; Vaishali, K.; Shastry, B.A. Effectiveness of structured exercise program on insulin resistance and quality of life in type 2 diabetes mellitus–A randomized controlled trial. *PLoS ONE* **2024**, *19*, e0302831. [CrossRef]
29. Kluding, P.M.; Pasnoor, M.; Singh, R.; D'Silva, L.J.; Yoo, M.; Billinger, S.A.; LeMaster, J.W.; Dimachkie, M.M.; Herbelin, L.; Wright, D.E. Safety of Aerobic Exercise in People With Diabetic Peripheral Neuropathy: Single-Group Clinical Trial. *Phys. Ther.* **2015**, *95*, 223–234. [CrossRef]
30. Taylor, J.D.; Fletcher, J.P.; Mathis, R.A.; Cade, W.T. Effects of Moderate- Versus High-Intensity Exercise Training on Physical Fitness and Physical Function in People With Type 2 Diabetes: A Randomized Clinical Trial. *Phys. Ther.* **2014**, *94*, 1720–1730. [CrossRef]
31. Cassidy, S.; Thoma, C.; Hallsworth, K.; Parikh, J.; Hollingsworth, K.G.; Taylor, R.; Jakovljevic, D.G.; Trenell, M.I. High intensity intermittent exercise improves cardiac structure and function and reduces liver fat in patients with type 2 diabetes: A randomised controlled trial. *Diabetologia* **2016**, *59*, 56–66. [CrossRef]

32. Dieli-Conwright, C.M.; Courneya, K.S.; Demark-Wahnefried, W.; Sami, N.; Lee, K.; Buchanan, T.A.; Spicer, D.V.; Tripathy, D.; Bernstein, L.; Mortimer, J.E. Effects of Aerobic and Resistance Exercise on Metabolic Syndrome, Sarcopenic Obesity, and Circulating Biomarkers in Overweight or Obese Survivors of Breast Cancer: A Randomized Controlled Trial. *J. Clin. Oncol.* **2018**, *36*, 875–883. [CrossRef] [PubMed]
33. Ekechukwu, N.I.; Anwara, S.U.; Mgbeojedo, U.G.; Chijioke, O.U.; Onwukwe, O.S.; Ezugwu, U.A.; Ekechukwu, E.N.D.; Okoronkwo, I.L. Effects of Structured Aerobic Exercise on Selected Clinical Profiles of Patients with Type 2 Diabetes Mellitus: A Systematic Review with Meta-Analysis. *Int. J. Med. Health Dev.* **2021**, *26*, 17–30. [CrossRef]
34. Hwang, M.-H.; Kim, S. Type 2 Diabetes: Endothelial dysfunction and Exercise. *J. Exerc. Nutr. Biochem.* **2014**, *18*, 239–247. [CrossRef] [PubMed]
35. Gordon, B.; Chen, S.; Durstine, J.L. The Effects of Exercise Training on the Traditional Lipid Profile and Beyond. *Curr. Sports Med. Rep.* **2014**, *13*, 253–259. [CrossRef]
36. De Nardi, A.T.; Tolves, T.; Lenzi, T.L.; Signori, L.U.; Silva, A.M.V.D. High-intensity interval training versus continuous training on physiological and metabolic variables in prediabetes and type 2 diabetes: A meta-analysis. *Diabetes Res. Clin. Pract.* **2018**, *137*, 149–159. [CrossRef] [PubMed]
37. Papagianni, G.; Panayiotou, C.; Vardas, M.; Balaskas, N.; Antonopoulos, C.; Tachmatzidis, D.; Didangelos, T.; Lambadiari, V.; Kadoglou, N.P.E. The anti-inflammatory effects of aerobic exercise training in patients with type 2 diabetes: A systematic review and meta-analysis. *Cytokine* **2023**, *164*, 156157. [CrossRef]
38. Westcott, W.L. Resistance Training is Medicine: Effects of Strength Training on Health. *Curr. Sports Med. Rep.* **2012**, *11*, 209–216. [CrossRef]
39. Lee, J.; Kim, D.; Kim, C. Resistance Training for Glycemic Control, Muscular Strength, and Lean Body Mass in Old Type 2 Diabetic Patients: A Meta-Analysis. *Diabetes Ther.* **2017**, *8*, 459–473. [CrossRef]
40. Qadir, R.; Sculthorpe, N.F.; Todd, T.; Brown, E.C. Effectiveness of Resistance Training and Associated Program Characteristics in Patients at Risk for Type 2 Diabetes: A Systematic Review and Meta-analysis. *Sports Med.-Open* **2021**, *7*, 38. [CrossRef]
41. Schroeder, E.C.; Franke, W.D.; Sharp, R.L.; Lee, D. Comparative effectiveness of aerobic, resistance, and combined training on cardiovascular disease risk factors: A randomized controlled trial. *PLoS ONE* **2019**, *14*, e0210292. [CrossRef]
42. Magalhães, J.P.; Santos, D.A.; Correia, I.R.; Hetherington-Rauth, M.; Ribeiro, R.; Raposo, J.F.; Matos, A.; Bicho, M.D.; Sardinha, L.B. Impact of combined training with different exercise intensities on inflammatory and lipid markers in type 2 diabetes: A secondary analysis from a 1-year randomized controlled trial. *Cardiovasc. Diabetol.* **2020**, *19*, 169. [CrossRef] [PubMed]
43. Liu, C.; Latham, N.K. Progressive resistance strength training for improving physical function in older adults. *Cochrane Database Syst. Rev.* **2009**, *3*, CD002759. [CrossRef] [PubMed]
44. Tavoian, D.; Russ, D.W.; Consitt, L.A.; Clark, B.C. Perspective: Pragmatic Exercise Recommendations for Older Adults: The Case for Emphasizing Resistance Training. *Front. Physiol.* **2020**, *11*, 799. [CrossRef] [PubMed]
45. Mann, S.; Beedie, C.; Jimenez, A. Differential Effects of Aerobic Exercise, Resistance Training and Combined Exercise Modalities on Cholesterol and the Lipid Profile: Review, Synthesis and Recommendations. *Sports Med.* **2014**, *44*, 211–221. [CrossRef]
46. Law, M.R.; Morris, J.K.; Wald, N.J. Use of blood pressure lowering drugs in the prevention of cardiovascular disease: Meta-analysis of 147 randomised trials in the context of expectations from prospective epidemiological studies. *BMJ* **2009**, *338*, b1665. [CrossRef]
47. Revello, K.; Fields, W. An Educational Intervention to Increase Nurse Adherence in Eliciting Patient Daily Goals. *Rehabil. Nurs.* **2015**, *40*, 320–326. [CrossRef]
48. Luhanga, E.T.; Hippocrate, A.A.E.; Suwa, H.; Arakawa, Y.; Yasumoto, K. Identifying and Evaluating User Requirements for Smartphone Group Fitness Applications. *IEEE Access* **2018**, *6*, 3256–3269. [CrossRef]
49. Marrero, D.G. Time to Get Moving: Helping Patients With Diabetes Adopt Exercise as Part of a Healthy Lifestyle. *Clin. Diabetes* **2005**, *23*, 154–159. [CrossRef]
50. Shan, R.; Sarkar, S.; Martin, S.S. Digital health technology and mobile devices for the management of diabetes mellitus: State of the art. *Diabetologia* **2019**, *62*, 877–887. [CrossRef]
51. Kiani, A.K.; Bonetti, G.; Donato, K.; Kaftalli, J.; Herbst, K.L.; Stuppia, L.; Fioretti, F.; Nodari, S.; Perrone, M.; Chiurazzi, P.; et al. Polymorphisms, diet and nutrigenomics. *J. Prev. Med. Hyg.* **2022**, *63* (Suppl. 3), E125–E141. [CrossRef]
52. Perrone, M.A.; Donatucci, B.; Salvati, A.; Gualtieri, P.; De Lorenzo, A.; Romeo, F.; Bernardini, S. Inflammation, oxidative stress and gene expression: The postprandial approach in professional soccer players to reduce the risk of muscle injuries and early atherosclerosis. *Med. Sport* **2019**, *72*, 234–243. [CrossRef]

MDPI AG
Grosspeteranlage 5
4052 Basel
Switzerland
Tel.: +41 61 683 77 34

Diabetology Editorial Office
E-mail: diabetology@mdpi.com
www.mdpi.com/journal/diabetology

www.ingramcontent.com/pod-product-compliance
Lightning Source LLC
Chambersburg PA
CBHW062038220926
51850CB00010B/2591
* 9 7 8 3 7 2 5 8 4 7 1 3 6 *